The Complete Air Fryer Encyclopedia [5 books in 1]

Plenty of Crave-Worthy Fried Recipes to Stay Healthy, Feel More Energetic and Thrive in a Meal

By

Mark

Machino

Table of Contents

Vegan Air Fryer Cookbook

The Complete Air Fryer Cookbook with Pictures

The Healthy Air Fryer Cookbook with Pictures

Breville Smart Air Fryer Oven Cookbook

AIR FRYER COOKBOOK FOR TWO

By

Mark

Machino

Table of Contents

Introduction:

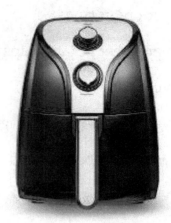

You have got the set of important knives, toaster oven, coffee machine, and quick pot along with the cutter you want to good care of. There may be a variety of things inside your kitchen, but maybe you wish to make more space for an air fryer. It's easy to crowd and load with the new cooking equipment even though you've a lot of them. However, an air fryer is something you will want to make space for.

The air fryer is identical to the oven in the way that it roasts and bakes, but the distinction is that elements of hating are placed over the top& are supported by a big, strong fan, producing food that is extremely crispy and, most importantly with little oil in comparison to the counterparts which are deeply fried. Usually, air fryers heat up pretty fast and, because of the centralized heat source & the fan size and placement, they prepare meals quickly & uniformly. The cleanup is another huge component of the air frying. Many baskets & racks for air fryers are dishwasher protected. We recommend a decent dish brush for those who are not dishwasher secure. It will go through all the crannies and nooks that facilitate the movement of air without making you crazy.

We have seen many rave reviews of this new trend, air frying. Since air frying, they argue, calls for fast and nutritious foods. But is the hype worth it? How do the air fryers work? Does it really fry food?

How do air fryers work?

First, let's consider how air fryer really works before we go to which type of air fryer is decent or any simple recipes. Just think of it; cooking stuff without oil is such a miracle. Then, how could this even be possible? Let's try to find out how to pick the best air fryer for your use now when you understand how the air fryer works.

How to pick the best air fryer

It is common to get lost when purchasing gadgets & electrical equipment, given that there're a wide range of choices available on the market. So, before investing in one, it is really ideal to have in mind the specifications and budget.

Before purchasing the air fryer, you can see the things you should consider:

Capacity/size: Air fryers are of various sizes, from one liter to sixteen liters. A three-liter capacity is fine enough for bachelors. Choose an air fryer that has a range of 4–6 liters for a family having two children. There is a restricted size of the basket which is used to put the food. You will have to prepare the meals in batches if you probably wind up using a tiny air fryer.

Timer: Standard air fryers arrive with a range timer of 30 minutes. For house cooking, it is satisfactory. Thought, if you are trying complex recipes which take a longer cooking time, pick the air fryer with a 1-hour timer.

Temperature: The optimum temperature for most common air fryers is 200 degrees C (400 f). You can quickly prepare meat dishes such as fried chicken, tandoori, kebabs etc.

The design, durability, brand value and controls are other considerations you might consider.

Now that you know which air fryer is best for you let's see the advantages of having an air fryer at your place.

What are the benefits of air fryers?

The benefits of air fryers are as follows:

Cooking with lower fat & will promote weight loss

Air fryers work with no oils and contain up to 80 percent lower fat than most fryers relative to a traditional deep fryer. Shifting to an air fryer may encourage loss of weight by decreasing fat & caloric intake for anyone who consumes fried food regularly and also has a problem with leaving the fast foods.

Faster time for cooking

Air frying is easier comparing with other cooking techniques, such as grilling or baking. Few air fryers need a preheat of 60 seconds, but others do not need a preheat any longer than a grill or an oven. So if there is a greater capacity or multiple compartments for the air fryer basket, you may make various dishes in one go.

Quick to clean

It's extremely easy to clean an air fryer. And after each use, air frying usually does not create enough of a mess except you cook fatty food such as steak or chicken wings. Take the air fryer out and clean it with soap & water in order to disinfect the air fryer.

Safer to be used

The air fryer is having no drawbacks, unlike hot plates or deep frying. Air fryers get hot, but splashing or spilling is not a risk.

Minimum use of electricity and environment friendly

Air fryers consume far less electricity than various electric ovens, saving your money & reducing carbon output.

Flexibility

Some of the air fryers are multi-functional. It's possible to heat, roast, steam, broil, fry or grill food.

Less waste and mess

Pan-fries or deep fryer strategies leave one with excess cooking oil, which is difficult to rid of and usually unsustainable. You can cook fully oil-less food with an air fryer. All the pieces have a coating of nonstick, dishwasher safe and nonstick coating.

Cooking without the use of hands

The air fryer includes a timer, & when it is full, it'll stop by itself so that you may feel secure while multitasking.

Feasible to use

It is very much convenient; you can use an air fryer whenever you want to. Few air fryers involve preheating, which is less than 5 minutes; with the air fryer, one may begin cooking immediately.

Reducing the possibility of the development of toxic acrylamide

Compared to making food in oil, air frying will decrease the potential of producing acrylamides. Acrylamide is a compound that, under elevated temperature cooking, appears in certain food and may have health impacts.

Chapter 1: Air fryer breakfast recipes

1. Air fryer breakfast frittata

Cook time: 20 minutes

Servings: 2 people

Difficulty: Easy

Ingredients:

- 1 pinch of cayenne pepper (not necessary)

- 1 chopped green onion

- Cooking spray

- 2 tbsp. diced red bell pepper

- ¼ pound fully cooked and crumbled breakfast sausages

- 4 lightly beaten eggs

- ½ cup shredded cheddar-Monterey jack cheese blend

Instructions:

1. Combine eggs, bell pepper, cheddar Monterey Jack cheese, sausages, cayenne and onion inside a bowl & blend to combine.

2. The air fryer should be preheated to 360 ° f (180° c). Spray a 6 by 2-inch non-stick cake pan along with a spray used in cooking.

3. Place the mixture of egg in the ready-made cake tray.

4. Cook for 18 - 20 minutes in your air fryer before the frittata is ready.

2. Air fryer banana bread

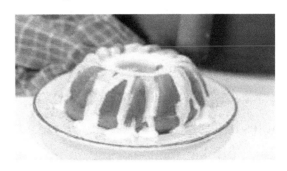

Cook time: 28 minutes

Serving: 8 people

Difficulty: Easy

Ingredients:

- 3/4 cup flour for all purposes

- 1/4 tbsp. salt

- 1 egg

- 2 mashed bananas overripe

- 1/4 cup sour cream

- 1/2 cup sugar

- 1/4 tbsp. baking soda

- 7-inch bundt pan

- 1/4 cup vegetable oil

- 1/2 tbsp. vanilla

Instructions:

1. In one tub, combine the dry ingredients and the wet ones in another. Mix the two slowly till flour is fully integrated, don't over mix.

2. With an anti-stick spray, spray and on a 7-inch bundt pan & then pour in the bowl.

3. Put it inside the air fryer basket & close. Placed it for 28 mins to 310 degrees

4. Remove when completed & permit to rest in the pan for about 5 mins.

5. When completed, detach and allow 5 minutes to sit in the pan. Then flip on a plate gently. Sprinkle melted icing on top, serve after slicing.

3. Easy air fryer omelet

Cook time: 8 minutes

Serving: 2 people

Difficulty: Easy

Ingredients:

- 1/4 cup shredded cheese

- 2 eggs

- Pinch of salt

- 1 teaspoon of McCormick morning breakfast seasoning – garden herb

- Fresh meat & veggies, diced

- 1/4 cup milk

Instructions:

1. In a tiny tub, mix the milk and eggs till all of them are well mixed.

2. Add a little salt in the mixture of an egg.

3. Then, in the mixture of egg, add the veggies.

4. Pour the mixture of egg in a greased pan of 6 by 3 inches.

5. Place your pan inside the air fryer container.

6. Cook for about 8 to 10 mins and at 350 f.

7. While you are cooking, slather the breakfast seasoning over the eggs & slather the cheese on the top.

8. With a thin spoon, loose the omelet from the pan and pass it to a tray.

9. Loosen the omelet from the sides of the pan with a thin spatula and pass it to a tray.

10. Its options to garnish it with additional green onions.

4. Air-fried breakfast bombs

Cook time: 20 mins

Serving: 2

Difficulty: easy

Ingredients:

- Cooking spray

- 1 tbsp. fresh chives chopped

- 3 lightly beaten, large eggs

- 4 ounces whole-wheat pizza dough freshly prepared

- 3 bacon slices center-cut

- 1 ounce 1/3-less-fat softened cream cheese

Instructions:

1. Cook the bacon in a standard size skillet for around 10 minutes, medium to very crisp. Take the bacon out of the pan; scatter.

Add the eggs to the bacon drippings inside the pan; then cook, stirring constantly, around 1 minute, until almost firm and yet loose. Place the eggs in a bowl; add the cream cheese, the chives, and the crumbled bacon.

2. Divide the dough into four identical sections. Roll each bit into a five-inch circle on a thinly floured surface. Place a quarter of the egg mixture in the middle of each circle of dough. Clean the underside of the dough with the help of water; wrap the dough all around the mixture of an egg to form a purse and pinch the dough.

3. Put dough purses inside the air fryer basket in one layer; coat really well with the help of cooking spray. Cook for 5 to 6 minutes at 350 degrees f till it turns to a golden brown; check after 4 mins.

5. Air fryer French toast

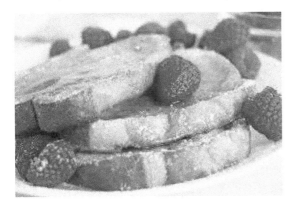

Cook time: 15 mins

Serving: 2 people

Difficulty: easy

Ingredients:

- 4 beaten eggs

- 4 slices of bread

- Cooking spray (non-stick)

Instructions:

1. Put the eggs inside a container or a bowl which is sufficient and big, so the pieces of bread will fit inside.

2. With a fork, mix the eggs and after that, place each bread slice over the mixture of an egg.

3. Turn the bread for one time so that every side is filled with a mixture of an egg.

4. After that, fold a big sheet of aluminum foil; this will keep the bread together. Switch the foil's side; this will ensure that the mixture of an egg may not get dry. Now put the foil basket in the air fryer basket. Make sure to allow space around the edges; this will let the circulation of hot air.

5. With the help of cooking spray, spray the surface of the foil basket and then put the bread over it. On top, you may add the excess mixture of an egg.

6. For 5 mins, place the time to 365 degrees f.

7. Turn the bread & cook it again for about 3 to 5 mins, until it's golden brown over the top of the French toast & the egg isn't runny.

8. Serve it hot, with toppings of your choice.

6. Breakfast potatoes in the air fryer

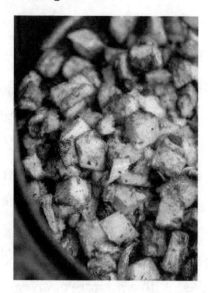

Cook time: 15 mins

Servings: 2

Difficulty: easy

Ingredients:

- 1/2 tbsp. kosher salt

- 1/2 tbsp. garlic powder

- Breakfast potato seasoning

- 1/2 tbsp. smoked paprika

- 1 tbsp. oil

- 5 potatoes medium-sized. Peeled & cut to one-inch cubes (Yukon gold works best)

- 1/4 tbsp. black ground pepper

Instructions:

1. At 400 degrees f, preheat the air fryer for around 2 to 3 minutes. Doing this will provide you the potatoes that are crispiest.

2. Besides that, brush your potatoes with oil and breakfast potato seasoning till it is fully coated.

3. Using a spray that's non-stick, spray on the air fryer. Add potatoes & cook for about 15 mins, shaking and stopping the basket for 2 to 3 times so that you can have better cooking.

4. Place it on a plate & serve it immediately.

7. Air fryer breakfast pockets

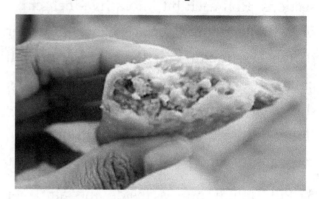

Cook time: 15 mins

Serving: 5 people

Difficulty: easy

Ingredients:

- 2-gallon zip lock bags

- Salt & pepper to taste

- 1/3 + 1/4 cup of whole milk

- 1 whole egg for egg wash

- Cooking spray

- 1-2 ounces of Velveeta cheese

- Parchment paper

- 1 lb. of ground pork

- 2 packages of Pillsbury pie crust

- 2 crusts to a package

- 4 whole eggs

Instructions:

1. Let the pie crusts out of the freezer.

2. Brown the pig and rinse it.

3. In a tiny pot, heat 1/4 cup of cheese and milk until it is melted.

4. Whisk four eggs, season with pepper and salt & add the rest of the milk.

5. Fumble the eggs in the pan until they are nearly fully cooked.

6. Mix the eggs, cheese and meat together.

7. Roll out the pie crust & cut it into a circle of about 3 to 4 inches (cereal bowl size).

8. Whisk 1 egg for making an egg wash.

9. Put around 2 tbsp. of the blend in the center of every circle.

10. Now, eggs wash the sides of the circle.

11. Create a moon shape by folding the circle.

12. With the help of a fork, folded edges must be crimped

13. Place the pockets inside parchment paper & put it inside a ziplock plastic bag overnight.

14. Preheat the air fryer for 360 degrees until it is ready to serve.

15. With a cooking spray, each pocket side must be sprayed.

16. Put pockets inside the preheated air fryer for around 15 mins or till they are golden brown.

17. Take it out from the air fryer & make sure it's cool before you serve it.

8. Air fryer sausage breakfast casserole

Cook time: 20 mins

Serving: 6 people

Difficulty: easy

Ingredients:

- 1 diced red bell pepper

- 1 lb. ground breakfast sausage

- 4 eggs

- 1 diced green bell pepper

- 1/4 cup diced sweet onion

- 1 diced yellow bell pepper

- 1 lb. hash browns

Instructions:

1. Foil line your air fryer's basket.

2. At the bottom, put some hash browns.

3. Cover it with the raw sausage.

4. Place the onions & peppers uniformly on top.

5. Cook for 10 mins at 355 degrees.

6. Open your air fryer & blend the casserole a little if necessary.

7. Break every egg inside the bowl and spill it directly over the casserole.

8. Cook for the next 10 minutes for 355 degrees.

9. Serve with pepper and salt for taste.

9. Breakfast egg rolls

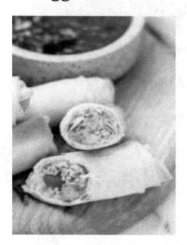

Cook time: 15 mins

Servings: 6 people

Difficulty: easy

Ingredients:

• Black pepper, to taste

• 6 large eggs

• Olive oil spray

• 2 tbsp. chopped green onions

• 1 tablespoon water

• 1/4 teaspoon kosher salt

• 2 tablespoons diced red bell pepper

• 1/2 pound turkey or chicken sausage

• 12 egg roll wrappers

• The salsa that is optional for dipping

Instructions:

1. Combine the water, salt and black pepper with the eggs.

2. Cook sausage in a non-stick skillet of medium size, make sure to let it cook in medium heat till there's no pink color left for 4 minutes, splitting into crumbles, then drain.

3. Stir in peppers and scallions & cook it for 2 minutes. Put it on a plate.

4. Over moderate flame, heat your skillet & spray it with oil.

5. Pour the egg mixture & cook stirring till the eggs are cooked and fluffy. Mix the sausage mixture.

6. Put one wrapped egg roll on a dry, clean work surface having corners aligned like it's a diamond.

7. Include an egg mixture of 1/4 cup on the lower third of your wrapper.

8. Gently raise the lower point closest to you & tie it around your filling.

9. Fold the right & left corners towards the middle & continue rolling into the compact cylinder.

10. Do this again with the leftover wrappers and fillings.

11. Spray oil on every side of your egg roll & rub it with hands to cover them evenly.

12. The air fryer must be preheated to 370 degrees f.

13. Cook the egg rolls for about 10 minutes in batches till it's crispy and golden brown.

14. Serve instantly with salsa, if required.

10. Air fryer breakfast casserole

Cook time: 45 mins

Servings: 6 people

Difficulty: medium

Ingredients:

- 1 tbsp. extra virgin olive oil
- Salt and pepper
- 4 bacon rashers
- 1 tbsp. oregano
- 1 tbsp. garlic powder
- 2 bread rolls stale
- 1 tbsp. parsley
- 320 grams grated cheese
- 4 sweet potatoes of medium size
- 3 spring onions
- 8 pork sausages of medium size
- 11 large eggs
- 1 bell pepper

Instructions:

1. Dice and peel the sweet potato in cubes. Mix the garlic, salt, oregano and pepper in a bowl with olive oil of extra virgin.

2. In an air fryer, put your sweet potatoes. Dice the mixed peppers, cut the sausages in quarters & dice the bacon.

3. Add the peppers, bacon and sausages over the sweet potatoes. Air fry it at 160c or 320 f for 15 mins.

4. Cube and slice the bread when your air fryer is heating & pound your eggs in a blending jug with the eggs, including some extra parsley along with pepper and salt. Dice the spring onion.

5. Check the potatoes when you hear a beep from the air fryer. A fork is needed to check on the potatoes. If you are unable to, then cook for a further 2 to 3 minutes. Mix the basket of the air fryer, include the spring onions & then cook it for an additional five minutes with the same temperature and cooking time.

6. Using the projected baking pans, place the components of your air fryer on 2 of them. Mix it while adding bread and cheese. Add your mixture of egg on them & they are primed for the actual air fry.

7. Put the baking pan inside your air fryer & cook for 25 minutes for 160 c or 320 f. If you planned to cook 2, cook 1 first and then the other one. Place a cocktail stick into the middle & then it's done if it comes out clear and clean.

11. Air fryer breakfast sausage ingredients

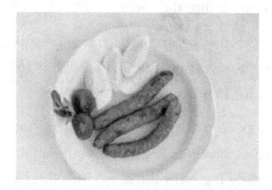

Cook time: 10 mins

Serving: 2 people

Difficulty: easy

Ingredients:

- 1 pound breakfast sausage

- Air fryer breakfast sausage ingredients

Instructions:

1. Insert your sausage links in the basket of an air fryer.

2. Cook your sausages or the sausage links for around 8 to 10 minutes at 360°.

12. Wake up air fryer avocado boats

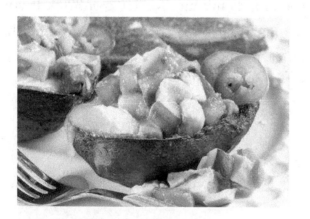

Cook time: 5 mins

Servings: 2

Difficulty: easy

Ingredients:

- 1/2 teaspoon salt

- 2 plum tomatoes, seeded & diced

- 1/4 teaspoon black pepper

- 1 tablespoon finely diced jalapeno (optional)

- 4 eggs (medium or large recommended)

- 1/4 cup diced red onion

- 2 avocados, halved & pitted

- 1 tablespoon lime juice

- 2 tablespoons chopped fresh cilantro

Instructions:

1. Squeeze the avocado fruit out from the skin with a spoon, leaving the shell preserved. Dice the avocado and put it in a bowl of medium-sized. Combine it with onion, jalapeno (if there is a need), tomato, pepper and cilantro. Refrigerate and cover the mixture of avocado until ready for usage.

2. Preheat the air-fryer for 350° f

3. Place the avocado shells on a ring made up of failing to make sure they don't rock when cooking. Just roll 2 three-inch-wide strips of aluminum foil into rope shapes to create them, and turn each one into a three-inch circle. In an air fryer basket, put every

avocado shell over a foil frame. Break an egg in every avocado shell & air fry for 5 - 7 minutes or when needed.

4. Take it out from the basket; fill including avocado salsa & serve.

12. Air fryer cinnamon rolls

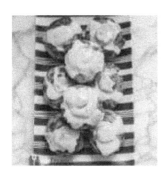

Cook time: 15 mins

Serving: 2 people

Difficulty: easy

Ingredients:

● 1 spray must non-stick cooking spray

● 1 can cinnamon rolls we used Pillsbury

Instructions:

1. put your cinnamon rolls inside your air fryer's basket, with the help of the rounds of
2. Parchment paper or by the cooking spray that is non-stick.

2. Cook at around 340 degrees f, 171 degrees for about 12 to 15 minutes, for one time.

3. Drizzle it with icing, place it on a plate and then serve.

13. Air-fryer all-American breakfast dumplings

Cook: 10 minutes

Servings: 1 person

Difficulty: easy

Ingredients:

● Dash salt

● 1/2 cup (about four large) egg whites or liquid egg fat-free substitute

● 1 tbsp. Pre-cooked real crumbled bacon

● 1 wedge the laughing cow light creamy Swiss cheese (or 1 tbsp. reduced-fat cream cheese)

● 8 wonton wrappers or gyoza

Instructions:

1. By using a non-stick spray, spray your microwave-safe bowl or mug. Include egg whites or any substitute, salt and cheese wedge. Microwave it for around 1.5 minutes, mixing in between until cheese gets well mixed and melted and the egg is set.

2. Mix the bacon in. Let it cool completely for about 5 minutes.

3. Cover a wrapper of gyoza with the mixture of an egg (1 tablespoon). Moist the corners with water & fold it in half, having the filling. Tightly push the corners to seal. Repeat this step to make seven more dumplings. Make sure to use a non-stick spray for spraying.

4. Insert the dumplings inside your air fryer in one single layer. (Save the leftover for another round if they all can't fit). Adjust the temperature to 375 or the closest degree. Cook it for around 5 mins or till it's crispy and golden brown.

Chapter 2: Air fryer seafood recipe

1. Air fryer 'shrimp boil'

Cook time: 15 mins

Servings: 2 people

Difficulty: easy

Ingredients:

- 2 tbsp. vegetable oil

- 1 lb. easy-peel defrosted shrimp

- 3 small red potatoes cut 1/2 inch rounds

- 1 tbsp. old bay seasoning

- 2 ears of corn cut into thirds

- 14 oz. smoked sausage, cut into three-inch pieces

Instructions:

1. Mix all the items altogether inside a huge tub & drizzle it with old bay seasoning, peppers, oil and salt. Switch to the air fryer basket attachment & place the basket over the pot.

2. Put inside your air fryer & adjust the setting of fish; make sure to flip after seven minutes.

3. Cautiously remove & then serve.

2. Air fryer fish & chips

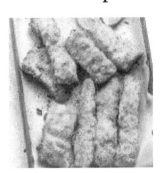

Cook time: 10 mins

Serving: 6 people

Difficulty: easy

Ingredients:

- Tartar sauce for serving

- ½ tbsp. garlic powder

- 1 pound cod fillet cut into strips

- Black pepper

- 2 cups panko breadcrumbs

- ½ cup all-purpose flour

- ¼ tbsp. salt

- Large egg beaten

- Lemon wedges for serving

- 2 teaspoons paprika

Instructions:

1. In a tiny tub, combine the flour, adding salt, paprika and garlic powder. Put your beaten egg in one bowl & your panko breadcrumbs in another bowl.

2. Wipe your fish dry with a towel. Dredge your fish with the mixture of flour, now the

egg & gradually your panko breadcrumbs, pushing down gently till your crumbs stick. Spray both ends with oil.

3. Fry at 400 degrees f. Now turn halfway for around 10 to 12 mins until it's lightly brown and crispy.

4. Open your basket & search for preferred crispiness with the help of a fork to know if it easily flakes off. You may hold fish for an extra 1 to 2 mins as required.

5. Serve instantly with tartar sauce and fries, if required.

3. Air-fryer scallops

Cook time: 20 mins

Servings: 2 people

Difficulty: easy

Ingredients:

- ¼ cup extra-virgin olive oil

- ½ tbsp. garlic finely chopped

- Cooking spray

- ½ teaspoons finely chopped garlic

- 8 large (1-oz.) Sea scallops, cleaned & patted very dry

- 1 tbsp. finely grated lemon zest

- ⅛ tbsp. salt

- 2 tbsps. Very finely chopped flat-leaf parsley

- 2 tbsp. capers, very finely chopped

- ¼ tbsp. ground pepper

Instructions:

1. Sprinkle the scallops with salt and pepper. Cover the air fryer basket by the cooking spray. Put your scallops inside the basket & cover them by the cooking spray. Put your basket inside the air fryer. Cook your scallops at a degree of 400 f till they attain the temperature of about 120 degrees f, which is an international temperature for 6 mins.

2. Mix capers, oil, garlic, lemon zest and parsley inside a tiny tub. Sprinkle over your scallops.

4. Air fryer tilapia

Cook time: 6 mins

Servings: 4 people

Difficulty: easy

Ingredients:

- 1/2 tbsp. paprika

- 1 tbsp. salt

- 2 eggs

- 4 fillets of tilapia

- 1 tbsp. garlic powder

- 1/2 teaspoon black pepper

- 1/2 cup flour

- 2 tbsp. lemon zest

- 1 tbsp. garlic powder

- 4 ounces parmesan cheese, grated

Instructions:

1. Cover your tilapia fillets:

Arrange three deep dishes. Out of these, put flour in one. Blend egg in second and make sure that the eggs are whisked in the last dish mix lemon zest, cheese, pepper, paprika and salt. Ensure that the tilapia fillets are dry, and after that dip, every fillet inside the flour & covers every side. Dip into your egg wash & pass them for coating every side of the fillet to your cheese mixture.

2. Cook your tilapia:

Put a tiny sheet of parchment paper in your bask of air fryer and put 1 - 2 fillets inside the baskets. Cook at 400°f for around 4 - 5 minutes till the crust seems golden brown, and the cheese completely melts.

5. Air fryer salmon

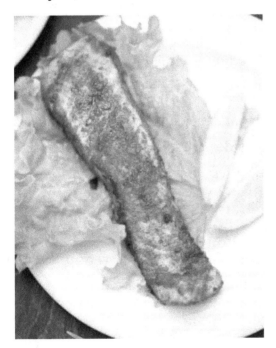

Cook time: 7 mins

Serving: 2 people

Difficulty: easy

Ingredients:

- 1/2 tbsp. salt
- 2 tbsp. olive oil
- 1/4 teaspoon ground black pepper
- 2 salmon fillets (about 1 1/2-inches thick)
- 1/2 teaspoon ginger powder
- 2 teaspoons smoked paprika
- 1 teaspoon onion powder
- 1/4 teaspoon red pepper flakes
- 1 tbsp. garlic powder
- 1 tablespoon brown sugar (optional)

Instructions:

1. Take the fish out of the refrigerator, check if there are any bones, & let it rest for 1 hour on the table.

2. Combine all the ingredients in a tub.

3. Apply olive oil in every fillet & then the dry rub solution.

4. Put the fillets in the Air Fryer basket.

5. set the air fryer for 7 minutes at the degree of 390 if your fillets have a thickness of 1-1/2-inches.

6. As soon as the timer stops, test fillets with a fork's help to ensure that they are ready to the perfect density. If you see that there is any need, then you cook it for a further few minutes. Your cooking time may vary with the temperature & size of the fish. It is best to set your air fryer for a minimum time, and then you may increase the time if there

is a need. This will prevent the fish from being overcooked.

6. Blackened fish tacos in the air fryer

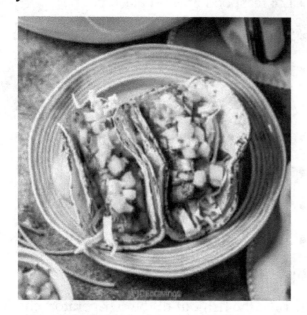

Cook time: 9 mins

Serving: 4 people

Difficulty: easy

Ingredients:

● 1 lb. Mahi mahi fillets (can use cod, catfish, tilapia or salmon)

● Cajun spices blend (or use 2-2.5 tbsp. store-bought Cajun spice blend)

● ¾ teaspoon salt

● 1 tbsp. paprika (regular, not smoked)

● 1 teaspoon oregano

● ½-¾ teaspoon cayenne (reduces or skips to preference)

● ½ teaspoon garlic powder

● ½ teaspoon onion powder

● ½ teaspoon black pepper

● 1 teaspoon brown sugar (skip for low-carb)

Additional ingredients for tacos:

● Mango salsa

● Shredded cabbage (optional)

● 8 corn tortillas

Instructions:

1. Get the fish ready

2. Mix cayenne, onion powder, brown sugar, salt, oregano, garlic powder, paprika and black pepper in a deep mixing tub.

3. Make sure to get the fish dry by using paper towels. Drizzle or brush the fish with a little amount of any cooking oil or olive oil. This allows the spices to stick to the fish.

4. Sprinkle your spice mix graciously on a single edge of your fish fillets. Rub the fish softly, so the ingredients stay on the fish.

5. Flip and brush the fish with oil on the other side & sprinkle with the leftover spices. Press the ingredients inside the fish softly.

6. Turn the air fryer on. Inside the basket put your fish fillets. Do not overlap the pan or overfill it. Close your basket.

7. Air fry the fish

8. Set your air fryer for 9 mins at 360°f. If you are using fillets which are thicker than an inch, then you must increase the cooking time to ten minutes. When the air fryer timer

stops, with the help of a fish spatula or long tongs, remove your fish fillets.

9. Assembling the tacos

10. Heat the corn tortillas according to your preference. Conversely, roll them inside the towel made up of wet paper & heat them in the microwave for around 20 to 30 seconds.

11. Stack 2 small fillets or insert your fish fillet. Add a few tablespoons of your favorite mango salsa or condiment & cherish the scorched fish tacos.

12. Alternatively, one can include a few cabbages shredded inside the tacos & now add fish fillets on the top.

7. Air fryer cod

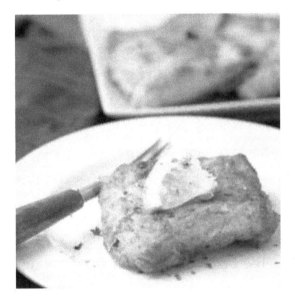

Cook time: 16 mins

Servings: 2 people

Difficulty: easy

Ingredients:

- 2 teaspoon of light oil for spraying

- 1 cup of plantain flour

- 0.25 teaspoon of salt

- 12 pieces of cod about 1 ½ pound

- 1 teaspoon of garlic powder

- 0.5 cup gluten-free flour blend

- 2 teaspoon of smoked paprika

- 4 teaspoons of Cajun seasoning or old bay

- Pepper to taste

Instructions:

1. Spray some oil on your air fryer basket & heat it up to 360° f.

2. Combine the ingredients in a tub & whisk them to blend. From your package, take the cod out and, with the help of a paper towel, pat dry.

3. Dunk every fish piece in the mixture of flour spice and flip it over & push down so that your fish can be coated.

4. Get the fish inside the basket of your air fryer. Ensure that there is room around every fish piece so that the air can flow round the fish.

5. Cook for around 8 minutes & open your air fryer so that you can flip your fish. Now cook another end for around 8 mins.

6. Now cherish the hot serving with lemon.

8. Air fryer miso-glazed Chilean sea bass

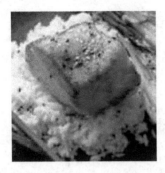

Cook time: 20 mins

Serving: 2 people

Difficulty: easy

Ingredients:

- 1/2 teaspoon ginger paste

- Fresh cracked pepper

- 1 tbsp. unsalted butter

- Olive oil for cooking

- 1 tbsp. rice wine vinegar

- 2 tbsp. miring

- 1/4 cup white miso paste

- 2 6 ounce Chilean sea bass fillets

- 4 tbsp. Maple syrup, honey works too.

Instructions:

1. Heat your air fryer to 375 degrees f. Apply olive oil onto every fish fillet and complete it with fresh pepper. Sprat olive oil on the pan of the air fryer and put the skin of the fish. Cook for about 12 to 15 minutes till you see the upper part change into golden brown color & the inner temperature now reached 135-degree f.

2. When the fish is getting cooked, you must have the butter melted inside a tiny saucepan in medium heat. When you notice that the butter melts, add maple syrup, ginger paste, miso paste, miring and rice wine vinegar, mix all of them till they are completely combined, boil them in a light flame and take the pan out instantly from the heat.

3. When your fish is completely done, brush the glaze and fish sides with the help of silicone pastry. Put it back inside your air fryer for around 1 to 2 extra minutes at 375 degrees f, till the glaze is caramelized. Complete it with green onion (sliced) & sesame seeds.

Instructions for oven

1. Heat the oven around 425 degrees f and put your baking sheet and foil sprayed with light olive oil. Bake it for about 20 to 25 minutes; this depends on how thick the fish is. The inner temperature must be around 130 degrees f when your fish is completely cooked.

2. Take out your fish, placed it in the oven & heat the broiler on a high flame. Now the fish must be brushed with miso glaze from the sides and the top & then put the fish inside the oven in the above rack. If the rack is very much near with your broiler, then place it a bit down, you might not want the fish to touch the broiler. Cook your fish for around 1 to 2 minutes above the broiler till you see it's getting caramelize. Make sure to

keep a check on it as it happens very quickly. Complete it with the help of green onions (sliced) and sesame seeds.

9. Air fryer fish tacos

Cook time: 35 mins

Serving: 6 people

Difficulty: Medium

Ingredients:

- ¼ teaspoon salt

- ¼ cup thinly sliced red onion

- 1 tbsp. water

- 2 tbsp. sour cream

- Sliced avocado, thinly sliced radishes, chopped fresh cilantro leaves and lime wedges

- 1 teaspoon lime juice

- ½ lb. skinless white fish fillets (such as halibut or mahi-mahi), cut into 1-inch strips

- 1 tbsp. mayonnaise

- 1 egg

- 1 package (12 bowls) old el Paso mini flour tortilla taco bowls, heated as directed on package

- 1 clove garlic, finely chopped

- ½ cup Progresso plain panko crispy bread crumbs

- 1 ½ cups shredded green cabbage

- 2 tbsp. old el Paso original taco seasoning mix (from 1-oz package)

Instructions:

1. Combine the sour cream, garlic, salt, mayonnaise and lime juice together in a medium pot. Add red onion and cabbage; flip to coat. Refrigerate and cover the mixture of cabbage until fit for serving.

2. Cut an 8-inch circle of parchment paper for frying. Place the basket at the bottom of the air fryer.

3. Place the taco-seasoning mix in a deep bowl. Beat the egg & water in another small bowl. Place the bread crumbs in another shallow dish. Coat the fish with your taco seasoning mix; dip inside the beaten egg, then cover with the mixture of bread crumbs, pressing to hold to it.

10. Air fryer southern fried catfish

Cook time: 13 mins

Servings: 4 people

Difficulty: easy

Ingredients:

- 1 lemon
- 1/4 teaspoon cayenne pepper
- Cornmeal seasoning mix
- 1/4 teaspoon granulated onion powder
- 1/2 cup cornmeal
- 1/2 teaspoon kosher salt
- 1/4 teaspoon chili powder
- 2 pounds catfish fillets
- 1/4 teaspoon garlic powder
- 1 cup milk
- 1/4 cup all-purpose flour
- 1/4 teaspoon freshly ground black pepper
- 2 tbsp. dried parsley flakes
- 1/2 cup yellow mustard

Instructions:

1. Add milk and put the catfish in a flat dish.

2. Slice the lemon in two & squeeze around two tbsp. of juice added into milk so that the buttermilk can be made.

3. Place the dish in the refrigerator & leave it for 15 minutes to soak the fillets.

4. Combine the cornmeal-seasoning mixture in a small bowl.

5. Take the fillets out from the buttermilk & pat them dry with the help of paper towels.

6. Spread the mustard evenly on both sides of the fillets.

7. Dip every fillet into a mixture of cornmeal & coat well to create a dense coating.

8. Place the fillets in the greased basket of the air fryer. Spray gently with olive oil.

9. Cook for around 10 minutes at 390 to 400 degrees. Turn over the fillets & spray them with oil & cook for another 3 to 5 mins.

11. Air fryer lobster tails with lemon butter

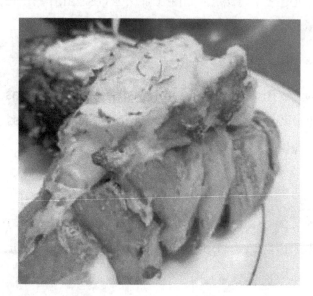

Cook time: 8 mins

Serving: 2 people

Difficulty: easy

Ingredients:

- 1 tbsp. fresh lemon juice

- 2 till 6 oz. Lobster tails, thawed

- Fresh chopped parsley for garnish (optional)

- 4 tbsp. melted salted butter

Instructions:

1. Make lemon butter combining lemon and melted butter. Mix properly & set aside.

2. Wash lobster tails & absorb the water with a paper towel. Butter your lobster tails by breaking the shell, take out the meat & place it over the shell.

3. Preheat the air fryer for around 5 minutes to 380 degrees. Place the ready lobster tails inside the basket of air fryer, drizzle with single tbsp. melted lemon butter on the meat of lobster. Cover the basket of the air fryer and cook for around 8 minutes at 380 degrees f, or when the lobster meat is not translucent. Open the air fryer halfway into the baking time, and then drizzle with extra lemon butter. Continue to bake until finished.

4. Remove the lobster tails carefully, garnish with crushed parsley if you want to, & plate. For dipping, serve with additional lemon butter.

12. Air fryer crab cakes with spicy aioli + lemon vinaigrette

Cook time: 20 mins

Servings: 2 people

Difficulty: easy

Ingredients:

For the crab cakes:

- 1. Avocado oil spray

- 16-ounce lump crab meat

- 1 egg, lightly beaten

- 2 tbsp. finely chopped red or orange pepper

- 1 tbsp. Dijon mustard

- 2 tbsp. finely chopped green onion

- 1/4 teaspoon ground pepper

- 1/4 cup panko breadcrumbs

- 2 tbsp. olive oil mayonnaise

For the aioli:

- 1/4 teaspoon cayenne pepper

- 1/4 cup olive oil mayonnaise

- 1 teaspoon white wine vinegar

- 1 teaspoon minced shallots

- 1 teaspoon Dijon mustard

For the vinaigrette:

- 2 tbsp. extra virgin olive oil

- 1 tbsp. white wine vinegar

- 4 tbsp. fresh lemon juice, about 1 ½ lemon

- 1 teaspoon honey

- 1 teaspoon lemon zest

To serve:

- Balsamic glaze, to taste

- 2 cups of baby arugula

Instructions:

1. Make your crab cake. Mix red pepper, mayonnaise, ground pepper, crab meat, onion, panko and Dijon in a huge bowl. Make sure to mix the ingredients well. Then add eggs & mix the mixture again till it's mixed well. Take around 1/4 cup of the mixture of crab into cakes which are around 1 inch thick. Spray with avocado oil gently.

2. Cook your crab cakes. Organize crab cakes in one layer in the air fryer. It depends on the air fryer how many batches will be required to cook them. Cook for 10 minutes at 375 degrees f. Take it out from your air fryer & keep it warm. Do this again if required.

3. Make aioli. Combine shallots, Dijon, vinegar, cayenne pepper and mayo. Put aside for serving until ready.

4. Make the vinaigrette. Combine honey, white vinegar, and lemon zest and lemon juice in a ting jar. Include olive oil & mix it well until mixed together.

5. Now serve. Split your arugula into 2 plates. Garnish with crab cakes. Drizzle it with vinaigrette & aioli. Include few drizzles of balsamic glaze if desired.

Chapter 3: Air Fryer Meat and Beef recipe

1. Air fryer steak

Cook time: 35 mins

Servings: 2

Difficulty: Medium

Ingredients:

- Freshly ground black pepper
- 1 tsp. freshly chopped chives
- 2 cloves garlic, minced
- 1(2 lb.) Bone-in rib eye
- 4 tbsp. Butter softened
- 1 tsp. Rosemary freshly chopped
- 2 tsp. Parsley freshly chopped
- 1 tsp. Thyme freshly chopped
- Kosher salt

Instructions:

1. In a tiny bowl, mix herbs and butter. Put a small layer of the wrap made up of plastic & roll in a log. Twist the ends altogether to make it refrigerate and tight till it gets hardened for around 20 minutes.

2. Season the steak with pepper and salt on every side.

3. Put the steak in the air-fryer basket & cook it around 400 degrees for 12 - 14 minutes, in medium temperature, depending on the thickness of the steak, tossing half-way through.

4. Cover your steak with the herb butter slice to serve.

2. Air-fryer ground beef wellington

Cook time: 20 mins

Serving: 2 people

Difficulty: easy

Ingredients:

- 1 large egg yolk
- 1 tsp. dried parsley flakes
- 2 tsp. flour for all-purpose
- 1/2 cup fresh mushrooms chopped
- 1 tbsp. butter
- 1/2 pound of ground beef
- 1 lightly beaten, large egg, it's optional
- 1/4 tsp. of pepper, divided
- 1/4 tsp. of salt
- 1 tube (having 4 ounces) crescent rolls refrigerated
- 2 tbsp. onion finely chopped
- 1/2 cup of half & half cream

Instructions:

1. Preheat the fryer to 300 degrees. Heat the butter over a moderate flame in a saucepan. Include mushrooms; stir, and cook for 5-6 minutes, until tender. Add flour & 1/8 of a tsp. of pepper when mixed. Add cream steadily. Boil it; stir and cook until

thickened, for about 2 minutes. Take it out from heat & make it aside.

2. Combine 2 tbsp. of mushroom sauce, 1/8 tsp. of the remaining pepper, onion and egg yolk in a tub. Crumble over the mixture of beef and blend properly. Shape it into two loaves. Unroll and divide the crescent dough into two rectangles; push the perforations to close. Put meatloaf over every rectangle. Bring together the sides and press to seal. Brush it with one beaten egg if necessary.

3. Place the wellingtons on the greased tray inside the basket of the air fryer in a single sheet. Cook till see the thermometer placed into the meatloaf measures 160 degrees, 18 to 22 minutes and until you see golden brown color.

Meanwhile, under low pressure, warm the leftover sauce; mix in the parsley. Serve your sauce, adding wellington.

3. Air-fried burgers

Cook time: 10 mins

Serving: 4 people

Difficulty: easy

Ingredients:

- 500 g of raw ground beef (1 lb.)
- 1 tsp. of Maggi seasoning sauce
- 1/2 tsp. of ground black pepper
- 1 tsp. parsley (dried)
- Liquid smoke (some drops)
- 1/2 tsp. of salt (salt sub)
- 1 tbsp. of Worcestershire sauce
- 1/2 tsp. of onion powder
- 1/2 tsp. of garlic powder

Instructions:

1. Spray the above tray, and set it aside. You don't have to spray your basket if you are having an air fryer of basket-type. The cooking temperature for basket types will be around 180 c or 350 f.

2. Mix all the spice things together in a little tub, such as the sauce of Worcestershire and dried parsley.

2. In a huge bowl, add it inside the beef.

3. Mix properly, and make sure to overburden the meat as this contributes to hard burgers.

4. Divide the mixture of beef into four, & the patties are to be shape off. Place your indent in the middle with the thumb to keep the patties from scrunching up on the center.

5. Place tray in the air fry; gently spray the surfaces of patties.

6. Cook for around 10 minutes over medium heat (or more than that to see that your food is complete). You don't have to turn your patties.

7. Serve it hot on a pan with your array of side dishes.

4. Air fryer meatloaf

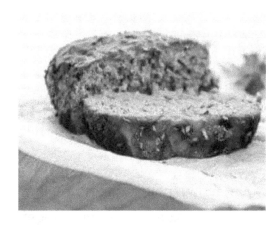

Cook time: 25 mins

Serving: 4 people

Difficulty: easy

Ingredients:

- 1/2 tsp. of Salt

- 1 tsp. of Worcestershire sauce

- 1/2 finely chopped, small onion

- 1 tbsp. of Yellow mustard

- 2 tbsp. of ketchup, divided

- 1 lb. Lean ground beef

- 1/2 tsp. Garlic powder

- 1/4 cup of dry breadcrumbs

- 1 egg, lightly beaten

- 1/4 tsp. Pepper

- 1 tsp. Italian seasoning

Instructions:

1. Put the onion, 1 tbsp. Ketchup, garlic powder, pepper, ground beef, egg, salt, breadcrumbs, Italian seasoning and Worcestershire sauce in a huge bowl.

2. Use hands to blend your spices with the meat equally, be careful you don't over-mix as it would make it difficult to over mix.

3. Shape meat having two inches height of 4 by 6, loaf. Switch your air fryer to a degree of 370 f & Put that loaf inside your air fryer.

4. Cook for fifteen min at a degree of 370 f.

5. In the meantime, mix the leftover 1 tbsp. of ketchup & the mustard in a tiny bowl.

6. Take the meatloaf out of the oven & spread the mixture of mustard over it.

7. Return the meatloaf to your air fryer & begin to bake at a degree of 370 degrees f till the thermometer placed inside the loaf measures 160 degrees f, around 8 to 10 further minutes.

8. Remove the basket from your air fryer when the meatloaf has touched 160 degrees f & then make the loaf stay inside the air fryer basket for around 5 to 10 minutes, after that slice your meatloaf.

5. Air fryer hamburgers

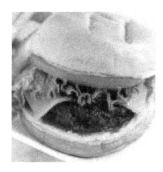

Cook time: 16 mins

Serving: 4 people

Difficulty: easy

Ingredients:

- 1 tsp. of onion powder
- 1 pound of ground beef (we are using 85/15)
- 4 pieces burger buns
- 1 tsp. salt
- 1/4 tsp. of black pepper
- 1 tsp. of garlic powder
- 1 tsp. of Worcestershire sauce

Instructions:

1. Method for standard ground beef:

2. Your air fryer must be preheated to 360 °.

3. In a bowl, put the unprocessed ground beef & add the seasonings.

4. To incorporate everything, make the of use your hands (or you can use a fork) & then shape the mixture in a ball shape (still inside the bowl).

5. Score the mixture of ground beef into 4 equal portions by having a + mark to split it.

Scoop out and turn each segment into a patty.

6. Place it in the air fryer, ensuring each patty has plenty of room to cook (make sure not to touch). If required, one can perform this in groups. We've got a bigger (5.8 quart) air fryer, and we did all of ours in a single batch.

7. Cook, turning half-way back, for 16 minutes. (Note: for bigger patties, you may have a need to cook longer.)

Process for Patties (pre-made):

1. In a tiny bowl, mix onion powder, pepper, garlic powder and salt, then stir till well mixed.

2. In a tiny bowl, pour in a few quantities of Worcestershire sauce. You may require A little more than one teaspoon (such as 1.5 tsp.), as some of it will adhere in your pastry brush.

3. Put patties on a tray & spoon or brush on a thin layer of your Worcestershire sauce.

4. Sprinkle with seasoning on every patty, saving 1/2 for another side.

5. With your hand, rub the seasoning to allow it to stick better.

6. Your air fryer should be preheated to 360 ° f.

7. Take out the basket when it's preheated & gently place your patties, seasoned one down, inside the basket.

8. Side 2 of the season, which is facing up the exact way as per above.

9. In an air fryer, put the basket back and cook for around 16 minutes, tossing midway through.

6. Air Fryer Meatloaf

Cook time: 25 mins

Serving: 4 people

Difficulty: Easy

Ingredients:

- Ground black pepper for taste

- 1 tbsp. of olive oil, or as required

- 1 egg, lightly beaten

- 1 tsp. of salt

- 1 pound of lean ground beef

- 1 tbsp. fresh thyme chopped

- 3 tbsp. of dry bread crumbs

- 1 finely chopped, small onion

- 2 thickly sliced mushrooms

Instructions:

1. Preheat your air fryer to a degree of 392 f (200°C).

2. Mix together egg, onion, salt, ground beef, pepper, bread crumbs and thyme in a tub. 3. Thoroughly knead & mix.

4. Transfer the mixture of beef in your baking pan & smooth out the surface. The mushrooms are to be pressed from the top & coated with the olive oil. Put the pan inside the basket of the air fryer & slide it inside your air fryer.

5. Set the timer of the air fryer for around 25 minutes & roast the meatloaf till it is nicely browned.

6. Make sure that the meatloaf stays for a minimum of 10 minutes, and after that, you can slice and serve.

7. Air Fryer Beef Kabobs

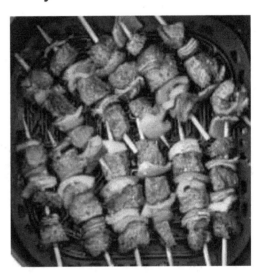

Cook time: 8 mins

Serving: 4 people

Difficulty: Easy

Ingredients:

- 1 big onion in red color or onion which you want

- 1.5 pounds of sirloin steak sliced into one-inch chunks

- 1 large bell pepper of your choice

For the marinade:

- 1 tbsp. of lemon juice

- Pinch of Salt & pepper

- 4 tbsp. of olive oil

- 1/2 tsp. of cumin

- 1/2 tsp. of chili powder

- 2 cloves garlic minced

Ingredients:

1. In a huge bowl, mix the beef & ingredients to marinade till fully mixed. Cover & marinate for around 30 minutes or up to 24 hours inside the fridge.

2. Preheat your air fryer to a degree of 400 f until prepared to cook. Thread the onion, pepper and beef onto skewers.

3. Put skewers inside the air fryer, which is already heated and the air fryer for about 8 to 10 minutes, rotating half-way until the outside is crispy and the inside is tender.

8. Air-Fried Beef and Vegetable Skewers

Cook time: 8 mins

Serving: 2

Difficulty: easy

Ingredients:

- 2 tbs. of olive oil

- 2 tsp. of fresh cilantro chopped

- Kosher salt & freshly black pepper ground

- 1 tiny yellow summer squash, sliced into one inch (of 2.5-cm) pieces

- 1/4 tsp. of ground coriander

- Lemon wedges to serve (optional)

- 1/8 tsp. of red pepper flakes

- 1 garlic clove, minced

- 1/2 tsp. of ground cumin

- 1/2 yellow bell pepper, sliced into one inch (that's 2.5-cm) pieces

- 1/2 red bell pepper, sliced into one inch (that's 2.5-cm) pieces

- 1/2 lb. (that's 250 g) boneless sirloin, sliced into one inch (of 2.5-cm) cubes

- 1 tiny zucchini, sliced into one inch (that's 2.5-cm) pieces

- 1/2 red onion, sliced into one inch (that's 2.5-cm) pieces

Ingredients:

1. Preheat your air fryer at 390 degrees f (199-degree c).

2. In a tiny bowl, mix together one tablespoon of cumin, red pepper flakes and coriander. Sprinkle the mixture of spices generously over the meat.

3. In a tub, mix together zucchini, oil, cilantro, bell peppers, summer squash, cilantro, onion and garlic. Season with black pepper and salt to taste.

4. Tightly thread the vegetables and meat onto the four skewers adding two layers rack of air fryer, rotating the bits and equally splitting them. Put the skewers over the rack & carefully set your rack inside the cooking basket. Put the basket inside the air fryer. Cook, without covering it for around 7 - 8 minutes, till the vegetables are crispy and

tender & your meat is having a medium-rare.

5. Move your skewers to a tray, and if you want, you can serve them with delicious lemon wedges.

9. Air fryer taco calzones

Cook time: 10 mins

Serving: 2 people

Difficulty: easy

Ingredients:

• 1 cup of taco meat

• 1 tube of Pillsbury pizza dough thinly crust

• 1 cup of shredded cheddar

Instructions:

1. Spread out the layer of your pizza dough over a clean table. Slice the dough into four squares with the help of a pizza cutter.

2. By the use of a pizza cutter, cut every square into a big circle. Place the dough pieces aside to create chunks of sugary cinnamon.

3. Cover 1/2 of every dough circle with around 1/4 cup of taco meat & 1/4 cup of shredded cheese.

4. To seal it firmly, fold the remaining over the cheese and meat and push the sides of your dough along with the help of a fork so that it can be tightly sealed. Repeat for all 4 calzones.

5. Each calzone much is gently picked up & spray with olive oil or pan spray. Organize them inside the basket of Air Fryer.

Cook your calzones at a degree of 325 for almost 8 to 10 minutes. Monitor them carefully when it reaches to 8 min mark. This is done so that there is no chance of overcooking.

6. Using salsa & sour cream to serve.

7. For the making of cinnamon sugary chunks, split the dough pieces into pieces having equal sides of around 2 inches long. Put them inside the basket of the air fryer & cook it at a degree of 325 for around 5 minutes. Instantly mix with the one ratio four sugary cinnamon mixtures.

10. Air Fryer Pot Roast

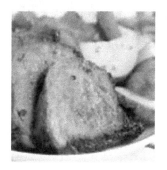

Cook time: 30 mins

Serving: 2 people

Difficulty: Medium

Ingredients:

• 1 tsp. of salt

• 3 tbsp. of brown sugar

• 1/2 cup of orange juice

- 1 tsp. of Worcestershire sauce

- 1/2 tsp. of pepper

- 3–4 pound thawed roast beef chuck roast

- 3 tbsp. of soy sauce

Instructions:

1. Combine brown sugar, Worcestershire sauce, soy sauce and orange juice.

2. Mix till the sugar is completely dissolved.

3. Spillover the roast & marinade for around 8 to 24 hours.

4. Put the roast in the basket of an air fryer.

5. Sprinkle the top with pepper and salt.

6. Air fry it at a degree of 400 f for around 30 minutes, turning it half-way through.

7. Allow it to pause for a period of 3 minutes.

8. Slice and serve into thick cuts.

Chapter 4: midnight snacks

1. Air fryer onion rings

Cook time: 7 mins

Serving: 2 people

Difficulty: easy

Ingredients:

• 2 beaten, large eggs

• Marinara sauce for serving

• 1 ½ tsp. of kosher salt

• ½ tsp. of garlic powder

• 1 medium yellow onion, cut into half in about (1 1/4 cm)

• 1 cup of flour for all-purpose (125 g)

• 1 ½ cups of panko breadcrumbs (172 g)

• 1 tsp. of paprika

• ⅛ tsp. of cayenne

• ½ tsp. of onion powder

• ½ tsp. black pepper freshly ground

Instructions:

1. Preheat your air fryer to 190°c (375°f).

2. Use a medium-size bowl to mix together onion powder, salt, paprika, cayenne, pepper, flour and garlic powder.

3. In 2 separate small cups, add your panko & eggs.

4. Cover onion rings with flour, then with the eggs, and afterward with the panko.

Working in lots, put your onion rings in one layer inside your air fryer & "fry" for 5 to 7 minutes or till you see golden brown color.

5. Using warm marinara sauce to serve.

2. Air fryer sweet potato chips

Cook time: 15 mins

Serving: 2

Difficulty: easy

Ingredients:

• 1 ½ tsp. of kosher salt

• 1 tsp. of dried thyme

• 1 large yam or sweet potato

• ½ tsp. of pepper

• 1 tbsp. of olive oil

Instructions:

1. Preheat your air fryer to a degree of 350 f (180 c).

2. Slice your sweet potato have a length of 3- to 6-mm (1⁄8-1⁄4-inch). In a medium tub, mix your olive oil with slices of sweet potato until well-seasoned. Add some pepper, thyme and salt to cover.

3. Working in groups, add your chips in one sheet & fry for around 14 minutes till you see a golden brown color and slightly crisp.

Fun.

3. Air fryer tortilla chips

Cook time: 5 mins

Serving: 2 people

Difficulty: easy

Ingredients:

- 1 tbsp. of olive oil

- Guacamole for serving

- 2 tsp. of kosher salt

- 12 corn of tortillas

- 1 tbsp. of McCormick delicious jazzy spice blend

Instructions:

1. Preheat your air fryer at a degree of 350 f (180 c).

2. Gently rub your tortillas with olive oil on every side.

3. Sprinkle your tortillas with delicious jazzy spice and salt mix on every side.

Slice every tortilla into six wedges.

4. Functioning in groups, add your tortilla wedges inside your air fryer in one layer & fry it for around 5 minutes or until you see golden brown color and crispy texture.

Serve adding guacamole

4. Air fryer zesty chicken wings

Cook time: 20 mins

Serving: 2 people

Difficulty: easy

Ingredients:

- 1 ½ tsp. of kosher salt

- 1 ½ lb. of patted dry chicken wings (of 680 g)

- 1 tbsp. of the delicious, zesty spice blend

Instructions:

1. Preheat your air fryer at 190°c (375°f).

2. In a tub, get your chicken wings mixed in salt & delicious zesty spice, which must be blend till well-seasoned.

3. Working in lots, add your chicken wings inside the air fryer in one layer & fry it for almost 20 minutes, turning it halfway through.

4. Serve it warm

5. Air fryer sweet potato fries

Cook time: 15 mins

Serving: 2 people

Difficulty: easy

Ingredients:

- 1/4 tsp. of sea salt

- 1 tbsp. of olive oil

- 2 (having 6-oz.) sweet potatoes, cut & peeled into sticks of 1/4-inch

- Cooking spray

- 1/4 tsp. of garlic powder

- 1 tsp. fresh thyme chopped

Instructions:

1. Mix together thyme, garlic powder, olive oil and salt in a bowl. Put sweet potato inside the mixture and mix well to cover.

2. Coat the basket of the air fryer gently with the help of cooking spray. Place your sweet potatoes in one layer inside the basket & cook in groups at a degree of 400 f until soft inside & finely browned from outside for around 14 minutes, rotating the fries halfway through the cooking process.

6. Air fryer churros with chocolate sauce

Cook time: 30 mins

Serving: 12

Difficulty: easy

Ingredients:

• 1/4 cup, adding 2 tbsp. Unsalted butter that's divided into half-cup (around 2 1/8 oz.)

• 3 tbsp. of heavy cream

• Half cup water

• 4 ounces of bitter and sweet finely chopped baking chocolate

• Flour for All-purpose

• 2 tsp. of ground cinnamon

• 2 large eggs

• 1/4 tsp. of kosher salt

• 2 tbsp. of vanilla kefir

• 1/3 cup of granulated sugar

Instruction:

1. Bring salt, water & 1/4 cup butter and boil it in a tiny saucepan with a medium-high flame. Decrease the heat to around medium-low flame; add flour & mix actively with a spoon made up of wood for around 30 seconds.

2. Stir and cook continuously till the dough is smooth. Do this till you see your dough continues to fall away from the sides of the pan & a film appears on the bottom of the pan after 2 to 3 minutes. Move the dough in a medium-sized bowl. Stir continuously for around 1 minute until slightly cooled. Add one egg from time to time while stirring continuously till you see it gets smoother after every addition. Move the mixture in the piping bag, which is fitted with having star tip of medium size. Chill it for around 30 minutes.

3. Pipe 6 (3" long) bits in one-layer inside a basket of the air fryer. Cook at a degree of 380 f for around 10 minutes. Repeat this step for the leftover dough.

4. Stir the sugar & cinnamon together inside a medium-size bowl. Use 2 tablespoons of melted butter to brush the cooked churros. Cover them with the sugar mixture.

5. Put the cream and chocolate in a tiny, microwaveable tub. Microwave with a high temperature for roughly 30 seconds until

molten and flat, stirring every 15 seconds. Mix in kefir.

6. Serve the churros, including chocolate sauce.

7. Whole-wheat pizzas in an air fryer

Cook time: 10 mins

Serving: 2 people

Difficulty: easy

Ingredients:

- 1 small thinly sliced garlic clove

- 1/4 ounce of Parmigiano-Reggiano shaved cheese (1 tbsp.)

- 1 cup of small spinach leaves (around 1 oz.)

- 1/4 cup marinara sauce (lower-sodium)

- 1-ounce part-skim pre-shredded mozzarella cheese (1/4 cup)

- 1 tiny plum tomato, sliced into 8 pieces

- 2 pita rounds of whole-wheat

Instructions:

1. Disperse marinara sauce equally on one side of every pita bread. Cover it each with half of the tomato slices, cheese, spinach leaves and garlic.

2. Put 1 pita in the basket of air-fryer & cook it at a degree of 350 f until the cheese is melted and the pita is crispy. Repeat with the leftover pita.

8. Air-fried corn dog bites

Cook time: 15 mins

Serving: 4 people

Difficulty: easy

Ingredients:

- 2 lightly beaten large eggs

- 2 uncured hot dogs of all-beef

- Cooking spray

- 12 bamboo skewers or craft sticks

- 8 tsp. of yellow mustard

- 1 1/2 cups cornflakes cereal finely crushed

- 1/2 cup (2 1/8 oz.) Flour for All-purpose

Instructions:

1. Split lengthwise every hot dog. Cut every half in three same pieces. Add a bamboo skewer or the craft stick inside the end of every hot dog piece.

2. Put flour in a bowl. Put slightly beaten eggs in another shallow bowl. Put crushed cornflakes inside another shallow bowl. Mix the hot dogs with flour; make sure to shake the surplus. Soak in the egg, helping you in dripping off every excess. Dredge inside the cornflakes crumbs, pushing to stick.

3. Gently coat the basket of the air fryer with your cooking spray. Put around six bites of corn dog inside the basket; spray the surface lightly with the help of cooking spray. Now cook at a degree of 375 f till the coating

shows a golden brown color and is crunchy for about 10 minutes, flipping the bites of corn dog halfway in cooking. Do this step with other bites of the corn dog.

4. Put three bites of corn dog with 2 tsp. of mustard on each plate to, and then serve immediately.

9. Crispy veggie quesadillas in an air fryer

Cook time: 20 mins

Serving: 4 people

Difficulty: easy

Instructions:

- Cooking spray

- 1/2 cup refrigerated and drained pico de gallo

- 4 ounces far educing cheddar sharp cheese, shredded (1 cup)

- 1 tbsp. of fresh juice (with 1 lime)

- 4(6-in.) whole-grain Sprouted flour tortillas

- 1/4 tsp. ground cumin

- 2 tbsp. fresh cilantro chopped

- 1 cup red bell pepper sliced

- 1 cup of drained & rinsed black beans canned, no-salt-added

- 1 tsp. of lime zest plus

- 1 cup of sliced zucchini

- 2 ounces of plain 2 percent fat reduced Greek yogurt

Instructions:

1. Put tortillas on the surface of your work. Sprinkle two tbsp. Shredded cheese on the half of every tortilla. Each tortilla must be top with cheese, having a cup of 1/4 each black beans, slices of red pepper equally and zucchini slices. Sprinkle equally with the leftover 1/2 cup of cheese. Fold the tortillas making a shape of a half-moon. Coat quesadillas lightly with the help of cooking spray & protect them with toothpicks.

2. Gently spray the cooking spray on the basket of the air fryer. Cautiously put two quesadillas inside the basket & cook it at a degree of 400 f till the tortillas are of golden brown color & slightly crispy, vegetables get softened, and the cheese if finally melted for around 10 minutes, rotating the quesadillas halfway while cooking. Do this step again with the leftover quesadillas.

3. As the quesadillas are cooking, mix lime zest, cumin, yogurt and lime juice altogether in a small tub. For serving, cut the quesadilla in slices & sprinkle it with cilantro. Serve it with a tablespoon of cumin cream and around 2 tablespoons of pico de gallo.

10. Air-fried curry chickpeas

Cook time: 10 mins

Serving: 4 people

Difficulty: easy

Ingredients:

- 2 tbsp. of curry powder

- Fresh cilantro thinly sliced

- 1(15-oz.) Can chickpeas (like garbanzo beans), rinsed & drained (1 1/2 cups)

- 1/4 tsp. of kosher salt

- 1/2 tbsp. of ground turmeric

- 1/2 tsp. of Aleppo pepper

- 1/4 tsp. of ground coriander

- 2 tbsp. of olive oil

- 1/4 tsp. and 1/8 tsp. of Ground cinnamon

- 2 tbsp. of vinegar (red wine)

- 1/4 tsp. of ground cumin

Instructions:

1. Smash chickpeas softly inside a tub with your hands (don't crush); remove chickpea skins.

2. Apply oil and vinegar to chickpeas, & toss for coating. Add turmeric, cinnamon, cumin, curry powder and coriander; whisk gently so that they can be mixed together.

3. Put chickpeas in one layer inside the bask of air fryer & cook at a degree of 400 f till it's crispy for around 15 mins; shake the chickpeas timely while cooking.

4. Place the chickpeas in a tub. Sprinkle it with cilantro, Aleppo pepper and salt; blend to coat.

11. Air fry shrimp spring rolls with sweet chili sauce.

Cook time: 20 mins

Serving: 4

Difficulty: easy

Ingredients:

- 1 cup of matchstick carrots

- 8 (8" square) wrappers of spring roll

- 2 1/2 tbsp. of divided sesame oil

- 4 ounces of peeled, deveined and chopped raw shrimp

- 1/2 cup of chili sauce (sweet)

- 1 cup of (red) bell pepper julienne-cut

- 2 tsp. of fish sauce

- 3/4 cup snow peas julienne-cut

- 2 cups of cabbage, pre-shredded

- 1/4 tsp. of red pepper, crushed

- 1 tbsp. of lime juice (fresh)

- 1/4 cup of fresh cilantro (chopped)

Instructions:

1. In a large pan, heat around 1 1/2 tsp. of oil until softly smoked. Add carrots, bell pepper and cabbage; Cook, stirring constantly, for 1 to 1 1/2 minutes, until finely wilted. Place it on a baking tray; cool for 5 minutes.

2. In a wide tub, place the mixture of cabbage, snow peas, cilantro, fish sauce, red pepper, shrimp and lime juice; toss to blend.

3. Put the wrappers of spring roll on the surface with a corner that is facing you. Add a filling of 1/4 cup in the middle of every wrapper of spring roll, extending from left-hand side to right in a three-inch wide strip.

4. Fold each wrapper's bottom corner over the filling, stuffing the corner tip under the filling. Fold the corners left & right over the filling. Brush the remaining corner softly with water; roll closely against the remaining corner; press gently to cover. Use 2 teaspoons of the remaining oil to rub the spring rolls.

5. Inside the basket of air fryer, put four spring rolls & cook at a degree of 390 f till it's golden, for 6 - 7 minutes, rotating the spring rolls every 5 minutes. Repeat with the leftover spring rolls. Use chili sauce to serve.

Chapter 5: Dessert recipes

1. Air fryer mores

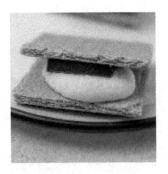

Cook time: 2 mins

Serving: 2 people

Difficulty: easy

Ingredients:

- 1 big marshmallow

- 2 graham crackers split in half

- 2 square, fine quality chocolate

Instructions:

1. Preheat the air fryer at a degree of 330 f.

2. When preheating, break 2 graham crackers into two to form four squares. Cut 1 big marshmallow into half evenly so that one side can be sticky.

3. Add every half of your marshmallow in a square of one graham cracker & push downwards to stick the marshmallow with graham cracker. You must now have two marshmallows coated with graham crackers & two regular graham crackers.

4. In one layer, put two graham crackers and marshmallows inside your air fryer & cook for about 2 minutes till you can see the marshmallow becoming toasted slightly.

5. Remove immediately and completely and add 1 chocolate square to the toasted marshmallow. Add the rest of the squares of the graham cracker and press down. Enjoy instantly.

2. Easy air fryer brownies

Cook time: 15 mins

Serving: 4 people

Difficulty: easy

Ingredients:

- 2 large eggs

- ½ cup flour for all-purpose

- ¼ cup melted unsalted butter

- 6 tbsp. of cocoa powder, unsweetened

- ¼ tsp. of baking powder

- ¾ cup of sugar

- ½ tsp. of vanilla extract

- 1 tbsp. of vegetable oil

- ¼ tsp. of salt

Instructions:

1. Get the 7-inch baking tray ready by gently greasing it with butter on all the sides and even the bottom. Put it aside

2. Preheat the air fryer by adjusting its temperature to a degree of 330 f & leaving it for around 5 minutes as you cook the brownie batter.

3. Add baking powder, cocoa powder, vanilla extract, flour for all-purpose, butter, vegetable oil, salt, eggs and sugar in a big tub & mix it unless well combined.

4. Add up all these for the preparation of the baking pan & clean the top.

5. Put it inside the air fryer & bake it for about 15 minutes or as long as a toothpick can be entered and comes out easily from the center.

6. Take it out and make it cool in the tray until you remove and cut.

3. Easy air fryer churros

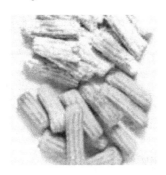

Cook time: 5 mins

Serving: 4 people

Difficulty: easy

Ingredients:

- 1 tbsp. of sugar
- Sifted powdered sugar & cinnamon or cinnamon sugar
- 1 cup (about 250ml) water
- 4 eggs
- ½ cup (113g) butter
- ¼ tsp. salt

- 1 cup (120g) all-purpose flour

Instructions:

1. Mix the ingredients bringing them to boil while stirring continuously.

2. Add flour & start mixing properly. Take it out from the heat & mix it till it gets smooth & the dough can be taken out from the pan easily.

3. Add one egg at one time and stir it until it gets smooth. Set it to cool.

4. Preheat your air fryer degree of 400 for 200 c.

5. Cover your bag of cake decorations with dough & add a star tip of 1/2 inch.

6. Make sticks which are having a length of 3 to 4 inches by moving your dough out from the bag in paper (parchment). You can now switch it inside your air fryer if you are ready to do so. If it is hard to handle the dough, put it inside the refrigerator for around 30 minutes.

7. Use cooking spray or coconut oil to spray the tray or the basket of your air fryer.

8. Add around 8 to 10 churros in a tray or inside the basket of the air fryer. Spray with oil.

9. Cook for 5 minutes at a degree of 400 for 200 c.

10. Until finished and when still hot, rill in regular sugar, cinnamon or sugar mixture.

11. Roll in the cinnamon-sugar blend, cinnamon or normal sugar until finished and when still high.

4. Air fryer sweet apples

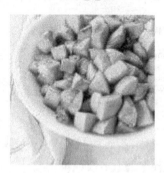

Cook time: 8 mins

Serving: 4 people

Difficulty: easy

Ingredients:

- ¼ cup of white sugar
- ⅓ Cup of water
- ¼ cup of brown sugar
- ½ tsp. of ground cinnamon
- 6 apples diced and cored
- ¼ tsp. of pumpkin pie spice
- ¼ tsp. of ground cloves

Instructions:

1. Put all the ingredients in a bowl that is oven safe & combine it with water and seasonings. Put the bowl inside the basket, oven tray or even in the toaster of an air fryer.

2. Air fry the mixture of apples at a degree of 350 f for around 6 minutes. Mix the apples & cook them for an extra 2 minutes. Serve it hot and enjoy.

5. Air fryer pear crisp for two

Cook time: 20 mins

Serving: 2

Difficulty: easy

Ingredients:

- ¾ tsp. of divided ground cinnamon
- 1 tbsp. of softened salted butter
- 1 tsp. of lemon juice
- 2 pears. Peeled, diced and cored
- 1 tbsp. of flour for all-purpose
- 2 tbsp. of quick-cooking oats
- 1 tbsp. of brown sugar

Instructions:

1. Your air fryer should be preheated at a degree of 360 f (180 c).

2. Mix lemon juice, 1/4 tsp. Cinnamon and pears in a bowl. Turn for coating and then split the mixture into 2 ramekins.

3. Combine brown sugar, oats, leftover cinnamon and flour in the tub. Using your fork to blend in the melted butter until the mixture is mushy. Sprinkle the pears.

4. Put your ramekins inside the basket of an air fryer & cook till the pears become bubbling and soft for around 18 - 20 minutes.

6. Keto chocolate cake – air fryer recipe

Cook time: 10 mins

Serving: 6 people

Difficulty: easy

Ingredients:

- 1 tsp. of vanilla extract

- 1/2 cup of powdered Swerve

- 1/3 cup of cocoa powder unsweetened

- 1/4 tsp. of salt

- 1 & 1/2 cups of almond flour

- 2 large eggs

- 1/3 cups of almond milk, unsweetened

- 1 tsp. of baking powder

Instructions:

1. In a big mixing tub, mix every ingredient until they all are well mixed.

2. Butter or spray your desired baking dish. We used bunt tins in mini size, but you can even get a 6-inch cake pan in the baskets of the air fryer.

3. Scoop batter equally inside your baking dish or dishes.

4. Set the temperature of the air fryer to a degree of 350 f & set a 10-minute timer. Your cake will be ready when the toothpick you entered comes out clear and clean.

Conclusion:

The air fryer seems to be a wonderful appliance that will assist you with maintaining your diet. You will also enjoy the flavor despite eating high amounts of oil if you prefer deep-fried food.

Using a limited quantity of oil, you will enjoy crunchy & crispy food without the additional adverse risk, which tastes exactly like fried food. Besides, the system is safe & easy to use. All you must do is choose the ingredients needed, and there will be nutritious food available for your family.

An air fryer could be something which must be considered if a person is attempting to eat a diet having a lower-fat diet, access to using the system to prepare a range of foods, & want trouble cooking experience.

Vegan Air Fryer Cookbook

By

Mark

Machino

Contents

Introduction

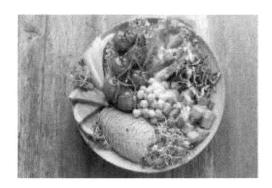

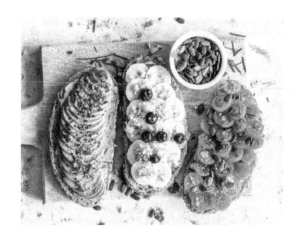

To have a good, satisfying life, a balanced diet is important. Tiredness and susceptibility to illnesses, many severe, arise from a lifestyle so full of junk food. Our community, sadly, does not neglect unsafe choices. People turn to immoral practices in order to satisfy desire, leading to animal torture. Two of the key explanations that people adhere to vegetarianism, a vegan-based diet that often excludes animal foods such as cheese, beef, jelly, and honey, are fitness and animal welfare.

It's essential for vegetarians to get the most nutrients out of any food, and that's where frying using an air fryer shines. The air fryer cooking will maintain as many nutrients as possible from beans and veggies, and the gadget makes it incredibly simple to cook nutritious food.

Although there are prepared vegan alternatives, the healthier choice, and far less pricey, is still to prepare your own recipes. This book provides the very first moves to being a vegan and offers 50 quick breakfast recipes, sides, snacks, and much more, so you have a solid base on which to develop.

This book will teach you all you need to thrive, whether you are either a vegan and only need more meal choices or have just begun contemplating transforming your diet.

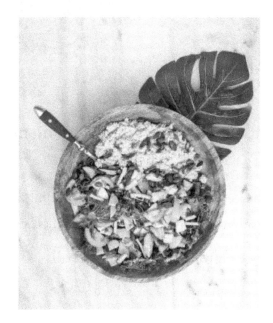

What is Cooking Vegan?

In recent decades, vegetarianism has become quite common, as individuals understand just how toxic the eating patterns of civilization have become. We are a society that enjoys meat, and, unfortunately, we go to dishonest measures to get the food we like. More citizens are choosing to give up beef and, unlike vegans, other livestock items due to various health issues, ethical issues, or both. Their diet moves to one focused on plants, whole grains, beans, fruit, seeds, nuts, and vegan varieties of the common dish.

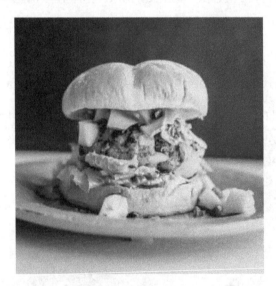

What advantages would veganism have?

There are a lot of advantages to a diet away from all animal items. Only a few includes:

- Healthier hair, skin, and nails

- High energy

- Fewer chances of flu and cold

- Fewer migraines

- Increased tolerance to cancer

- Strengthened fitness of the heart

Although research has proven that veganism will contribute to reducing BMI, it must not be followed for the mere sake of weight reduction. "Vegan" does not indicate "lower-calorie," and if you wish to reduce weight, other healthier activities, including exercising and consuming water, can complement the diet.

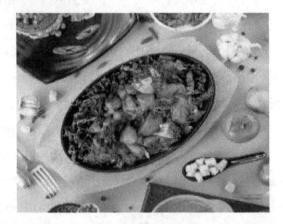

Air Fryer

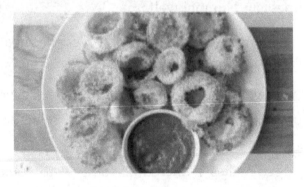

A common kitchen gadget used to create fried foods such as beef, baked goods and potato chips is an air fryer. It provides a crunchy, crisp coating by blowing hot air across the food. This also leads to a chemical reaction commonly known as the Maillard effect, which happens in the presence of heat in between reducing sugar and amino acid.

This adds to shifts in food color and taste. Due to the reduced amount of calories and fat, air-fried items are marketed as a healthier substitute to deep-fried foods.

Rather than fully soaking the food in fat, air-frying utilizes just a teaspoon to create a flavor and feel equivalent to deep-fried foods.

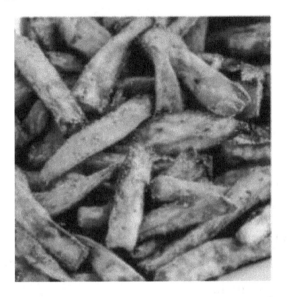

The flavor and appearance of the fried food in the air are similar to the deep fryer outcomes: On the surface, crispy; from the inside, soft. You do need to use a limited amount of oil, though, or any at all (based on what you're baking). But indeed, contrary to deep frying, if you agree to use only 1-2 teaspoons of plant-based oil with spices and you stuck to air-frying vegetables rather than anything else, air frying is certainly a better option.

The secret to weight loss, decreased likelihood of cardiovascular illness and better long-term wellbeing as we mature is any gadget that assists you and your friends in your vegetarian game.

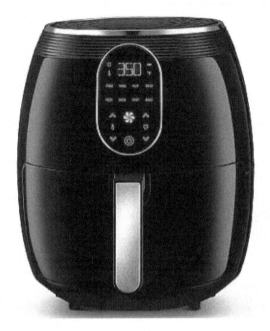

Air fryer's Working Process:

The air fryer is a worktop kitchen gadget that operates in the same manner as a traditional oven. To become acquainted with the operating theory of the traditional oven, you will need a little study. The air fryer uses rotating hot air to fry and crisp your meal, close to the convection oven. In a traditional convection oven, the airflow relies on revolving fans, which blast hot air around to produce an even or equalized temperature dispersal throughout the oven.

This is compared to the upward airflow of standard ovens, where the warm place is typically the oven's tip. And although the air fryer is not quite like the convection oven, it is a great approximation of it in the field of airflow for most components. The gadget has an air inlet at the top that lets air in and a hot air outlet at the side. All of these features are used to monitor the temperature within the air fryer. Temperatures will rise to 230 ° C, based on the sort of air fryer you're buying.

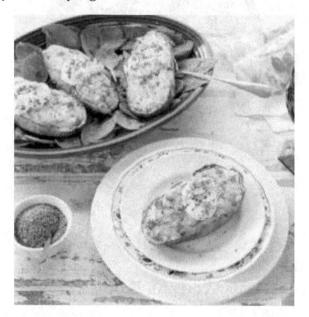

In conjunction with any grease, this hot air is used for cooking the food in the bowl within the device, if you like. Yes, if you want a taste of the oil, you should apply more oil. To jazz up the taste of the meal, simply add a little more to the blend. But the key concept behind the air fryer is to reduce the consumption of calories and fat without reducing the amount of taste.

Using air frying rather than deep frying saves between 70-80 calories, according to researchers. The growing success of recipes for air fryers is simply attributed to its impressive performance. It is simple to use and less time-consuming than conventional ovens.

This is more or less a lottery win for people searching for healthy alternative to deep-frying, as demonstrated by its widespread popularity in many homes today. In contrast to conventional ovens or deep frying, the air fryer creates crispy, crunchy, wonderful, and far fewer fatty foods in less duration. For certain individuals like us; this is what distinguishes air fryer recipes.

Tips for using an Air Fryer

1. The food is cooked easily. Air fried, unlike conventional cooking techniques, cut the cooking time a great deal. Therefore, to stop burning the food or getting a not-so-great flavor, it is best to hold a close eye on the gadget. Notice, remember that the smaller the food on the basket, the shorter the cooking period, which implies that the food cooks quicker.

2. You may need to reduce the temperature at first. Bear in mind that air fryers depend on the flow of hot air, which heats up rapidly. This ensures that it's better, to begin with, a low temperature so that the food cooks equally. It is likely that when the inside is already cooking, the exterior of the food is all cooked and begins to become dark or too dry.

3. When air fryers are in operation, they create some noise. If you are new to recipes for air fryers, you may have to realize that air fryers create noise while working. When it's in service, a whirring tone emanates from the device. However, the slight

annoyance pales in contrast to the various advantages of having an air fryer.

4. Hold the grate within the container at all hours. As previously mentioned, the air fryer has a container inside it, where the food is put and permitted to cook. This helps hot air to flow freely around the food, allowing for even cooking.

5. Don't stuff the air fryer with so much food at once. If you plan to make a meal for one guy, with only one batch, you would most definitely be able to get your cooking right. If you're cooking for two or more individuals, you can need to plan the food in groups. With a 4 - 5 quart air fryer, you can always need to cook in groups, depending on the size and sort of air fryer you have. This not only means that your device works longer but also keeps your food from cooking unevenly. You shouldn't have to turn the air fryer off as you pull out the basket since it simply turns off on its own until the basket is out. Often, make sure the drawer is completely retracted; otherwise, the fryer would not turn back on.

6. Take the basket out of the mix and mix the ingredients. You might need to move the food around or switch it over once every few minutes, based on the dish you're preparing and the time it takes to prepare your dinner.

The explanation for this is that even cooking can be done. Certain recipes involve the foods in the basket to shake and shuffle throughout the cooking phase. And an easy-to-understand checklist is given for each recipe to direct you thru the cycle.

7. The air fryer does not need cooking mist. It isn't needed. In order to prevent the urge to use non-stick frying spray in the container, you must deliberately take care of this. The basket is now coated with a non-stick covering, so what you need to do is fill your meal inside the container and push it back in.

Outcome

You can create nutritious meals very simply and fast, right in the comfort of your house. There are many excellent recipes for producing healthier meals and nutritious foods, which you can notice in the air fryer recipes illustrated in this book. However, you'll need to pay careful attention to the ingredients and know-how to easily use the air fryer to do this. To get straightforward guidance on installation and usage, you can need to refer to the company's manual.

CHAPTER 1: Breakfast Recipes

1. Toasted French toast

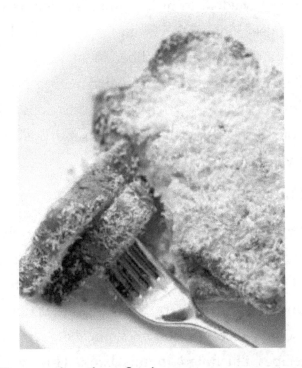

Preparation time: 2 minutes

Cooking time: 5 minutes

Servings: 1 people

Ingredients:

- ½ Cup of Unsweetened Shredded Coconut
- 1 Tsp. Baking Powder
- ½ Cup Lite Culinary Coconut Milk
- 2 Slices of Gluten-Free Bread (use your favorite)

Directions:

1. Stir together the baking powder and coconut milk in a large rimmed pot.

2. On a tray, layout your ground coconut.

3. Pick each loaf of your bread and dip it in your coconut milk for the very first time, and then pass it to the ground coconut, let it sit for a few minutes, then cover the slice entirely with the coconut.

4. Place the covered bread loaves in your air fryer, cover it, adjust the temperature to about 350 ° F and set the clock for around 4 minutes.

5. Take out from your air fryer until done, and finish with some maple syrup of your choice. French toast is done. Enjoy!

2. Vegan Casserole

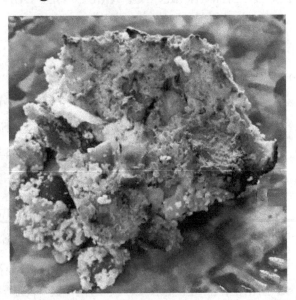

Preparation time: 10-12 minutes

Cooking time: 15-20 minutes

Servings: 2-3 people

Ingredients:

- 1/2 cup of cooked quinoa
- 1 tbsp. of lemon juice
- 2 tbsp. of water
- 2 tbsp. of plain soy yogurt
- 2 tbsp. of nutritional yeast
- 7 ounces of extra-firm tofu about half a block, drained but not pressed
- 1/2 tsp. of ground cumin
- 1/2 tsp. of red pepper flakes
- 1/2 tsp. of freeze-dried dill
- 1/2 tsp. of black pepper
- 1/2 tsp. of salt
- 1 tsp. of dried oregano
- 1/2 cup of diced shiitake mushrooms
- 1/2 cup of diced bell pepper I used a combination of red and green
- 2 small celery stalks chopped
- 1 large carrot chopped
- 1 tsp. of minced garlic
- 1 small onion diced
- 1 tsp. of olive oil

Directions:

1. Warm the olive oil over medium-low heat in a big skillet. Add your onion and garlic and simmer till the onion is transparent (for about 3 to 6 minutes). Add your bell pepper, carrot, and celery and simmer for another 3 minutes. Mix the oregano, mushrooms, pepper, salt, cumin, dill, and red pepper powder. Mix completely and lower the heat to low. If the vegetables tend to cling, stir regularly and add in about a teaspoon of water.

2. Pulse the nutritional yeast, tofu, water, yogurt, and some lemon juice in a food mixer until fluffy. To your skillet, add your tofu mixture. Add in half a cup of cooked quinoa. Mix thoroughly.

3. Move to a microwave-proof plate or tray that works for your air fryer basket.

4. Cook for around 15 minutes at about 350°F (or 18 to 20 minutes at about 330°F, till it turns golden brown).

5. Please take out your plate or tray from your air fryer and let it rest for at least five minutes before eating.

3. Vegan Omelet

Preparation time: 15 minutes

Cooking time: 16 minutes

Servings: 3 people

Ingredients:

- ½ cup of grated vegan cheese
- 1 tbsp. of water
- 1 tbsp. of brags
- 3 tbsp. of nutritional yeast

- ¼ tsp. of basil

- ¼ tsp. of garlic powder

- ¼ tsp. of onion powder

- ¼ tsp. of pepper

- ½ tsp. of cumin

- ½ tsp. of turmeric

- ¼ tsp. of salt

- ¼ cup of chickpea flour (or you may use any bean flour)

- ½ cup of finely diced veggies (like chard, kale, dried mushrooms, spinach, watermelon radish etc.)

- half a piece of tofu (organic high in protein kind)

Directions:

4. Blend all your ingredients in a food blender or mixer, excluding the vegetables and cheese.

5. Move the batter from the blender to a container and combine the vegetables and cheese in it. Since it's faster, you could use both hands to combine it.

6. Brush the base of your air fryer bucket with some oil.

7. Put a couple of parchment papers on your counter. On the top of your parchment paper, place a cookie cutter of your desire.

8. In your cookie cutter, push 1/6 of the paste. Then raise and put the cookie cutter on a different section of your parchment paper.

9. Redo the process till you have about 6 pieces using the remainder of the paste.

10. Put 2 or 3 of your omelets at the base of your air fryer container. Using some oil, brush the topsides of the omelets.

11. Cook for around 5 minutes at about 370 °, turn and bake for another 4 minutes or more if needed. And redo with the omelets that remain.

12. Offer with sriracha mayo or whatever kind of dipping sauce you prefer. Or use them for a sandwich at breakfast.

4. Waffles with Vegan chicken

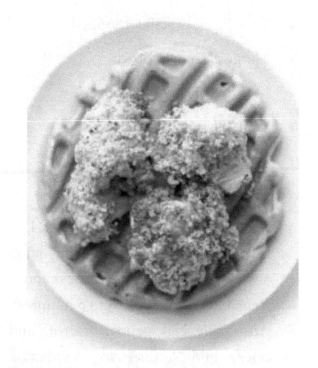

Preparation time: 10 minutes

Cooking time: 15 minutes

Servings: 2 people

Ingredients:

Fried Vegan Chicken:

- ¼ to ½ teaspoon of Black Pepper
- ½ teaspoon of Paprika
- ½ teaspoon of Onion Powder
- ½ teaspoon of Garlic Powder
- 2 teaspoon of Dried Parsley
- 2 Cups of Gluten-Free Panko
- ¼ Cup of Cornstarch
- 1 Cup of Unsweetened Non-Dairy Milk
- 1 Small Head of Cauliflower

Yummy Cornmeal Waffles:

- ½ teaspoon of Pure Vanilla Extract
- ¼ Cup of Unsweetened Applesauce
- ½ Cup of Unsweetened Non-Dairy Milk
- 1 to 2 TB Erythritol (or preferred sweetener)
- 1 teaspoon Baking Powder
- ¼ Cup of Stoneground Cornmeal
- ⅔ Cup of Gluten-Free All-Purpose Flour

Toppings:

- Vegan Butter
- Hot Sauce
- Pure Maple Syrup

Directions:

For making your Vegan Fried Chicken:

1. Dice the cauliflower (you wouldn't have to be careful in this) into big florets and put it aside.
2. Mix the cornstarch and milk in a tiny pot.
3. Throw the herbs, panko, and spices together in a big bowl or dish.
4. In the thick milk mixture, soak your cauliflower florets, then cover the soaked bits in the prepared panko mix before putting the wrapped floret into your air fryer bucket.
5. For the remaining of your cauliflower, redo the same process.
6. Set your air fryer clock for around 15 minutes to about 400 ° F and let the cauliflower air fry.

For making you're Waffles:

1. Oil a regular waffle iron and warm it up.
2. Mix all your dry ingredients in a pot, and then blend in your wet ingredients until you have a thick mixture.
3. To create a big waffle, utilize ½ of the mixture and redo the process to create another waffle for a maximum of two persons.

To Organize:

1. Put on dishes your waffles, place each with ½ of the cooked cauliflower, now drizzle with the hot sauce, syrup, and any extra toppings that you want. Serve warm!

5. Tempeh Bacon

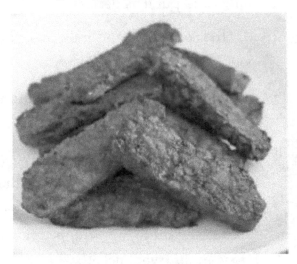

Preparation time: 15 minutes plus 2 hour marinating time

Cooking time: 10 minutes

Servings: 4 people

Ingredients:

- ½ teaspoon of freshly grated black pepper
- ½ teaspoon of onion powder
- ½ teaspoon of garlic powder
- 1 ½ teaspoon of smoked paprika
- 1 teaspoon of apple cider vinegar
- 1 tablespoon of olive oil (plus some more for oiling your air fryer)
- 3 tablespoon of pure maple syrup
- ¼ cup of gluten-free, reduced-sodium tamari
- 8 oz. of gluten-free tempeh

Directions:

1. Break your Tempeh cube into two parts and boil for about 10 minutes, some more if required. To the rice cooker bowl, add a cup of warm water. Then, put the pieces of tempeh into the steamer basket of the unit. Close the cover, push the button for heat or steam cooking (based on your rice cooker's type or brand), and adjust the steaming timer for around 10 minutes.

2. Let the tempeh cool completely before taking it out of the rice cooker or your steamer basket for around 5 minutes.

3. Now make the sauce while cooking the tempeh. In a 9" x 13" baking tray, incorporate all the rest of your ingredients and mix them using a fork. Then set it aside and ready the tempeh.

4. Put the tempeh steamed before and cooled on a chopping board, and slice into strips around 1/4' wide. Put each slice gently in the sauce. Then roll over each slice gently. Seal and put in the fridge for two to three hours or even overnight, rotating once or twice during the time.

5. Turn the bits gently one more time until you are about to create the tempeh bacon. And if you would like, you may spoon over any leftover sauce.

6. Put your crisper plate/tray into the air fryer if yours came with one instead of a built-in one. Oil the base of your crisper tray or your air fryer basket slightly with some olive oil or using an olive oil spray that is anti-aerosol.

7. Put the tempeh slices in a thin layer gently in your air fryer bucket. If you have a tiny air fryer, you will have to air fry it in two or multiple rounds. Air fry for around 10-15 minutes at about 325 ° F before the slices are lightly golden but not burnt. You may detach your air fryer container to inspect it and make sure it's not burnt. It normally takes about 10 minutes.

6. Delicious Potato Pancakes

Preparation time: 5 minutes

Cooking time: 15 minutes

Servings: 4 people

Ingredients:

- black pepper according to taste
- 3 tablespoon of flour
- ¼ teaspoon of pepper
- ¼ teaspoon of salt
- ½ teaspoon of garlic powder
- 2 tablespoon of unsalted butter
- ¼ cup of milk
- 1 beaten egg
- 1 medium onion, chopped

Directions:

1. Preheat the fryer to about 390° F and combine the potatoes, garlic powder, eggs, milk, onion, pepper, butter, and salt in a small bowl; add in the flour and make a batter.

2. Shape around 1/4 cup of your batter into a cake.

3. In the fryer's cooking basket, put the cakes and cook for a couple of minutes.

4. Serve and enjoy your treat!

CHAPTER 2: Air Fryer Main Dishes

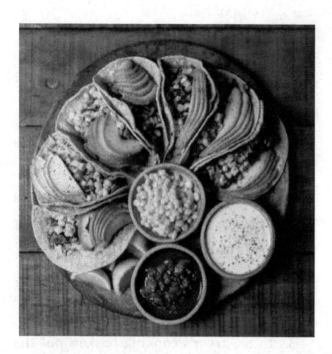

1. Mushroom 'n Bell Pepper Pizza

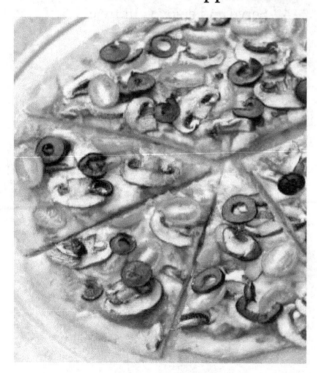

Servings: 10 people

Ingredients:

- salt and pepper according to taste
- 2 tbsp. of parsley
- 1 vegan pizza dough
- 1 shallot, chopped
- 1 cup of oyster mushrooms, chopped
- ¼ red bell pepper, chopped

Directions:

1. Preheat your air fryer to about 400°F.
2. Cut the pie dough into small squares. Just set them aside.
3. Put your bell pepper, shallot, oyster mushroom, and parsley all together into a mixing dish.
4. According to taste, sprinkle with some pepper and salt.
5. On top of your pizza cubes, put your topping.
6. Put your pizza cubes into your air fryer and cook for about 10 minutes.

Preparation time: 5 minutes

Cooking time: 10 minutes

2. Veggies Stuffed Eggplants

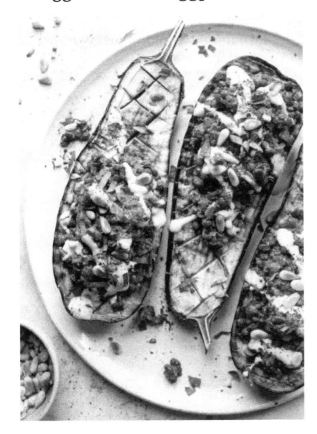

Preparation time: 5 minutes

Cooking time: 14 minutes

Servings: 5 people

Ingredients:

- 2 tbsp. of tomato paste
- Salt and ground black pepper, as required
- ½ tsp. of garlic, chopped
- 1 tbsp. of vegetable oil
- 1 tbsp. of fresh lime juice
- ½ green bell pepper, seeded and chopped
- ¼ cup of cottage cheese, chopped
- 1 tomato, chopped
- 1 onion, chopped
- 10 small eggplants, halved lengthwise

Directions:

1. Preheat your air fryer to about 320°F and oil the container of your air fryer.

2. Cut a strip longitudinally from all sides of your eggplant and scrape out the pulp in a medium-sized bowl.

3. Add lime juice on top of your eggplants and place them in the container of your Air Fryer.

4. Cook for around a couple of minutes and extract from your Air Fryer.

5. Heat the vegetable oil on medium-high heat in a pan and add the onion and garlic.

6. Sauté for around 2 minutes and mix in the tomato, salt, eggplant flesh, and black pepper.

7. Sauté and add bell pepper, tomato paste, cheese, and cilantro for roughly 3 minutes.

8. Cook for around a minute and put this paste into your eggplants.

9. Shut each eggplant with its lids and adjust the Air Fryer to 360°F.

10. Organize and bake for around 5 minutes in your Air Fryer Basket.

11. Dish out on a serving tray and eat hot.

3. Air-fried Falafel

Preparation time: 10 minutes

Cooking time: 25 minutes

Servings: 6 people

Ingredients:

- Salt and black pepper according to taste
- 1 teaspoon of chili powder
- 2 teaspoon of ground coriander
- 2 teaspoon of ground cumin
- 1 onion, chopped
- 4 garlic cloves, chopped
- Juice of 1 lemon
- 1 cup of fresh parsley, chopped
- ½ cup of chickpea flour

Directions:

1. Add flour, coriander, chickpeas, lemon juice, parsley, onion, garlic, chili, cumin, salt, turmeric, and pepper to a processor and mix until mixed, not too battery; several chunks should be present.

2. Morph the paste into spheres and hand-press them to ensure that they are still around.

3. Spray using some spray oil and place them in a paper-lined air fryer bucket; if necessary, perform in groups.

4. Cook for about 14 minutes at around 360°F, rotating once mid-way through the cooking process.

5. They must be light brown and crispy.

4. Almond Flour Battered Wings

Preparation time: 10 minutes

Cooking time: 25 minutes

Servings: 4 people

Ingredients:

- Salt and pepper according to taste
- 4 tbsp. of minced garlic
- 2 tbsp. of stevia powder
- 16 pieces of vegan chicken wings
- ¾ cup of almond flour
- ¼ cup of butter, melted

Directions:

1. Preheat your air fryer for about 5 minutes.

2. Mix the stevia powder, almond flour, vegan chicken wings, and garlic in a mixing dish. According to taste, sprinkle with some black pepper and salt.

3. Please put it in the bucket of your air fryer and cook at about 400°F for around 25 minutes.

4. Ensure you give your fryer container a shake midway through the cooking process.

5. Put in a serving dish after cooking and add some melted butter on top. Toss it to coat it completely.

5. Spicy Tofu

Preparation time: 5 minutes

Cooking time: 13 minutes

Servings: 3 people

Ingredients:

- Salt and black pepper, according to taste
- 1 tsp. of garlic powder
- 1 tsp. of onion powder
- 1½ tsp. of paprika
- 1½ tbsp. of avocado oil
- 3 tsp. of cornstarch
- 1 (14-ounces) block extra-firm tofu, pressed and cut into ¾-inch cubes

Directions:

1. Preheat your air fryer to about 390°F and oil the container of your air fryer with some spray oil.
2. In a medium-sized bowl, blend the cornstarch, oil, tofu, and spices and mix to cover properly.
3. In the Air Fryer basket, place the tofu bits and cook for around a minute, flipping twice between the cooking times.
4. On a serving dish, spread out the tofu and enjoy it warm.

6. Sautéed Bacon with Spinach

Preparation time: 5 minutes

Cooking time: 9 minutes

Servings: 2 people

Ingredients:

- 1 garlic clove, minced
- 2 tbsp. of olive oil
- 4-ounce of fresh spinach
- 1 onion, chopped
- 3 meatless bacon slices, chopped

Directions:

1. Preheat your air fryer at about 340° F and oil the air fryer's tray with some olive oil or cooking oil spray.
2. In the Air Fryer basket, put garlic and olive oil.
3. Cook and add in the onions and bacon for around 2 minutes.
4. Cook and mix in the spinach for approximately 3 minutes.
5. Cook for 4 more minutes and plate out in a bowl to eat.

7. Garden Fresh Veggie Medley

Preparation time: 5 minutes

Cooking time: 15 minutes

Servings: 4 people

Ingredients:

- 1 tbsp. of balsamic vinegar
- 1 tbsp. of olive oil
- 2 tbsp. of herbs de Provence
- 2 garlic cloves, minced
- 2 small onions, chopped
- 3 tomatoes, chopped
- 1 zucchini, chopped
- 1 eggplant, chopped
- 2 yellow bell peppers seeded and chopped
- Salt and black pepper, according to taste.

Directions:

1. Preheat your air fryer at about 355° F and oil up the air fryer basket.

2. In a medium-sized bowl, add all the ingredients and toss to cover completely.

3. Move to the basket of your Air Fryer and cook for around 15 minutes.

4. After completing the cooking time, let it sit in the air fryer for around 5 minutes and plate out to serve warm.

8. Colorful Vegetable Croquettes

Preparation time: 5 minutes

Cooking time: 10 minutes

Servings: 4 people

Ingredients:

- 1/2 cup of parmesan cheese, grated
- 2 eggs
- 1/4 cup of coconut flour
- 1/2 cup of almond flour
- 2 tbsp. of olive oil
- 3 tbsp. of scallions, minced
- 1 clove garlic, minced
- 1 bell pepper, chopped
- 1/2 cup of mushrooms, chopped
- 1/2 tsp. of cayenne pepper
- Salt and black pepper, according to taste.
- 2 tbsp. of butter
- 4 tbsp. of milk
- 1/2 pound of broccoli

Directions:

1. Boil your broccoli in a medium-sized saucepan for up to around 20 minutes. With butter, milk, black pepper, salt, and cayenne pepper, rinse the broccoli and mash it.

2. Add in the bell pepper, mushrooms, garlic, scallions, and olive oil and blend properly. Form into patties with the blend.

3. Put the flour in a deep bowl; beat your eggs in a second bowl; then put the parmesan cheese in another bowl.

4. Dip each patty into your flour, accompanied by the eggs and lastly the parmesan cheese, push to hold the shape.

5. Cook for around 16 minutes, turning midway through the cooking period, in the preheated Air Fryer at about 370° F. Bon appétit!

9. Cheesy Mushrooms

Preparation time: 3 minutes

Cooking time: 8 minutes

Servings: 4 people

Ingredients:

- 1 tsp. of dried dill
- 2 tbsp. of Italian dried mixed herbs
- 2 tbsp. of olive oil
- 2 tbsp. of cheddar cheese, grated
- 2 tbsp. of mozzarella cheese, grated
- Salt and freshly ground black pepper, according to taste
- 6-ounce of button mushrooms stemmed

Directions:

Preheat the air fryer at around 355° F and oil your air fryer basket.

In a mixing bowl, combine the Italian dried mixed herbs, mushrooms, salt, oil, and black pepper and mix well to cover.

In the Air Fryer bucket, place the mushrooms and cover them with some cheddar cheese and mozzarella cheese.

To eat, cook for around 8 minutes and scatter with dried dill.

10. Greek-style Roasted Vegetables

Preparation time: 10 minutes

Cooking time: 25 minutes

Servings: 3 people

Ingredients:

- 1/2 cup of Kalamata olives, pitted
- 1 (28-ounce) canned diced tomatoes with juice
- 1/2 tsp. of dried basil
- Sea salt and freshly cracked black pepper, according to taste
- 1 tsp. of dried rosemary
- 1 cup of dry white wine
- 2 tbsp. of extra-virgin olive oil
- 2 bell peppers, cut into 1-inch chunks
- 1 red onion, sliced
- 1/2 pound of zucchini, cut into 1-inch chunks
- 1/2 pound of cauliflower, cut into 1-inch florets
- 1/2 pound of butternut squash, peeled and cut into 1-inch chunks

Directions:

1. Add some rosemary, wine, olive oil, black pepper, salt, and basil along with your vegetables toss until well-seasoned.

2. Onto a lightly oiled baking dish, add 1/2 of the canned chopped tomatoes; scatter to fill the base of your baking dish.

3. Add in the vegetables and add the leftover chopped tomatoes to the top. On top of tomatoes, spread the Kalamata olives.

4. Bake for around 20 minutes at about 390° F in the preheated Air Fryer, turning the dish midway through your cooking cycle. Serve it hot and enjoy it!

11. Vegetable Kabobs with Simple Peanut Sauce

Preparation time: 10 minutes

Cooking time: 30 minutes

Servings: 4 people

Ingredients:

- 1/3 tsp. of granulated garlic
- 1 tsp. of dried rosemary, crushed
- 1 tsp. of red pepper flakes, crushed
- Sea salt and ground black pepper, according to your taste.
- 2 tbsp. of extra-virgin olive oil
- 8 small button mushrooms, cleaned

- 8 pearl onions, halved
- 2 bell peppers, diced into 1-inch pieces
- 8 whole baby potatoes, diced into 1-inch pieces

Peanut Sauce:

- 1/2 tsp. of garlic salt
- 1 tbsp. of soy sauce
- 1 tbsp. of balsamic vinegar
- 2 tbsp. of peanut butter

Directions:

1. For a few minutes, dunk the wooden chopsticks in water.

2. String the vegetables onto your chopsticks; drip some olive oil all over your chopsticks with the vegetables on it; dust with seasoning.

3. Cook for about 1 minute at 400°F in the preheated Air Fryer.

Peanut Sauce:

1. In the meantime, mix the balsamic vinegar with some peanut butter, garlic salt and some soy sauce in a tiny dish. Offer the kabobs with a side of peanut sauce. Eat warm!

12. Hungarian Mushroom Pilaf

Preparation time: 10 minutes

Cooking time: 50 minutes

Servings: 4 people

Ingredients:

- 1 tsp. of sweet Hungarian paprika
- 1/2 tsp. of dried tarragon
- 1 tsp. of dried thyme
- 1/4 cup of dry vermouth
- 1 onion, chopped
- 2 garlic cloves
- 2 tbsp. of olive oil
- 1 pound of fresh porcini mushrooms, sliced
- 2 tbsp. of olive oil
- 3 cups of vegetable broth
- 1 ½ cups of white rice

Directions:

1. In a wide saucepan, put the broth and rice, add some water, and bring it to a boil.

2. Cover with a lid and turn the flame down to a low temperature and proceed to cook for the next 18 minutes or so. After cooking, let it rest for 5 to 10 minutes, and then set aside.

3. Finally, in a lightly oiled baking dish, mix the heated, fully cooked rice with the rest of your ingredients.

4. Cook at about 200° degrees for around 20 minutes in the preheated Air Fryer, regularly monitoring to even cook.

5. In small bowls, serve. Bon appétit!

13. Chinese cabbage Bake

Preparation time: 15 minutes

Cooking time: 35 minutes

Servings: 4 people

Ingredients:

- 1 cup of Monterey Jack cheese, shredded
- 1/2 tsp. of cayenne pepper
- 1 cup of cream cheese
- 1/2 cup of milk
- 4 tbsp. of flaxseed meal
- 1/2 stick butter
- 2 garlic cloves, sliced
- 1 onion, thickly sliced
- 1 jalapeno pepper, seeded and sliced
- Sea salt and freshly ground black pepper, according to taste.
- 2 bell peppers, seeded and sliced
- 1/2 pound of Chinese cabbage, roughly chopped

Directions:

1. Heat the salted water in a pan and carry it to a boil. For around 2 to 3 minutes, steam the Chinese cabbage. To end the cooking process, switch the Chinese cabbage to cold water immediately.

2. Put your Chinese cabbage in a lightly oiled casserole dish. Add in the garlic, onion, and peppers.

3. Next, over low fire, melt some butter in a skillet. Add in your flaxseed meal steadily and cook for around 2 minutes to create a paste.

4. Add in the milk gently, constantly whisking until it creates a dense mixture. Add in your cream cheese. Sprinkle some cayenne pepper, salt, and black pepper. To the casserole tray, transfer your mixture.

5. Cover with some Monterey Jack cheese and cook for about 2 minutes at around 390° F in your preheated Air Fryer. Serve it warm.

14. Brussels sprouts With Balsamic Oil

Preparation time: 5 minutes

Cooking time: 15 minutes

Servings: 4 people

Ingredients:

- 2 tbsp. of olive oil
- 2 cups of Brussels sprouts, halved
- 1 tbsp. of balsamic vinegar
- ¼ tsp. of salt

Directions:

1. For 5 minutes, preheat your air fryer.

2. In a mixing bowl, blend all of your ingredients to ensure the zucchini fries are very well coated. Put the fries in the basket of an air fryer.

3. Close it and cook it at about 350°F for around 15 minutes.

15. Aromatic Baked Potatoes with Chives

Preparation time: 15 minutes

Cooking time: 45 minutes

Servings: 2 people

Ingredients:

- 2 tbsp. of chives, chopped
- 2 garlic cloves, minced
- 1 tbsp. of sea salt
- 1/4 tsp. of smoked paprika
- 1/4 tsp. of red pepper flakes
- 2 tbsp. of olive oil
- 4 medium baking potatoes, peeled

Directions:

1. Toss the potatoes with your seasoning, olive oil, and garlic.

2. Please put them in the basket of your Air Fryer. Cook at about 400° F for around 40 minutes just until the potatoes are fork soft in your preheated Air Fryer.

3. Add in some fresh minced chives to garnish. Bon appétit!

16. Easy Vegan "chicken"

Preparation time: 10 minutes

Cooking time: 20 minutes

Servings: 4 people

Ingredients:

- 1 tsp. of celery seeds
- 1/2 tsp. of mustard powder
- 1 tsp. of cayenne pepper
- 1/4 cup of all-purpose flour
- 1/2 cup of cornmeal
- 8 ounces of soy chunks
- Sea salt and ground black pepper, according to taste.

Directions:

1. In a skillet over medium-high flame, cook the soya chunks in plenty of water. Turn off the flame and allow soaking for several minutes. Drain the remaining water, wash, and strain it out.

2. In a mixing bowl, combine the rest of the components. Roll your soy chunks over the breading paste, pressing lightly to stick.

3. In the slightly oiled Air Fryer basket, place your soy chunks.

4. Cook at about 390° for around 10 minutes in your preheated Air Fryer, rotating them over midway through

the cooking process; operate in batches if required. Bon appétit!

17. Paprika Vegetable Kebab's

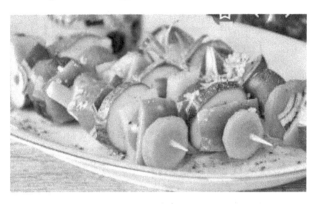

Preparation time: 10 minutes

Cooking time: 20 minutes

Servings: 4 people

Ingredients:

- 1/2 tsp. of ground black pepper
- 1 tsp. of sea salt flakes
- 1 tsp. of smoked paprika
- 1/4 cup of sesame oil
- 2 tbsp. of dry white wine
- 1 red onion, cut into wedges
- 2 cloves garlic, pressed
- 1 tsp. of whole grain mustard
- 1 fennel bulb, diced
- 1 parsnip, cut into thick slices
- 1 celery, cut into thick slices

Directions:

1. Toss all of the above ingredients together in a mixing bowl to

uniformly coat. Thread the vegetables alternately onto the wooden skewers.

2. Cook for around 15 minutes at about 380° F on your Air Fryer grill plate.

3. Turn them over midway during the cooking process.

4. Taste, change the seasonings if needed and serve steaming hot.

18. Spiced Soy Curls

Preparation time: 5 minutes

Cooking time: 10 minutes

Servings: 2 people

Ingredients:

- 1 tsp. of poultry seasoning
- 2 tsp. of Cajun seasoning
- ¼ cup of fine ground cornmeal
- ¼ cup of nutritional yeast
- 4 ounces of soy curls
- 3 cups of boiling water
- Salt and ground white pepper, as needed

Directions:

1. Dip the soy curls for around a minute or so in hot water in a heat-resistant tub.

2. Drain your soy coils using a strainer and force the excess moisture out using a broad spoon.

3. Mix the cornmeal, nutritional yeast, salt, seasonings, and white pepper well in a mixing bowl.

4. Transfer your soy curls to the bowl and coat well with the blend. Let the air-fryer temperature to about 380° F. Oil the basket of your air fryers.

5. Adjust soy curls in a uniform layer in the lined air fryer basket. Cook for about 10 minutes in the air fryer, turning midway through the cycle.

6. Take out the soy curls from your air fryer and put them on a serving dish. Serve it steaming hot.

19. Cauliflower & Egg Rice Casserole

Preparation time: 5 minutes

Cooking time: 15 minutes

Servings: 4 people

Ingredients:

- 2 eggs, beaten
- 1 tablespoon of soy sauce
- Salt and black pepper according to taste.
- ½ cup of chopped onion
- 1 cup of okra, chopped
- 1 yellow bell pepper, chopped
- 2 teaspoon of olive oil

Directions:

1. Preheat your air fryer to about 380° F. Oil a baking tray with spray oil. Pulse

the cauliflower till it becomes like thin rice-like capsules in your food blender.

2. Now add your cauliflower rice to a baking tray mix in the okra, bell pepper, salt, soy sauce, onion, and pepper and combine well.

3. Drizzle a little olive oil on top along with the beaten eggs. Put the tray in your air fryer and cook for about a minute. Serve it hot.

20. Hollandaise Topped Grilled Asparagus

Preparation time: 2 minutes

Cooking time: 15 minutes

Servings: 6 people

Ingredients:

- A punch of ground white pepper
- A pinch of mustard powder
- 3 pounds of asparagus spears, trimmed
- 3 egg yolks
- 2 tbsp. of olive oil
- 1 tsp. of chopped tarragon leaves
- ½ tsp. of salt
- ½ lemon juice
- ½ cup of butter, melted
- ¼ tsp. of black pepper

Directions:

1. Preheat your air fryer to about 330° F. In your air fryer, put the grill pan attachment.

2. Mix the olive oil, salt, asparagus, and pepper into a Ziploc bag. To mix all, give everything a quick shake. Load onto the grill plate and cook for about 15 minutes.

3. In the meantime, beat the lemon juice, egg yolks, and salt in a double boiler over a moderate flame until velvety.

4. Add in the melted butter, mustard powder, and some white pepper. Continue whisking till the mixture is creamy and thick. Serve with tarragon leaves as a garnish.

5. Pour the sauce over the asparagus spears and toss to blend.

21. Crispy Asparagus Dipped In Paprika-garlic Spice

Preparation time: 2 minutes

Cooking time: 15 minutes

Servings: 5 people

Ingredients:

- ¼ cup of almond flour
- ½ tsp. of garlic powder
- ½ tsp. of smoked paprika
- 10 medium asparagus, trimmed
- 2 large eggs, beaten
- 2 tbsp. of parsley, chopped

- Salt and pepper according to your taste

Directions:

1. For about 5 minutes, preheat your air fryer.

2. Mix the almond flour, garlic powder, parsley, and smoked paprika in a mixing dish. To taste, season with some salt and black pepper.

3. Soak your asparagus in the beaten eggs, and then dredge it in a combination of almond flour.

4. Put in the bowl of your air fryer. Close the lid. At about 350°F, cook for around a minute.

22. Eggplant Gratin with Mozzarella Crust

Preparation time: 10 minutes

Cooking time: 30 minutes

Servings: 2 people

Ingredients:

- 1 tablespoon of breadcrumbs
- ¼ cup of grated mozzarella cheese
- Cooking spray
- Salt and pepper according to your taste
- ¼ teaspoon of dried marjoram
- ¼ teaspoon of dried basil
- 1 teaspoon of capers

- 1 tablespoon of sliced pimiento-stuffed olives
- 1 clove garlic, minced
- ⅓ cup of chopped tomatoes
- ¼ cup of chopped onion
- ¼ cup of chopped green pepper
- ¼ cup of chopped red pepper

Directions:

1. Put the green pepper, eggplant, onion, red pepper, olives, tomatoes, basil marjoram, garlic, salt, capers, and pepper in a container and preheat your air fryer to about 300° F.

2. Lightly oil a baking tray with a spray of cooking olive oil.

3. Fill your baking with the eggplant combination and line it with the vessel.

4. Place some mozzarella cheese on top of it and top with some breadcrumbs. Put the dish in the frying pan and cook for a few minutes.

23. Asian-style Cauliflower

Preparation time: 10 minutes

Cooking time: 25 minutes

Servings: 4 people

Ingredients:

- 2 tbsp. of sesame seeds
- 1/4 cup of lime juice

- 1 tbsp. of fresh parsley, finely chopped
- 1 tbsp. of ginger, freshly grated
- 2 cloves of garlic, peeled and pressed
- 1 tbsp. of sake
- 1 tbsp. of tamari sauce
- 1 tbsp. of sesame oil
- 1 onion, peeled and finely chopped
- 2 cups of cauliflower, grated

Directions:

1. In a mixing bowl, mix your onion, cauliflower, tamari sauce, sesame oil, garlic, sake, and ginger; whisk until all is well integrated.

2. Air-fry it for around a minute at about 400° F.

3. Pause your Air Fryer. Add in some parsley and lemon juice.

4. Cook for an extra 10 minutes at about 300° degrees F in the air fryer.

5. In the meantime, in a non-stick pan, toast your sesame seeds; swirl them continuously over medium-low heat. Serve hot on top of the cauliflower with a pinch of salt and pepper.

24. Two-cheese Vegetable Frittata

Preparation time: 15 minutes

Cooking time: 35 minutes

Servings: 2 people

Ingredients:

- ⅓ cup of crumbled Feta cheese
- ⅓ cup of grated Cheddar cheese
- Salt and pepper according to taste
- ⅓ cup of milk
- 4 eggs, cracked into a bowl
- 2 teaspoon of olive oil
- ¼ lb. of asparagus, trimmed and sliced thinly
- ¼ cup of chopped chives
- 1 small red onion, sliced
- 1 large zucchini, sliced with a 1-inch thickness
- ⅓ cup of sliced mushrooms

Directions:

1. Preheat your air fryer to about 380° F. Set aside your baking dish lined with some parchment paper. Put salt, milk, and pepper into the egg bowl; whisk evenly.

2. Put a skillet on the stovetop over a moderate flame, and heat your olive oil. Add in the zucchini, asparagus, baby spinach, onion, and mushrooms; stir-fry for around 5 minutes. Transfer the vegetables into your baking tray, and finish with the beaten egg.

3. Put the tray into your air fryer and finish with cheddar and feta cheese.

4. For about 15 minutes, cook. Take out your baking tray and add in some fresh chives to garnish.

25. Rice & Beans Stuffed Bell Peppers

Preparation time: 10 minutes

Cooking time: 15 minutes

Servings: 5 people

Ingredients:

- 1 tbsp. of Parmesan cheese, grated

- ½ cup of mozzarella cheese, shredded

- 5 large bell peppers, tops removed and seeded

- 1½ tsp. of Italian seasoning

- 1 cup of cooked rice

- 1 (15-ounces) can of red kidney beans, rinsed and drained

- 1 (15-ounces) can of diced tomatoes with juice

- ½ small bell pepper, seeded and chopped

Directions:

1. Combine the tomatoes with juice, bell pepper, rice, beans, and Italian seasoning in a mixing dish. Using the rice mixture, fill each bell pepper uniformly.

2. Preheat the air fryer to 300° F. Oil the basket of your air fryer with some spray oil. Put the bell peppers in a uniform layer in your air fryer basket.

3. Cook for around 12 minutes in the air fryer. In the meantime, combine the Parmesan and mozzarella cheese in a mixing dish.

4. Remove the peppers from the air fryer basket and top each with some cheese mix. Cook for another 3 -4 minutes in the air fryer

5. Take the bell peppers from the air fryer and put them on a serving dish. Enable to cool slowly before serving. Serve it hot.

26. Parsley-loaded Mushrooms

Preparation time: 5 minutes

Cooking time: 15 minutes

Servings: 2 people

Ingredients:

- 2 tablespoon of parsley, finely chopped

- 2 teaspoon of olive oil

- 1 garlic clove, crushed

- 2 slices white bread

- salt and black pepper according to your taste

Directions:

1. Preheat the air fryer to about 360° F. Crush your bread into crumbs in a food blender. Add the parsley, garlic, and pepper; blend with the olive oil and mix.

2. Remove the stalks from the mushrooms and stuff the caps with breadcrumbs. In your air fryer basket, position the mushroom heads. Cook for a few minutes, just until golden brown and crispy.

27. Cheesy Vegetable Quesadilla

Preparation time: 2 minutes

Cooking time: 15 minutes

Servings: 1 people

Ingredients:

- 1 teaspoon of olive oil
- 1 tablespoon of cilantro, chopped
- ½ green onion, sliced
- ¼ zucchini, sliced
- ¼ yellow bell pepper, sliced
- ¼ cup of shredded gouda cheese

Directions:

1. Preheat your air fryer to about 390° F. Oil a basket of air fryers with some cooking oil.

2. Put a flour tortilla in your air fryer basket and cover it with some bell pepper, Gouda cheese, cilantro, zucchini, and green onion. Take the other tortilla to cover and spray with some olive oil.

3. Cook until slightly golden brown, for around 10 minutes. Cut into 4 slices for serving when ready. Enjoy!

28. Creamy 'n Cheese Broccoli Bake

Preparation time: 10 minutes

Cooking time: 30 minutes

Servings: 2 people

Ingredients:

- 1/4 cup of water
- 1-1/2 teaspoons of butter, or to taste
- 1/2 cup of cubed sharp Cheddar cheese
- 1/2 (14 ounces) can evaporate milk, divided
- 1/2 large onion, coarsely diced
- 1 tbsp. of dry bread crumbs, or to taste
- salt according to taste
- 2 tbsp. of all-purpose flour
- 1-pound of fresh broccoli, coarsely diced

Directions:

1. Lightly oil the air-fryer baking pan with cooking oil. Add half of the milk and flour into a pan and simmer at about 360° F for around 5 minutes.

2. Mix well midway through the cooking period. Remove the broccoli and the extra milk. Cook for the next 5 minutes after fully blending.

3. Mix in the cheese until it is fully melted. Mix the butter and bread crumbs well in a shallow tub. Sprinkle the broccoli on top.

4. At about 360° F, cook for around 20 minutes until the tops are finely golden brown. Enjoy and serve warm.

29. Sweet & Spicy Parsnips

Preparation time: 12 minutes

Cooking time: 44 minutes

Servings: 6 people

Ingredients:

- ¼ tsp. of red pepper flakes, crushed

- 1 tbsp. of dried parsley flakes, crushed

- 2 tbsp. of honey

- 1 tbsp. of n butter, melted

- 2 pounds of a parsnip, peeled and cut into 1-inch chunks

- Salt and ground black pepper, according to your taste.

Directions:

1. Let the air-fryer temperature to about 355° F. Oil the basket of your air fryers. Combine the butter and parsnips in a big dish.

2. Transfer the parsnip pieces into the lined air fryer basket arranges them in a uniform layer. Cook for a few minutes in the fryer.

3. In the meantime, combine the leftover ingredients in a large mixing bowl.

4. Move the parsnips into the honey mixture bowl after around 40 minutes and toss them to coat properly.

5. Again, in a uniform layer, organize the parsnip chunks into your air fryer basket.

6. Air-fry for another 3-4 minutes. Take the parsnip pieces from the air fryer and pass them onto the serving dish. Serve it warm.

30. Zucchini with Mediterranean Dill Sauce

Preparation time: 20 minutes

Cooking time: 60 minutes

Servings: 4 people

Ingredients:

- 1/2 tsp. of freshly cracked black peppercorns

- 2 sprigs thyme, leaves only, crushed

- 1 sprig rosemary, leaves only, crushed

- 1 tsp. of sea salt flakes

- 2 tbsp. of melted butter

- 1 pound of zucchini, peeled and cubed

For your Mediterranean Dipping:

- 1 tbsp. of olive oil

- 1 tbsp. of fresh dill, chopped

- 1/3 cup of yogurt

- 1/2 cup of mascarpone cheese

Directions:

1. To start, preheat your Air Fryer to 350° F. Now, add ice cold water to the container with your potato cubes and let them sit in the bath for about 35 minutes.

2. Dry your potato cubes with a hand towel after that. Whisk together the sea salt flakes, melted butter, thyme, rosemary, and freshly crushed peppercorns in a mixing container. This butter/spice mixture can be rubbed onto the potato cubes.

3. In the cooking basket of your air fryer, air-fry your potato cubes for around 18 to 20 minutes or until cooked completely; ensure you shake the potatoes at least once during cooking to cook them uniformly.

4. In the meantime, by mixing the rest of the ingredients, create the Mediterranean dipping sauce. To dip and eat, serve warm potatoes with Mediterranean sauce!

31. Zesty Broccoli

Preparation time: 10 minutes

Cooking time: 15 minutes

Servings: 4 people

Ingredients:

- 1 tbsp. of butter

- 1 large crown broccoli, chopped into bite-sized pieces

- 1 tbsp. of white sesame seeds

- 2 tbsp. of vegetable stock

- ½ tsp. of red pepper flakes, crushed

- 3 garlic cloves, minced

- ½ tsp. of fresh lemon zest, grated finely

- 1 tbsp. of pure lemon juice

Directions:

1. Preheat the Air fryer to about 355° F and oil an Air fryer pan with cooking spray. In the Air fryer plate, combine the vegetable stock, butter, and lemon juice.

2. Move the mixture and cook for about 2 minutes into your Air Fryer. Cook for a minute after incorporating the broccoli and garlic.

3. Cook for a minute with lemon zest, sesame seeds, and red pepper flakes. Remove the dish from the oven and eat immediately.

32. Chewy Glazed Parsnips

Preparation time: 15 minutes

Cooking time: 44 minutes

Servings: 6 people

Ingredients:

- ¼ tsp. of red pepper flakes, crushed
- 1 tbsp. of dried parsley flakes, crushed
- 2 tbsp. of maple syrup
- 1 tbsp. of butter, melted
- 2 pounds of parsnips, skinned and chopped into 1-inch chunks

Directions:

1. Preheat the Air fryer to about 355° F and oil your air fryer basket. In a wide mixing bowl, combine the butter and parsnips and toss well to cover. Cook for around 40 minutes with the parsnips in the Air fryer basket.

2. In the meantime, combine in a wide bowl the rest of your ingredients. Move this mix to your basket of the air fryer and cook for another 4 minutes or so. Remove the dish from the oven and eat promptly.

33. Hoisin-glazed Bok Choy

Preparation time: 5 minutes

Cooking time: 10 minutes

Servings: 4 people

Ingredients:

- 1 tbsp. of all-purpose flour
- 2 tbsp. of sesame oil
- 2 tbsp. of hoisin sauce
- 1/2 tsp. of sage
- 1 tsp. of onion powder
- 2 garlic cloves, minced
- 1 pound of baby Bok choy, roots removed, leaves separated

Directions:

1. In a lightly oiled Air Fryer basket, put the onion powder, garlic, Bok Choy, and sage. Cook for around 3 minutes at about 350° F in a preheated Air Fryer.

2. Whisk together the sesame oil, hoisin sauce, and flour in a deep mixing dish. Drizzle over the Bok choy with the gravy. Cook for an extra minute. Bon appétit!

34. Green Beans with Okra

Preparation time: 10 minutes

Cooking time: 20 minutes

Servings: 2 people

Ingredients:

- 3 tbsp. of balsamic vinegar

- ¼ cup of nutritional yeast

- ½ (10-ounces) of bag chilled cut green beans

- ½ (10-ounces) of bag chilled cut okra

- Salt and black pepper, according to your taste.

Directions:

1. Preheat your Air fryer to about 400° F and oil the air fryer basket.

2. In a wide mixing bowl, toss together the salt, green beans, okra, vinegar, nutritional yeast, and black pepper.

3. Cook for around 20 minutes with the okra mixture in your Air fryer basket. Dish out into a serving plate and eat warm.

35. Celeriac with some Greek Yogurt Dip

Preparation time: 12 minutes

Cooking time: 25 minutes

Servings: 2 people

Ingredients:

- 1/2 tsp. of sea salt

- 1/2 tsp. of ground black pepper, to taste

- 1 tbsp. of sesame oil

- 1 red onion, chopped into 1 1/2-inch piece

- 1/2 pound of celeriac, chopped into 1 1/2-inch piece

Spiced Yogurt:

- 1/2 tsp. of chili powder

- 1/2 tsp. of mustard seeds

- 2 tbsp. of mayonnaise

- 1/4 cup of Greek yogurt

Directions:

1. In the slightly oiled cooking basket, put the veggies in one uniform layer. Pour sesame oil over the veggies.

2. Season with a pinch of black pepper and a pinch of salt. Cook for around 20 minutes at about 300° F, tossing the basket midway through your cooking cycle.

3. In the meantime, whisk all the leftover ingredients into the sauce. Spoon the sauce over the veggies that have been cooked. Bon appétit!

36. Wine & Garlic Flavored Vegetables

Preparation time: 7-10 minutes

Cooking time: 15 minutes

Servings: 4 people

Ingredients:

- 4 cloves of garlic, minced

- 3 tbsp. of red wine vinegar

- 1/3 cup of olive oil

- 1 red onion, diced

- 1 package frozen diced vegetables
- 1 cup of baby Portobello mushrooms, diced
- 1 tsp. of Dijon mustard
- 1 ½ tbsp. of honey
- Salt and pepper according to your taste
- ¼ cup of chopped fresh basil

Directions:

1. Preheat the air fryer to about 330° F. In the air fryer, put the grill pan attachment.

2. Combine the veggies and season with pepper, salt, and garlic in a Ziploc container. To mix all, give everything a strong shake. Dump and cook for around 15 minutes on the grill pan.

3. Additionally, add the remainder of the ingredients into a mixing bowl and season with some more salt and pepper. Drizzle the sauce over your grilled vegetables.

37. Spicy Braised Vegetables

Preparation time: 10 minutes

Cooking time: 25 minutes

Servings: 4 people

Ingredients:

- 1/2 cup of tomato puree
- 1/4 tsp. of ground black pepper

- 1/2 tsp. of fine sea salt
- 1 tbsp. of garlic powder
- 1/2 tsp. of fennel seeds
- 1/4 tsp. of mustard powder
- 1/2 tsp. of porcini powder
- 1/4 cup of olive oil
- 1 celery stalk, chopped into matchsticks
- 2 bell peppers, deveined and thinly diced
- 1 Serrano pepper, deveined and thinly diced
- 1 large-sized zucchini, diced

Directions:

1. In your Air Fryer cooking basket, put your peppers, zucchini, sweet potatoes, and carrot.

2. Drizzle with some olive oil and toss to cover completely; cook for around 15 minutes in a preheated Air Fryer at about 350°F.

3. Make the sauce as the vegetables are frying by quickly whisking the remaining ingredients (except the tomato ketchup). Slightly oil up a baking dish that fits your fryer.

4. Add the cooked vegetables to the baking dish, along with the sauce, and toss well to cover.

5. Turn the Air Fryer to about 390° F and cook for 2-4 more minutes with the vegetables. Bon appétit!

CHAPTER 3: Air Fryer Snack Side Dishes and Appetizer Recipes

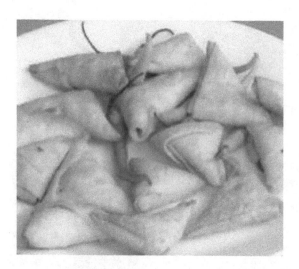

1. Crispy 'n Tasty Spring Rolls

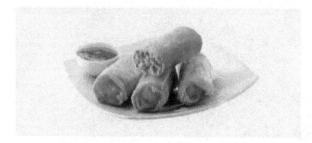

Preparation time: 5 minutes

Cooking time: 15 minutes

Servings: 4 people

Ingredients:

- 8 spring roll wrappers
- 1 tsp. of nutritional yeast
- 1 tsp. of corn starch + 2 tablespoon water
- 1 tsp. of coconut sugar
- 1 tbsp. of soy sauce
- 1 medium carrot, shredded
- 1 cup of shiitake mushroom, sliced thinly
- 1 celery stalk, chopped
- ½ tsp. of ginger, finely chopped

Directions:

1. Mix your carrots, celery stalk, soy sauce, coconut sugar, ginger, and nutritional yeast with each other in a mixing dish.
2. Have a tbsp. of your vegetable mix and put it in the middle of your spring roll wrappers.
3. Roll up and secure the sides of your wraps with some cornstarch.
4. Cook for about 15 minutes or till your spring roll wraps is crisp in a preheated air fryer at 200F.

2. Spinach & Feta Crescent Triangles

Preparation time: 10 minutes

Cooking time: 20 minutes

Servings: 4 people

Ingredients:

- ¼ teaspoon of salt
- 1 teaspoon of chopped oregano
- ¼ teaspoon of garlic powder
- 1 cup of crumbled feta cheese
- 1 cup of steamed spinach

Directions:

1. Preheat your air fryer to about 350 F, and then roll up the dough over a level surface that is gently floured.

2. In a medium-sized bowl, mix the spinach, feta, salt, oregano, and ground garlic cloves. Split your dough into four equal chunks.

3. Split the mix of feta/spinach among the four chunks of dough. Fold and seal your dough using a fork.

4. Please put it on a baking tray covered with parchment paper, and then put it in your air fryer.

5. Cook until nicely golden, for around 1 minute.

3. Healthy Avocado Fries

Preparation time: 5 minutes

Cooking time: 20 minutes

Servings: 2 people

Ingredients:

- ¼ cup of aquafaba
- 1 avocado, cubed
- Salt as required

Directions:

1. Mix the aquafaba, crumbs, and salt in a mixing bowl.

2. Preheat your air fryer to about 390°F and cover the avocado pieces uniformly in the crumbs blend.

3. Put the ready pieces in the cooking bucket of your air fryer and cook for several minutes.

4. Twice-fried Cauliflower Tater Tots

Preparation time: 5 minutes

Cooking time: 16 minutes

Servings: 12 people

Ingredients:

- 3 tbsp. Of oats flaxseed meal + 3 tbsp. of water)
- 1-pound of cauliflower, steamed and chopped
- 1 tsp. of parsley, chopped
- 1 tsp. of oregano, chopped
- 1 tsp. of garlic, minced
- 1 tsp. of chives, chopped
- 1 onion, chopped
- 1 flax egg (1 tablespoon 3 tablespoon desiccated coconuts)
- ½ cup of nutritional yeast
- salt and pepper according to taste
- ½ cup of bread crumbs

Directions:

1. Preheat your air fryer to about 390 degrees F.

2. To extract extra moisture, place the steamed cauliflower onto a ring and a paper towel.

3. Put and mix the remainder of your ingredients, excluding your bread crumbs, in a small mixing container.

4. Use your palms, blend it until well mixed and shapes into a small ball.

5. Roll your tater tots over your bread crumbs and put them in the bucket of your air fryer.

6. For a minute, bake. Raise the cooking level to about 400 F and cook for the next 10 minutes.

5. Cheesy Mushroom & Cauliflower Balls

Preparation time: 10 minutes

Cooking time: 50 minutes

Servings: 4 people

Ingredients:

- Salt and pepper according to taste
- 2 sprigs chopped fresh thyme
- ¼ cup of coconut oil
- 1 cup of Grana Padano cheese
- 1 cup of breadcrumbs
- 2 tablespoon of vegetable stock
- 3 cups of cauliflower, chopped
- 3 cloves garlic, minced
- 1 small red onion, chopped
- 3 tablespoon of olive oil

Directions:

1. Over moderate flame, put a pan. Add some balsamic vinegar. When the oil is heated, stir-fry your onion and garlic till they become transparent.

2. Add in the mushrooms and cauliflower and stir-fry for about 5 minutes. Add in your stock, add thyme and cook till your cauliflower has consumed the stock. Add pepper, Grana Padano cheese, and salt.

3. Let the mix cool down and form bite-size spheres of your paste. To harden, put it in the fridge for about 30 minutes.

4. Preheat your air fryer to about 350°F.

5. Add your coconut oil and breadcrumbs into a small bowl and blend properly.

6. Take out your mushroom balls from the fridge, swirl the breadcrumb paste once more, and drop the balls into your breadcrumb paste.

7. Avoid overcrowding, put your balls into your air fryer's container and cook for about 15 minutes, flipping after every 5 minutes to ensure even cooking.

8. Serve with some tomato sauce and brown sugar.

6. Italian Seasoned Easy Pasta Chips

Preparation time: 5 minutes

Cooking time: 10 minutes

Servings: 2 people

Ingredients:

- 2 cups of whole wheat bowtie pasta
- 1 tbsp. of olive oil
- 1 tbsp. of nutritional yeast
- 1 ½ tsp. of Italian seasoning blend
- ½ tsp. of salt

Directions:

1. Put the accessory for the baking tray into your air fryer.

2. Mix all the ingredients in a medium-sized bowl, offer it a gentle stir.

3. Add the mixture to your air fryer basket.

4. Close your air fryer and cook at around 400°degrees F for about 10 minutes.

7. Thai Sweet Potato Balls

Preparation time: 10 minutes

Cooking time: 50 minutes

Servings: 4 people

Ingredients:

- 1 cup of coconut flakes
- 1 tsp. of baking powder
- 1/2 cup of almond meal
- 1/4 tsp. of ground cloves
- 1/2 tsp. of ground cinnamon
- 2 tsp. of orange zest
- 1 tbsp. of orange juice
- 1 cup of brown sugar
- 1 pound of sweet potatoes

Directions:

1. Bake your sweet potatoes for around 25 to 30 minutes at about 380° F till they become soft; peel and mash them in a medium-sized bowl.

2. Add orange zest, orange juice, brown sugar, ground cinnamon, almond meal, cloves, and baking powder. Now blend completely.

3. Roll the balls around in some coconut flakes.

4. Bake for around 15 minutes or until fully fried and crunchy in the preheated Air Fryer at about 360° F.

5. For the rest of the ingredients, redo the same procedure. Bon appétit!

8. Barbecue Roasted Almonds

Preparation time: 5 minutes

Cooking time: 20 minutes

Servings: 6 people

Ingredients:

- 1 tbsp. of olive oil

- 1/4 tsp. of smoked paprika
- 1/2 tsp. of cumin powder
- 1/4 tsp. of mustard powder
- 1/4 tsp. of garlic powder
- Sea salt and ground black pepper, according to taste
- 1 ½ cups of raw almonds

Directions:

1. In a mixing pot, mix all your ingredients.

2. Line the container of your Air Fryer with some baking parchment paper. Arrange the covered almonds out in the basket of your air fryer in a uniform layer.

3. Roast for around 8 to 9 minutes at about 340°F, tossing the bucket once or twice. If required, work in groups.

4. Enjoy!

9. Croissant Rolls

Preparation time: 2 minutes

Cooking time: 6 minutes

Servings: 8 people

Ingredients:

- 4 tbsp. of butter, melted
- 1 (8-ounces) can croissant rolls

Directions:

1. Adjust the air-fryer temperature to about 320°F. Oil the basket of your air fryers.

2. Into your air fryer basket, place your prepared croissant rolls.

3. Airs fry them for around 4 minutes or so.

4. Flip to the opposite side and cook for another 2-3 minutes.

5. Take out from your air fryer and move to a tray.

6. Glaze with some melted butter and eat warm.

10. Curry' n Coriander Spiced Bread Rolls

Preparation time: 5 minutes

Cooking time: 15 minutes

Servings: 5 people

Ingredients:

- salt and pepper according to taste
- 5 large potatoes, boiled
- 2 sprigs, curry leaves
- 2 small onions, chopped
- 2 green chilies, seeded and chopped
- 1 tbsp. of olive oil
- 1 bunch of coriander, chopped
- ½ tsp. of turmeric

- 8 slices of vegan wheat bread, brown sides discarded
- ½ tsp. of mustard seeds

Directions:

1. Mash your potatoes in a bowl and sprinkle some black pepper and salt according to taste. Now set aside.

2. In a pan, warm up the olive oil over medium-low heat and add some mustard seeds. Mix until the seeds start to sputter.

3. Now add in the onions and cook till they become transparent. Mix in the curry leaves and turmeric powder.

4. Keep on cooking till it becomes fragrant for a couple of minutes. Take it off the flame and add the mixture to the potatoes.

5. Mix in the green chilies and some coriander. This is meant to be the filling.

6. Wet your bread and drain excess moisture. In the center of the loaf, put a tbsp. of the potato filling and gently roll the bread so that the potato filling is fully enclosed within the bread.

7. Brush with some oil and put them inside your air fryer basket.

8. Cook for around 15 minutes in a preheated air fryer at about 400°F.

9. Ensure that the air fryer basket is shaken softly midway through the cooking period for an even cooking cycle.

11. Scrumptiously Healthy Chips

Preparation time: 5 minutes

Cooking time: 10 minutes

Servings: 2 people

Ingredients:

- 2 tbsp. of olive oil
- 2 tbsp. of almond flour
- 1 tsp. of garlic powder
- 1 bunch kale
- Salt and pepper according to taste

Directions:

1. For around 5 minutes, preheat your air fryer.

2. In a mixing bowl, add all your ingredients, add the kale leaves at the end and toss to completely cover them.

3. Put in the basket of your fryer and cook until crispy for around 10 minutes.

12. Kid-friendly Vegetable Fritters

Preparation time: 5 minutes

Cooking time: 20 minutes

Servings: 4 people

Ingredients:

- 2 tbsp. of olive oil

- 1/2 cup of cornmeal
- 1/2 cup of all-purpose flour
- 1/2 tsp. of ground cumin
- 1 tsp. of turmeric powder
- 2 garlic cloves, pressed
- 1 carrot, grated
- 1 sweet pepper, seeded and chopped
- 1 yellow onion, finely chopped
- 1 tbsp. of ground flaxseeds
- Salt and ground black pepper, according to taste
- 1 pound of broccoli florets

Directions:

1. In salted boiling water, blanch your broccoli until al dente, for around 3 to 5 minutes. Drain the excess water and move to a mixing bowl; add in the rest of your ingredients to mash the broccoli florets.

2. Shape the paste into patties and position them in the slightly oiled Air Fryer basket.

3. Cook for around 6 minutes at about 400° F, flipping them over midway through the cooking process; if needed, operate in batches.

4. Serve hot with some Vegenaise of your choice. Enjoy it!

13. Avocado Fries

Preparation time: 10 minutes

Cooking time: 50 minutes

Servings: 4 people

Ingredients:

- 2 avocados, cut into wedges
- 1/2 cup of parmesan cheese, grated
- 2 eggs
- Sea salt and ground black pepper, according to taste.
- 1/2 cup of almond meal
- 1/2 head garlic (6-7 cloves)

Sauce:

- 1 tsp. of mustard
- 1 tsp. of lemon juice
- 1/2 cup of mayonnaise

Directions:

1. On a piece of aluminum foil, put your garlic cloves and spray some cooking spray on it. Wrap your garlic cloves in the foil.

2. Cook for around 1-2 minutes at about 400°F in your preheated Air Fryer. Inspect the garlic, open the foil's top end, and keep cooking for an additional 10-12 minutes.

3. Once done, let them cool for around 10 to 15 minutes; take out the cloves by pressing them out of their skin; mash your garlic and put them aside.

4. Mix the salt, almond meal, and black pepper in a small dish.

5. Beat the eggs until foamy in a separate bowl.

6. Put some parmesan cheese in the final shallow dish.

7. In your almond meal blend, dip the avocado wedges, dusting off any excess.

8. In the beaten egg, dunk your wedges; eventually, dip in some parmesan cheese.

9. Spray your avocado wedges on both sides with some cooking oil spray.

10. Cook for around 8 minutes in the preheated Air Fryer at about 395° F, flipping them over midway thru the cooking process.

11. In the meantime, mix the ingredients of your sauce with your cooked crushed garlic.

12. Split the avocado wedges between plates and cover with the sauce before serving. Enjoy!

14. Crispy Wings with Lemony Old Bay Spice

Preparation time: 10 minutes

Cooking time: 25 minutes

Servings: 4 people

Ingredients:

- Salt and pepper according to taste
- 3 pounds of vegan chicken wings
- 1 tsp. of lemon juice, freshly squeezed
- 1 tbsp. of old bay spices
- ¾ cup of almond flour
- ½ cup of butter

Directions:

1. For about 5 minutes, preheat your air fryer. Mix all your ingredients in a mixing dish, excluding the butter. Put in the bowl of an air fryer.

2. Preheat the oven to about 350°F and bake for around 25 minutes. Rock the fryer container midway thru the cooking process, also for cooking.

3. Drizzle with some melted butter when it's done frying. Enjoy!

15. Cold Salad with Veggies and Pasta

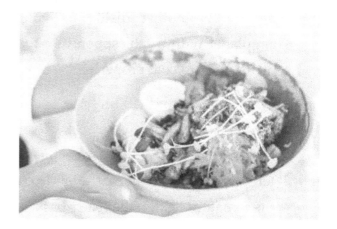

Preparation time: 30 minutes

Cooking time: 1 hour 35 minutes

Servings: 12 people

Ingredients:

- ½ cup of fat-free Italian dressing
- 2 tablespoons of olive oil, divided
- ½ cup of Parmesan cheese, grated
- 8 cups of cooked pasta
- 4 medium tomatoes, cut in eighths
- 3 small eggplants, sliced into ½-inch thick rounds
- 3 medium zucchinis, sliced into ½-inch thick rounds
- Salt, according to your taste.

Directions:

1. Preheat your Air fryer to about 355° F and oil the inside of your air fryer basket. In a dish, mix 1 tablespoon of olive oil and zucchini and swirl to cover properly.

2. Cook for around 25 minutes your zucchini pieces in your Air fryer basket. In another dish, mix your eggplants with a tablespoon of olive oil and toss to coat properly.

3. Cook for around 40 minutes your eggplant slices in your Air fryer basket. Re-set the Air Fryer temperature to about 320° F and put the tomatoes next in the ready basket.

4. Cook and mix all your air-fried vegetables for around 30 minutes. To serve, mix in the rest of the ingredients and chill for at least 2 hours, covered.

16. Zucchini and Minty Eggplant Bites

Preparation time: 15 minutes

Cooking time: 35 minutes

Servings: 8 people

Ingredients:

- 3 tbsp. of olive oil
- 1 pound of zucchini, peeled and cubed
- 1 pound of eggplant, peeled and cubed
- 2 tbsp. of melted butter
- 1 ½ tsp. of red pepper chili flakes
- 2 tsp. of fresh mint leaves, minced

Directions:

1. In a large mixing container, add all of the ingredients mentioned above.

2. Roast the zucchini bites and eggplant in your Air Fryer for around 30 minutes at about 300° F, flipping once or twice during the cooking cycle. Serve with some dipping sauce that's homemade.

17. Stuffed Potatoes

Preparation time: 15 minutes

Cooking time: 31 minutes

Servings: 4 people

Ingredients:

- 3 tbsp. of canola oil

- ½ cup of Parmesan cheese, grated

- 2 tbsp. of chives, chopped

- ½ of brown onion, chopped

- 1 tbsp. of butter

- 4 potatoes, peeled

Directions:

1. Preheat the Air fryer to about 390° F and oil the air fryer basket. Coat the canola oil on the potatoes and place them in your Air Fryer Basket.

2. Cook for around 20 minutes before serving on a platter. Halve each potato and scrape out the middle from each half of it.

3. In a frying pan, melt some butter over medium heat and add the onions. Sauté in a bowl for around 5 minutes and dish out.

4. Combine the onions with the middle of the potato, chives and half of the cheese. Stir well and uniformly cram the onion potato mixture into the potato halves.

5. Top and layer the potato halves in your Air Fryer basket with the leftover cheese. Cook for around 6 minutes before serving hot.

18. Paneer Cutlet

Preparation time: 5 minutes

Cooking time: 15 minutes

Servings: 1 people

Ingredients:

- ½ teaspoon of salt

- ½ teaspoon of oregano

- 1 small onion, finely chopped

- ½ teaspoon of garlic powder

- 1 teaspoon of butter

- ½ teaspoon of chai masala

- 1 cup of grated cheese

Directions:

1. Preheat the air fryer to about 350° F and lightly oil a baking dish. In a mixing bowl, add all ingredients and stir well. Split the mixture into cutlets and put them in an oiled baking dish.

2. Put the baking dish in your air fryer and cook your cutlets until crispy, around a minute or so.

19. Spicy Roasted Cashew Nuts

Preparation time: 10 Minutes

Cooking time: 20 Minutes

Servings: 4

Ingredients:

- 1/2 tsp. of ancho chili powder

- 1/2 tsp. of smoked paprika

- Salt and ground black pepper, according to taste

- 1 tsp. of olive oil

- 1 cup of whole cashews

Directions:

1. In a mixing big bowl, toss all your ingredients.

2. Line parchment paper to cover the Air Fryer container. Space out the spiced cashews in your basket in a uniform layer.

3. Roast for about 6 to 8 minutes at 300 degrees F, tossing the basket once or twice during the cooking process. Work in batches if needed. Enjoy!

CHAPTER 4: Deserts

1. Almond-apple Treat

Preparation time: 5 minutes

Cooking time: 15 minutes

Servings: 4 people

Ingredients:

- 2 tablespoon of sugar
- ¾ oz. of raisins
- 1 ½ oz. of almonds

Directions:

1. Preheat your air fryer to around 360° F.

2. Mix the almonds, sugar, and raisins in a dish. Blend using a hand mixer.

3. Load the apples with a combination of the almond mixture. Please put them in the air fryer basket and cook for a few minutes. Enjoy!

2. Pepper-pineapple With Butter-sugar Glaze

Preparation time: 5 minutes

Cooking time: 10 minutes

Servings: 2 people

Ingredients:

- Salt according to taste.
- 2 tsp. of melted butter
- 1 tsp. of brown sugar

- 1 red bell pepper, seeded and julienned
- 1 medium-sized pineapple, peeled and sliced

Directions:

1. To about 390°F, preheat your air fryer. In your air fryer, put the grill pan attachment.

2. In a Ziploc bag, combine all ingredients and shake well.

3. Dump and cook on the grill pan for around 10 minutes to ensure you turn the pineapples over every 5 minutes during cooking.

3. True Churros with Yummy Hot Chocolate

Preparation time: 10 minutes

Cooking time: 25 minutes

Servings: 3 people

Ingredients:

- 1 tsp. of ground cinnamon
- 1/3 cup of sugar
- 1 tbsp. of cornstarch
- 1 cup of milk
- 2 ounces of dark chocolate
- 1 cup of all-purpose flour
- 1 tbsp. of canola oil
- 1 tsp. of lemon zest
- 1/4 tsp. of sea salt

- 2 tbsp. of granulated sugar
- 1/2 cup of water

Directions:

1. To create the churro dough, boil the water in a pan over a medium-high flame; then, add the salt, sugar, and lemon zest and fry, stirring continuously, until fully dissolved.

2. Take the pan off the heat and add in some canola oil. Stir the flour in steadily, constantly stirring until the solution turns to a ball.

3. With a broad star tip, pipe the paste into a piping bag. In the oiled Air Fryer basket, squeeze 4-inch slices of dough. Cook for around 6 minutes at a temperature of 300° F.

4. Make the hot cocoa for dipping in the meantime. In a shallow saucepan, melt some chocolate and 1/2 cup of milk over low flame.

5. In the leftover 1/2 cup of milk, mix the cornstarch and blend it into the hot chocolate mixture. Cook for around 5 minutes on low flame.

6. Mix the sugar and cinnamon; roll your churros in this combination. Serve with a side of hot cocoa. Enjoy!

Conclusion

These times, air frying is one of the most common cooking techniques and air fryers have become one of the chef's most impressive devices. In no time, air fryers can help you prepare nutritious and tasty meals! To prepare unique dishes for you and your family members, you do not need to be a master in the kitchen.

Everything you have to do is buy an air fryer and this wonderful cookbook for air fryers! Soon, you can make the greatest dishes ever and inspire those around you.

Cooked meals at home with you! Believe us! Get your hands on an air fryer and this handy set of recipes for air fryers and begin your new cooking experience. Have fun!

The Complete Air Fryer Cookbook with Pictures

By Mark Machino

Contents

INTRODUCTION:

The aim of this cookbook is to provide the easiness for those who are professional or doing job somewhere. But with earning, it is also quite necessary to cook food easily & timely instead of ordering hygienic or costly junk food. As we know, after doing office work, no one can cook food with the great effort. For the ease of such people, there are a lot of latest advancements in kitchen accessories. The most popular kitchen appliances usually helps to make foods or dishes like chicken, mutton, beef, potato chips and many other items in less time and budget. There are a lot of things that should be considered when baking with an air fryer. One of the most important tips is to make sure you have all of your equipment ready for the bake. It is best to be prepared ahead of time and this includes having pans, utensils, baking bags, the air fryer itself, and the recipe book instead of using stove or oven. With the help of an air fryer, you can make various dishes for a single person as well as the entire family timely and effortlessly. As there is a famous proverb that "Nothing can be done on its own", it indicates that every task takes time for completion. Some tasks take more time and effort and some requires less time and effort for their completion. Therefore, with the huge range of advancements that come to us are just for our ease. By using appliances like an air fryer comes for the comfort of professional people who are busy in earning their livelihood. In this book, you can follow the latest, delicious, and quick, about 70 recipes that will save your time and provide you healthy food without any great effort.

Chapter # 1:

An Overview & Benefits of an Air Fryer

Introduction:

The most popular kitchen appliance that usually helps to make foods or dishes like chicken, mutton, beef, potato chips and many other items in less time and budget.

Today, everything is materialistic, every person is busy to earn great livelihood. Due to a huge burden of responsibilities, they have no time to cook food on stove after doing hard work. Because, traditionally cooking food on the stove takes more time and effort. Therefore, there are a vast variety of Kitchen appliances. The kitchen appliances are so much helpful in making or cooking food in few minutes and in less budget. You come to home from job, and got too much tired. So, you can cook delicious food in an Air Fryer efficiently and timely as compared to stove. You can really enjoy the food without great effort and getting so much tired.

The Air Fryer Usability:

Be prepared to explore all about frying foods that you learned. To crisp, golden brown excellence (yes, French-fried potatoes and potato chips!), air fryers will fry your favourite foods using minimum or no oil. You can not only make commonly fried foods such as chips and French fries of potatoes, however it is also ideal for proteins, vegetables such as drummettes and chicken wings, coquettes & feta triangles as well as appetizers. And cookies are perfectly cooked in an air fryer, such as brownies and blondies.

The Air Fryer Works as:

- Around 350-375°F (176-190°C) is the ideal temperature of an Air Fryer

- To cook the surface of the food, pour over a food oil at the temperature mentioned above. The oil can't penetrate because it forms a type of seal.

- Simultaneously, the humidity within the food turns into steam that helps to actually cook the food from the inside. It is cleared that the steam helps to maintain the oil out of the food.

- The oil flows into the food at a low temperature, rendering it greasy.

- It oxidizes the oil and, at high temperatures, food will dry out.

On the other hand, an air fryer is similar to a convection oven, but in a diverse outfit, food preparation done at very high temperatures whereas, inside it, dry air circulates around the food at the same time, while making it crisp without putting additional fat, it makes it possible for cooking food faster.

What necessary to Search for in an Air Fryer?

As we know, several different sizes and models of air fryers are available now. If you're cooking for a gathering, try the extra-large air fryer, that can prepare or fry a whole chicken, other steaks or six servings of French fries.

Suppose, you've a fixed counter space, try the Large Air Fryer that uses patented machinery to circulate hot air for sufficient, crispy results. The latest air fryer offers an extra compact size with identical capacity! and tar equipment, which ensures that food is cooking evenly (no further worries of build-ups). You will be able to try all the fried foods you enjoy, with no embarrassment.

To increase the functionality of an air fryer, much more, you can also purchase a wide range of different accessories, including a stand, roasting pan, muffin cups, and mesh baskets. Check out the ingredients of our air fryer we created, starting from buttermilk with black pepper seasoning to fry chicken or Sichuan garlic seasoning suitable for Chinese cuisine.

We will read about the deep fryer, with tips and our favourite recipes like burgers, chicken wings, and many more.

Most Common - Five Guidelines for an Air Fryer usage:

1. Shake the food.

Open the air fryer and shake the foods efficiently because the food is to "fry" in the machine's basket—Light dishes like Sweet French fries and Garlic chips will compress. Give Rotation to the food every 5-10 mins for better performance

2. Do not overload.

Leave enough space for the food so that the air circulates efficiently; so that's gives you crunchy effects. Our kitchen testing cooks trust that the snacks and small batches can fry in air fryer.

3. Slightly spray to food.

Gently spray on food by a cooking spray bottle and apply a touch of oil on food to make sure the food doesn't stick to the basket.

4. Retain an Air fry dry.

Beat food to dry before start cooking (even when marinated, e.g.) to prevent splashing & excessive smoke. Likewise, preparing high-fat foods such as chicken steaks or wings, be assured to remove the grease from the lower part of machine regularly.

5. Other Most Dominant cooking techniques.

The air fryer is not just for deep frying; It is also perfect for further safe methods of cooking like baking, grilling, roasting and many more. Our kitchen testing really loves using the unit for cooking salmon in air fryer!

An Air Fryer Helps to reduce fat content

Generally, food cooked in deep fryer contains higher fat level than preparing food in other cooking appliances. For Example; a fried chicken breast contains about 30% more fat just like a fat level in roasted chicken

Many Manufacturers claimed, an Air fryer can reduce fat from fried food items up-to 75%. So, an air fryer requires less amount of fat than a deep fryer. As, many dishes cooked in deep fryer consume 75% oil (equal to 3 cups) and an air fryer prepare food by applying the oil in just about 1 tablespoon (equal to 15ml).

One research tested the potato chips prepared in air fryer characteristics then observed: the air frying method produces a final product with slightly lower fat but same moisture content and color. So, there is a major impact on anyone's health, an excessive risk of illnesses such as inflammation, infection and heart disease has been linked to a greater fat intake from vegetable oils.

Air Fryer provides an Aid in Weight Loss

The dishes prepared deep fryer are not just having much fat but also more in calories that causes severe increase in weight. Another research of 33,542 Spanish grown-ups indicates that a greater usage of fried food linked with a higher occurrence of obesity. Dietetic fat has about twice like many calories per gram while other macro-nutrients such as carbohydrates, vitamins and proteins, averaging in at 9 calories throughout each and every gram of oil or fat.

By substituting to air fryer is an easy way to endorse in losing weight and to reduce calories and it will be done only by taking food prepared in air fryer.

Air Fried food may reduce the potentially harmful chemicals

Frying foods can produce potentially hazardous compounds such as acrylamide, in contrast to being higher in fat and calories. An acrylamide is a compound that is formed in carbohydrate- rich dishes or foods during highly-heated cooking methods such as frying. Acrylamide is known as a "probable carcinogen" which indicates as some research suggests that it could be associated with the development of cancer. Although the findings are conflicting, the link between dietary acrylamide and a greater risk of kidney, endometrial and ovarian cancers has been identified in some reports. Instead of cooking food in a deep fryer, air frying your food may aid the acrylamide content. Some researches indicates that air-frying method may cut the acrylamide by 90% by comparing deep frying method. All other extremely harmful chemicals produced by high-heat cooking are polycyclic aromatic hydrocarbons, heterocyclic amines and aldehydes and may be associated with a greater risk of cancer. That's why, the air fried food may help to reduce the chance of extremely dangerous chemicals or compounds and maintain your health.

Chapter # 2:

70 Perfectly Portioned Air Fryer Recipes for Busy People in Minimum Budget

1. Air fried corn, zucchini and haloumi fritters

Ingredients

- Coarsely grated block haloumi - 225g
- Coarsely grated Zucchini - 2 medium sized
- Frozen corn kernels - 150g (1 cup)
- Lightly whisked eggs - 2
- Self-raising flour - 100g
- Extra virgin olive oil - to drizzle
- Freshly chopped oregano leaves - 3 tablespoons
- Fresh oregano extra sprigs - to serve
- Yoghurt - to serve

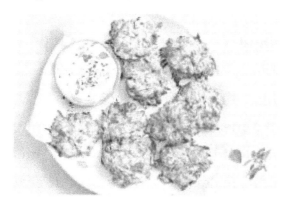

Method

1. Use your palms to squeeze out the extra liquid from the zucchini and place them in a bowl. Add the corn and haloumi and stir for combining them. Then add the eggs, oregano and flour. Add seasoning and stir until fully mixed.

2. Set the temperature of an air fryer to 200 C. Put spoonsful of the mixture of zucchini on an air fryer. Cook until golden and crisp, for 8 minutes. Transfer to a dish that is clean. Again repeat this step by adding the remaining mixture in 2 more batches.

3. Take a serving plate and arrange soft fritters on it. Take yoghurt in a small serving bowl. Add seasoning of black pepper on the top of yoghurt. Drizzle with olive oil. At the end, serve this dish with extra oregano.

2. Air fryer fried rice

Ingredients

- Microwave long grain rice - 450g packet
- Chicken tenderloins - 300g
- Rindless bacons - 4 ranchers
- Light Soy sauce - 2 tablespoons
- Oyster sauce - 2 tablespoons
- Sesame oil - 1 tablespoon
- Fresh finely grated ginger - 3 tablespoons
- Frozen peas - 120g (3/4 cup)

- Lightly whisked eggs - 2
- Sliced green shallots - 2
- Thin sliced red chilli - 1
- Oyster sauce - to drizzle

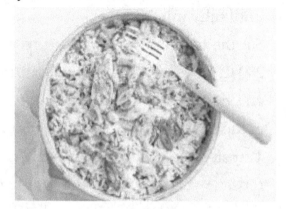

Method

1. Set the 180°C temperature of an air fryer. Bacon and chicken is placed on the rack of an air fryer. Cook them until fully cooked for 8-10 minutes. Shift it to a clean plate and set this plate aside to cool. Then, slice and chop the bacon and chicken.

2. In the meantime, separate the rice grains in the packet by using your fingers. Heat the rice for 60 seconds in a microwave. Shift to a 20cm ovenproof, round high-sided pan or dish. Apply the sesame oil, soy sauce, ginger, oyster sauce and 10ml water and mix well.

3. Put a pan/dish in an air fryer. Cook the rice for 5 minutes till them soft. Then whisk the chicken, half of bacon and peas in the eggs. Completely cook the eggs in 3 minutes. Mix and season the

top of half shallot with white pepper and salt.

4. Serve with the seasoning of chilli, remaining bacon and shallot and oyster sauce.

3. Air fried banana muffins

Ingredients

- Ripe bananas - 2
- Brown sugar - 60g (1/3 cup)
- Olive oil - 60ml (1/4 cup)
- Buttermilk - 60ml (1/4 cup)
- Self-raising flour - 150g (1 cup)
- Egg - 1
- Maple syrup - to brush or to serve

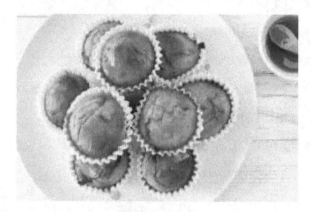

Method

1. Mash the bananas in a small bowl using a fork. Until needed, set aside.

2. In a medium cup, whisk the flour and sugar using a balloon whisk. In the middle, make a well. Add the buttermilk, oil and egg. Break up the egg with the help of a whisk. Stir by using wooden spoon until the mixture is mixed. Stir the banana through it.

3. Set the temperature of an air fryer at 180C. Splits half of the mixture into 9 cases of patties. Remove the rack from the air fryer and pass the cases to the rack carefully. Switch the rack back to the fryer. Bake the muffins completely by cooking them for 10 minutes. Move to the wire rack. Repeat this step on remaining mixture to produce 18 muffins.

4. Brush the muffin tops with maple syrup while they're still warm. Serve, if you like, with extra maple syrup.

4. Air fried Nutella brownies

Ingredients

- Plain flour - 150g (1 cup)
- Castor white sugar - 225g (1 cup)
- Lightly whisked eggs - 3
- Nutella - 300g (1 cup)
- Cocoa powder - to dust

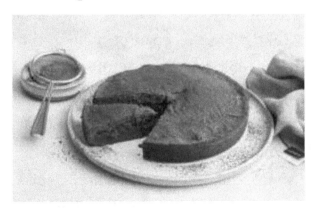

Method

1. Apply butter in a 20cm circular cake pan. Cover the base by using baking paper.

2. Whisk the flour and sugar together in a bowl by using balloon whisk. In the middle, make a well. Add the Nutella and egg in the middle of bowl by making a well. Stir with a large metal spoon until mixed. Move this mixture to the previously prepared pan and smooth the surface of the mixture by using metal spoon.

3. Pre - heat an air fryer to 160C. Bake the brownie about 40 minutes or until a few crumbs stick out of a skewer inserted in the middle. Fully set aside to cool.

4. Garnish the top of the cake by dusting them with cocoa powder, and cut them into pieces. Brownies are ready to be served.

5. Air fried celebration bites

Ingredients

- Frozen shortcrust partially thawed pastry - 4 sheets
- Lightly whisked eggs - 1
- Unrapped Mars Celebration chocolates - 24
- Icing sugar - to dust
- Cinnamon sugar - to dust
- Whipped cream - to serve

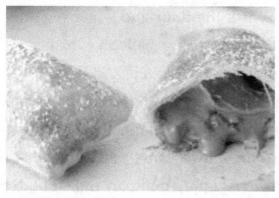

Method

1. Slice each pastry sheet into 6 rectangles. Brush the egg gently. One chocolate is placed in the middle of each rectangular piece of pastry. Fold the pastry over to cover the chocolate completely. Trim the pastry, press and seal the sides. Place it on a tray containing baking paper. Brush the egg on each pastry and sprinkle cinnamon sugar liberally.

2. In the air-fryer basket, put a sheet of baking paper, making sure that the paper is 1 cm smaller than the basket to allow airflow. Put six pockets in the basket by taking care not to overlap. Cook for 8-9 minutes at 190°C until pastries are completely cooked with golden color. Shift to a dish. Free pockets are then used again.

3. Sprinkle Icing sugar on the top of tasty bites. Serve them with a whipped cream to intensify its flavor.

6. Air fried nuts and bolts

Ingredients

- Dried farfalle pasta - 2 cups
- Extra virgin olive oil - 60ml (1/4th cup)
- Brown sugar - 2 tablespoons
- Onion powder - 1 tablespoon
- Smoked paprika - 2 tablespoons
- Chili powder - 1/2 tablespoon
- Garlic powder - 1/2 tablespoon
- Pretzels - 1 cup
- Raw macadamias - 80g (1/2 cup)
- Raw cashews - 80g (1/2 cup)
- Kellog's Nutri-grain cereal - 1 cup
- Sea salt - 1 tablespoon

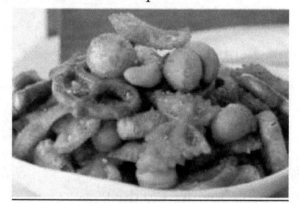

Method

1. Take a big saucepan of boiling salted water, cook the pasta until just ready and soft. Drain thoroughly. Shift pasta to a tray and pat with a paper towel to dry. Move the dried pasta to a wide pot.

2. Mix the sugar, oil, onion, paprika, chili and garlic powders together in a clean bowl. Add half of this mixture in the bowl containing pasta. Toss this bowl slightly for the proper coating of mixture over pasta.

3. Set the temperature at 200C of an Air Fryer. Put the pasta in air fryer's pot. After cooking for 5 minutes, shake the pot and cook for more 5-7 minutes, until they look golden and crispy. Shift to a wide bowl.

4. Take the pretzels in a bowl with the nuts and apply the remaining mixture of spices. Toss this bowl for the proper coating. Put in air fryer's pot and cook at 180C for 3-4 minutes. Shake this pot and cook for more 2-3 minutes until it's golden in color. First add pasta and then add the cereal. Sprinkle salt on it and toss to mix properly. Serve this dish after proper cooling.

7. Air fried coconut shrimps

Ingredients

- Plain flour - 1/2 cup
- Eggs - 2
- Bread crumbs - 1/2 cup
- Black pepper powder - 1.5 teaspoons
- Sweetless flaked coconut - 3/4 cup
- Uncooked, deveined and peeled shrimp - 12 ounces
- Salt - 1/2 teaspoon
- Honey - 1/4 cup
- Lime juice - 1/4 cup
- Finely sliced serrano chili - 1
- Chopped cilantro - 2 teaspoons
- Cooking spray

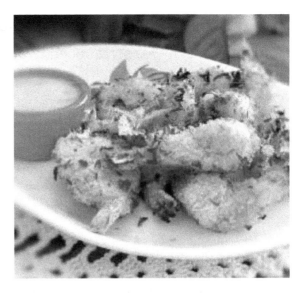

Method

1. Stir the pepper and flour in a clean bowl together. Whisk the eggs in another bowl and h panko and coconut in separate bowl. Coat the shrimps with flour mixture by holding each shrimp by tail and shake off the extra flour. Then coat the floured shrimp with egg and allow it to drip off excess. Give them the final coat of coconut mixture and press them to stick. Shift on a clean plate. Spray shrimp with cooking oil.

2. Set the temperature of the air-fryer to 200C. In an air fryer, cook half of the shrimp for 3 minutes. Turn the shrimp and cook further for more 3 minutes until color changes in golden. Use 1/4 teaspoon of salt for seasoning. Repeat this step for the rest of shrimps.

3. In the meantime, prepare a dip by stirring lime juice, serrano chili and honey in a clean bowl.

4. Serve fried shrimps with sprinkled cilantro and dip.

8. Air fried Roasted Sweet and Spicy Carrots

Ingredients

- Cooking oil
- Melted butter - 1 tablespoon
- Grated orange zest - 1 teaspoon
- Carrots - 1/2 pound
- Hot honey - 1 tablespoon
- Cardamom powder - 1/2 teaspoon
- Fresh orange juice - 1 tablespoon
- Black pepper powder - to taste
- Salt - 1 pinch

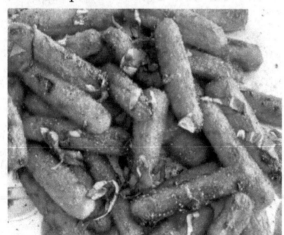

Method

1. Set the temperature of an air to 200C. Lightly coat its pot with cooking oil.

2. Mix honey, cardamom and orange zest in a clean bowl. Take 1 tablespoon of this sauce in another bowl and place aside.

Coat carrots completely by tossing them in remaining sauce. Shift carrots to an air fryer pot.

3. Air fry the carrots and toss them after every 6 minutes. Cook carrots for 15-20 minutes until they are fully cooked and roasted. Combine honey butter sauce with orange juice to make sauce. Coat carrots with this sauce. Season with black pepper and salt and serve this delicious dish.

9. Air fried Chicken Thighs

Ingredients

- Boneless chicken thighs - 4
- Extra virgin olive oil - 2 teaspoons
- Smoked paprika - 1 teaspoon
- Salt - 1/2 teaspoon
- Garlic powder - 3/4 teaspoon
- Black pepper powder - 1/2 teaspoon

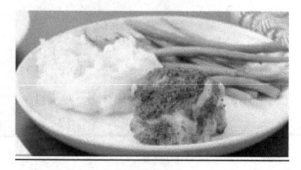

Method

1. Set the temperature of an air fryer to 200C.

2. Dry chicken thighs by using tissue paper. Brush olive oil on the skin side of

each chicken thigh. Shift the single layer of chicken thighs on a clean tray.

3. Make a mixture of salt, black pepper, paprika and garlic powder in a clean bowl. Use a half of this mixture for the seasoning of 4 chicken thighs on both sides evenly. Then shift single layer of chicken thighs in an air fryer pot by placing skin side up.

4. Preheat the air fryer and maintain its temperature to 75C. Fry chicken for 15-18 minutes until its water become dry and its color changes to brown. Serve immediately.

10. Air fried French Fries

Ingredients

- Peeled Potatoes - 1 pound
- Vegetable oil - 2 tablespoon
- Cayenne pepper - 1 pinch
- Salt - 1/2 teaspoon

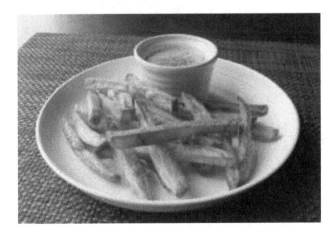

Method

1. Lengthwise cut thick slices of potato of 3/8 inches.

2. Soak sliced potatoes for 5 minutes in water. Drain excess starch water from soaked potatoes after 5 minutes. Place these potatoes in boiling water pan for 8-10 minutes.

3. Remove water from the potatoes and dry them completely. Cool them for 10 minutes and shift in a clean bowl. Add some oil and fully coat the potatoes with cayenne by tossing.

4. Set the temperature of an air fryer to 190C. Place two layers of potatoes in air fryer pot and cook them for 10-15 minutes. Toss fries continuously and cook for more 10 minutes until their color changes to golden brown. Season fries with salt and serve this appetizing dish immediately.

11. Air fried Mini Breakfast Burritos

Ingredients

- Mexican style chorizo - 1/4 cup
- Sliced potatoes - 1/2 cup
- Chopped serrano pepper - 1
- 8-inch flour tortillas - 4
- Bacon grease - 1 tablespoon
- Chopped onion - 2 tablespoon
- Eggs - 2
- Cooking avacado oil - to spray
- Salt - to taste
- Black pepper powder - to taste

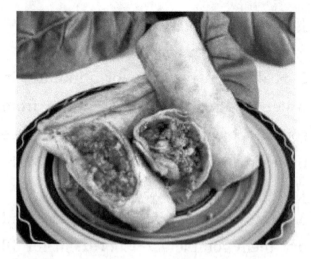

Method

1. Take chorizo in a large size pan and cook on medium flame for 8 minutes with continuous stirring until its color change into reddish brown. Shift chorizo in a clean plate and place separate.

2. Take bacon grease in same pan and melt it on medium flame. Place sliced potatoes and cook them for 10 minutes with constant stirring. Add serrano pepper and onion meanwhile. Cook for more 2-5 minutes until potatoes are fully cooked, onion and serrano pepper become soften. Then add chorizo and eggs and cook for more 5 minutes until potato mixture is fully incorporated. Use pepper and salt for seasoning.

3. In the meantime, heat tortillas in a large pan until they become soft and flexible. Put 1/3 cup of chorizo mixture at the center of each tortilla. Filling is covered by rolling the upper and lower side of tortilla and give shape of burrito.

Spray cooking oil and place them in air fryer pot.

4. Fry these burritos at 200C for 5 minutes. Change the side's continuously and spray with cooking oil. Cook in air fryer for 3-4 minutes until color turns into light brown. Shift burritos in a clean dish and serve this delicious dish.

12. Air fried Vegan Tator Tots

Ingredients

- Frozen potato nuggets (Tator Tots) - 2 cups
- Buffalo wing sauce - 1/4 cup
- Vegan ranch salad - 1/4 cup

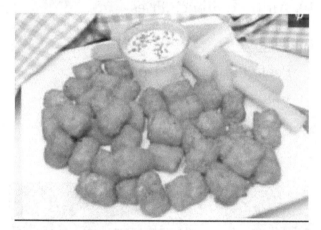

Method

1. Set the temperature of an air fryer to 175C.

2. Put frozen potato nuggets in air fryer pot and cook for 6-8 minutes with constant shake.

3. Shift potatoes to a large-sized bowl and add wing sauce. Combine evenly

by tossing them and place them again in air fryer pot.

4. Cook more for 8-10 minutes without disturbance. Shift to a serving plate. Serve with ranch dressing and enjoy this dish.

13. Air fried Roasted Cauliflower

Ingredients

- Cauliflower florets - 4 cups
- Garlic - 3 cloves
- Smoked paprika - 1/2 teaspoon
- Peanut oil - 1 tablespoon
- Salt - 1/2 teaspoon

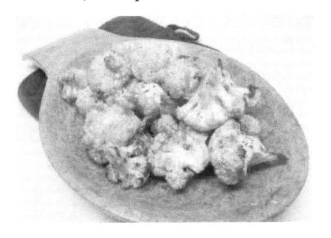

Method

1. Set the temperature of an air fryer to 200C.

2. Smash garlic cloves with a knife and mix with salt, oil and paprika. Coat cauliflower in this mixture.

3. Put coated cauliflower in air fryer pot and cook around 10-15 minutes with stirring after every 5 minutes. Cook according to desired color and crispiness and serve immediately.

14. Air fried Cinnamon-Sugar Doughnuts

Ingredients

- White sugar - 1/2 cup
- Brown sugar - 1/4 cup
- Melted butter - 1/4 cup
- Cinnamon powder - 1 teaspoon
- Ground nutmeg - 1/4 TEASPOON
- Packed chilled flaky biscuit dough - 1 (16.3 ounce)

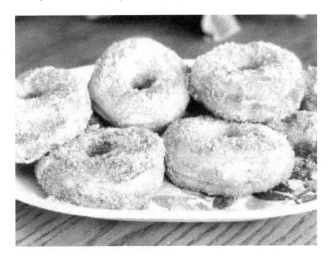

Method

1. Put melted butter in a clean bowl. Add brown sugar, white sugar, nutmeg and cinnamon and mix.

2. Divide and cut biscuit dough into many single biscuits and give them the shape of doughnuts using a biscuit cutter. Shift doughnuts in an air fryer pot.

3. Air fry the doughnuts for 5-6 minutes at 175C until color turns into golden brown. Turn the side of doughnuts and cook for more 1-3 minutes.

4. Shift doughnuts from air fryer to a clean dish and dip them in melted butter. Then completely coat these doughnuts in sugar and cinnamon mixture and serve frequently.

15. Air Fried Broiled Grapefruit

Ingredients

- Chilled red grapefruit - 1
- Melted butter - 1 tablespoon
- Brown sugar - 2 tablespoon
- Ground cinnamon - 1/2 teaspoon
- Aluminium foil

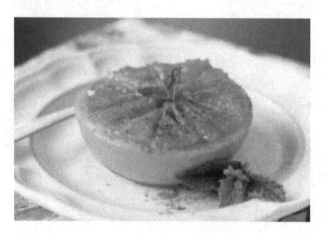

Method

1. Set the temperature of an air fryer to 200C.

2. Cut grapefruit crosswise to half and also cut a thin slice from one end of grapefruit for sitting your fruit flat on a plate.

3. Mix brown sugar in melted butter in a small sized bowl. Coat the cut side of the grapefruit with this mixture. Dust the little brown sugar over it.

4. Take 2 five inch pieces of aluminium foil and put the half grapefruit on each piece. Fold the sides evenly to prevent juice leakage. Place them in air fryer pot.

5. Broil for 5-7 minutes until bubbling of sugar start in an air fryer. Before serving, sprinkle cinnamon on grapefruit.

16. Air Fried Brown Sugar and Pecan Roasted Apples

Ingredients

- Apples - 2 medium
- Chopped pecans - 2 tablespoons
- Plain flour - 1 teaspoon
- Melted butter - 1 tablespoon
- Brown sugar - 1 tablespoon
- Apple pie spice - 1/4 teaspoon

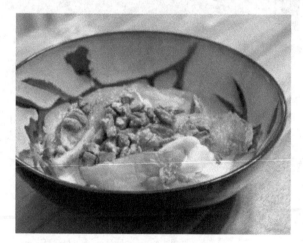

Method

1. Set the temperature of an air fryer to 180C.

2. Mix brown sugar, pecan, apple pie spice and flour in a clean bowl. Cut apples in wedges and put them in another bowl and coat them with melted

butter by tossing. Place a single layer in an air fryer pot and add mixture of pecan on the top.

3. Cook apples for 12-15 minutes until they get soft.

17. Air Fried Breaded Sea Scallops

Ingredients

- Crushed butter crackers - 1/2 cup
- Seafood seasoning - 1/2 teaspoon
- Sea scallops - 1 pound
- Garlic powder - 1/2 teaspoon
- Melted butter - 2 tablespoons
- Cooking oil - for spray

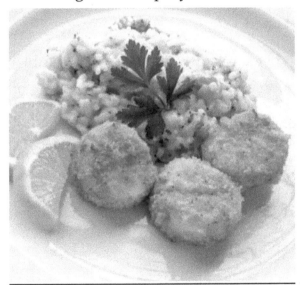

Method

1. Set the temperature of an air fryer to 198C.

2. Combine garlic powder, seafood seasoning and cracker crumbs in a clean bowl. Take melted butter in another bowl.

3. Coat each scallop with melted butter. Then roll them in breading until

completely enclose. Place them on a clean plate and repeat this step with rest of the scallops.

4. Slightly spray scallops with cooking oil and place them on the air fryer pot at equal distance. You may work in 2-3 batches.

5. Cook them for 2-3 minutes in preheated air fryer. Use a spatula to change the side of each scallop. Cook for more 2 minutes until they become opaque. Dish out in a clean plate and serve immediately.

18. Air Fried Crumbed Fish

Ingredients

- Flounder fillets - 4
- Dry bread crumbs - 1 cup
- Egg - 1
- Sliced lemon - 1
- Vegetable oil - 1/4 cup

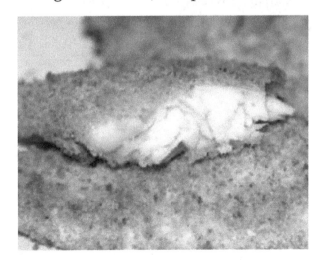

Method

1. Set the temperature of an air fryer to 180C.

2. Combine oil and bread crumbs in a clean bowl and mix them well.

3. Coat each fish fillets with beaten egg, then evenly dip them in the crumbs mixture.

4. Place coated fillets in preheated air fryer and cook for 10-12 minutes until fish easily flakes by touching them with fork. Shift prepared fish in a clean plate and serve with lemon slices.

19. Air Fried Cauliflower and Chickpea Tacos

Ingredients

- Cauliflower - 1 small
- Chickpeas - 15 ounce
- Chili powder - 1 teaspoon
- Cumin powder - 1 teaspoon
- Lemon juice - 1 tablespoon
- Sea salt - 1 teaspoon
- Garlic powder - 1/4 teaspoon
- Olive oil - 1 tablespoon

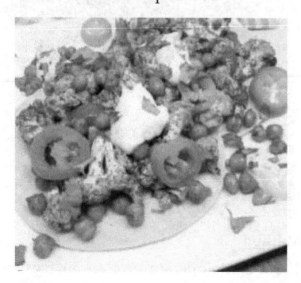

Method

1. Set the temperature of an air fryer to 190C.

2. Mix lime juice, cumin, garlic powder, salt, olive oil and chili powder in a clean bowl. Now coat well the cauliflower and chickpeas in this mixture by constant stirring.

3. Put cauliflower mixture in an air fryer pot. Cook for 8-10 minutes with constant stirring. Cook for more 10 minutes and stir for final time. Cook for more 5 minutes until desired crispy texture is attained.

5. Place cauliflower mixture by using spoon and serve.

20. Air Fried Roasted Salsa

Ingredients

- Roma tomatoes - 4
- Seeded Jalapeno pepper - 1
- Red onion - 1/2
- Garlic - 4 cloves
- Cilantro - 1/2 cup
- Lemon juice - 1
- Cooking oil - to spray
- Salt - to taste

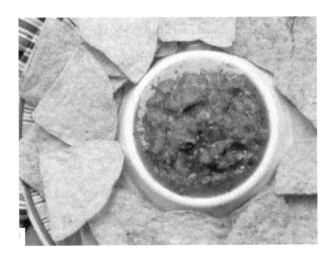

Method

1. Set the temperature of an air fryer to 200C.

2. Put tomatoes, red onion and skin side down of jalapeno in an air fryer pot. Brush lightly these vegetables with cooking oil for roasting them easily.

3. Cook vegetables in an air fryer for 5 minutes. Then add garlic cloves and again spray with cooking oil and fry for more 5 minutes.

4. Shift vegetables to cutting board and allow them to cool for 8-10 minutes.

5. Separate skins of jalapeno and tomatoes and chop them with onion into large pieces. Add them to food processor bowl and add lemon juice, cilantro, garlic and salt. Pulsing for many times until all the vegetables are evenly chopped. Cool them for 10-15 minutes and serve this delicious dish immediately.

21. Air Fried Flour Tortilla Bowls

Ingredients

- Flour tortilla - 1 (8 inch)
- Souffle dish - 1 (4 1/2 inch)

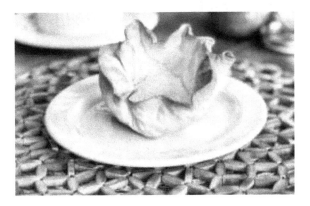

Method

1. Set the temperature of an air fryer to 190C.

2. Take tortilla in a large pan and heat it until it become soft. Put tortilla in the souffle dish by patting down side and fluting up from its sides of dish.

3. Air fry tortilla for 3-5 minutes until its color change into golden brown.

4. Take out tortilla bowl from the dish and put the upper side in the pot. Air fry again for more 2 minutes until its color turns into golden brown. Dish out and serve.

22. Air Fried Cheese and Mini Bean Tacos

Ingredients

- Can Refried beans - 16 ounce

- American cheese - 12 slices
- Flour tortillas - 12 (6 inch)
- Taco seasoning mix - 1 ounce
- Cooking oil - to spray

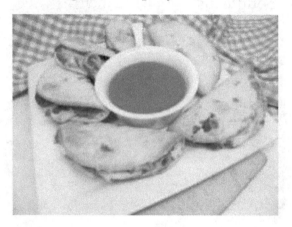

Method

1. Set the temperature of an air fryer to 200C.

2. Combine refried beans and taco seasoning evenly in a clean bowl and stir.

3. Put 1 slice of cheese in the center of tortilla and place 1 tablespoon of bean mixture over cheese. Again place second piece of cheese over this mixture. Fold tortilla properly from upper side and press to enclose completely. Repeat this step for the rest of beans, cheese and tortillas.

4. Spray cooking oil on the both sides of tacos. Put them in an air fryer at equal distance. Cook the tacos for 3 minutes and turn it side and again cook for more 3 minutes. Repeat this step for the rest of

tacos. Transfer to a clean plate and serve immediately.

23. Air Fried Lemon Pepper Shrimp

Ingredients

- Lemon - 1
- Lemon pepper - 1 teaspoon
- Olive oil - 1 tablespoon
- Garlic powder - 1/4 teaspoon
- Paprika - 1/4 teaspoon
- Deveined and peeled shrimps - 12 ounces
- Sliced lemon – 1

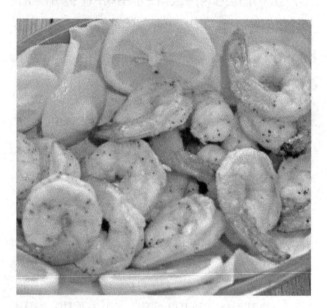

Method

1. Set the temperature of an air fryer to 200C.

2. Mix lemon pepper, garlic powder, and olive oil, paprika and lemon juice in a clean bowl. Coat shrimps by this mixture by tossing.

3. Put shrimps in an air fryer and cook for 5-8 minutes until its color turn to pink. Dish out cooked shrimps and serve with lemon slices.

24. Air Fried Shrimp a la Bang Bang

Ingredients

- Deveined raw shrimps - 1 pound
- Sweet chili sauce - 1/4 cup
- Plain flour - 1/4 cup
- Green onions - 2
- Mayonnaise - 1/2 cup
- Sriracha sauce - 1 tablespoon
- Bread crumbs - 1 cup
- Leaf lettuce - 1 head

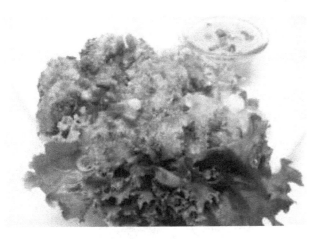

Method

1. Set the temperature of an air fryer to 200C

2. Make a bang bang sauce by mixing chili sauce, mayonnaise and sriracha sauce in a clean bowl. Separate some sauce for dipping in a separate small bowl.

3. Place bread crumbs and flour in two different plates. Coat shrimps with mayonnaise mixture, then with flour and then bread crumbs. Set coated shrimps on a baking paper.

4. Place them in an air fryer pot and cook for 10-12 minutes. Repeat this step for the rest of shrimps. Transfer shrimps to a clean dish and serve with green onions and lettuce.

25. Air Fried Spicy Bay Scallops

Ingredients

- Bay scallops - 1 pound
- Chili powder - 2 teaspoons
- Smoked paprika- 2 teaspoons
- Garlic powder - 1 teaspoon
- Olive oil - 2 teaspoons
- Black pepper powder - 1/4 teaspoon
- Cayenne red pepper - 1/8 teaspoon

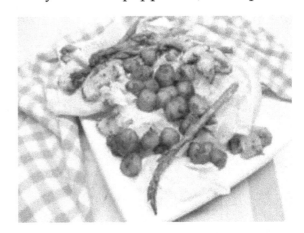

Method

1. Set the temperature of an air fryer to 200C

2. Mix smoked paprika, olive oil, bay scallops, garlic powder, pepper, chili powder and cayenne pepper in a clean bowl and stir properly. Shift this mixture to an air fryer.

3. Air fry for 6-8 minutes with constant shaking until scallops are fully cooked. Transfer this dish in a clean plate and serve immediately.

26. Air Fried Breakfast Fritatta

Ingredients

- Fully cooked breakfast sausages - 1/4 pound
- Cheddar Monterey Jack cheese - 1/2 cup
- Green onion - 1
- Cayenne pepper - 1 pinch
- Red bell pepper - 2 tablespoons
- Eggs - 4
- Cooking oil - to spray

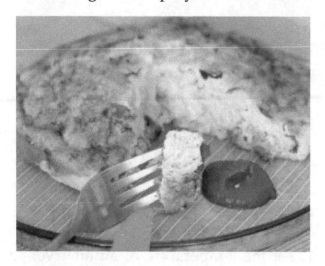

Method

1. Set the temperature of an air fryer to 180C.

2. Mix eggs, sausages, Cheddar Monterey Jack cheese, onion, bell pepper and cayenne in a clean bowl and stir to mix properly.

3. Spray cooking oil on a clean non-stick cake pan. Put egg mixture in the cake pan. Air fry for 15-20 minutes until fritatta is fully cooked and set. Transfer it in a clean plate and serve immediately.

27. Air Fried Roasted Okra

Ingredients

- Trimmed and sliced Okra - 1/2 pound
- Black pepper powder - 1/8 teaspoon
- Olive oil - 1 teaspoon
- Salt - 1/4 teaspoon

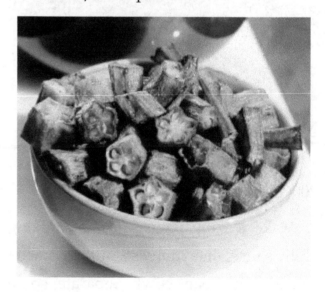

Method

1. Set the temperature of an air fryer to 175C.

2. Mix olive oil, black pepper, salt and okra in a clean bowl and stir to mix properly.

3. Make a single layer of this mixture in an air fryer pot. Air fry for 5-8 minutes with constant stirring. Cook for more 5 minutes and again toss. Cook for more 3 minutes and dish out in a clean plate and serve immediately.

28. Air Fried Rib-Eye Steak

Ingredients

- Rib-eye steak - 2 (1 1/2 inch thick)
- Olive oil - 1/4 cup
- Grill seasoning - 4 teaspoons
- Reduced sodium soy sauce - 1/2 cup

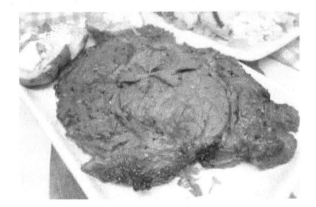

Method

1. Mix olive oil, soy sauce, seasoning and steaks in a clean bowl and set aside meat for marination.

2. Take out steaks and waste the remaining mixture. Remove excess oil from steak by patting.

3. Add 1 tablespoon water in an air fryer pot for the prevention from smoking during cooking of steaks.

3. Set the temperature of an air fryer to 200C. Place steaks in an air fryer pot. Air fry for 7-8 minutes and turn its side after every 8 minutes. Cook for more 7 minutes until it is rarely medium. Cook for final 3 minutes for a medium steak and dish out in a clean plate and serve immediately.

29. Air Fried Potato Chips

Ingredients

- Large potatoes - 2
- Olive oil - to spray
- Fresh parsley - optional
- Sea salt - 1/2 teaspoon

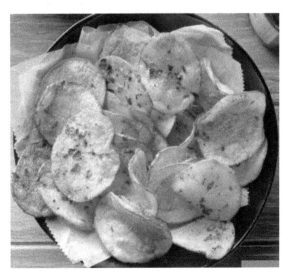

Method

1. Set the temperature of an air fryer to 180C.

2. Peel off the potatoes and cut them into thin slices. Shift the slices in a bowl containing ice chilled water and soak for 10 minutes. Drain potatoes, again add chilled water and soak for more 15 minutes.

3. Remove water from potatoes and allow to dry by using paper towel. Spray potatoes with cooking oil and add salt according to taste.

4. Place a single layer of potatoes slices in an oiled air fryer pot and cook for 15-18 minutes until color turns to golden brown and crispy. Stir constantly and turn its sides after every 5 minutes.

5. Dish out these crispy chips and serve with parsley.

30. Air Fried Tofu

Ingredients

- Packed tofu - 14 ounces
- Olive oil - 1/4 cup
- Reduced sodium soy sauce - 3 tablespoons
- Crushed red pepper flakes - 1/4 teaspoon
- Green onions - 2
- Cumin powder - 1/4 teaspoon
- Garlic - 2 cloves

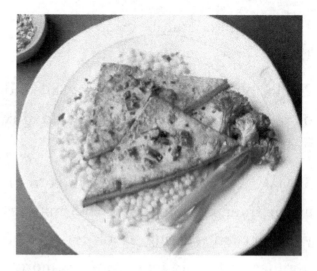

Method

1. Set the temperature of an air fryer to 200C.

2. Mix olive oil, soy sauce, onions, garlic, cumin powder and red pepper flakes in a deep bowl to make marinade mixture.

3. Cut 3/8 inches' thick slices of tofu lengthwise and then diagonally. Coat tofu with marinade mixture. Place them in refrigerate for 4-5 minutes and turn them after every 2 minutes.

4. Place tofu in buttered air fryer pot. Put remaining marinade over each tofu. Cook for 5-8 minutes until color turns to golden brown. Dish out cooked tofu and serve immediately.

31. Air Fried Acorn Squash Slices

Ingredients

- Medium sized acorn squash - 2
- Soft butter - 1/2 cup
- Brown sugar - 2/3 cup

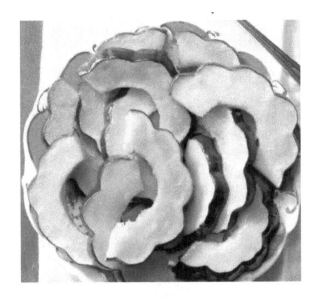

- Black pepper - 1/4 teaspoon

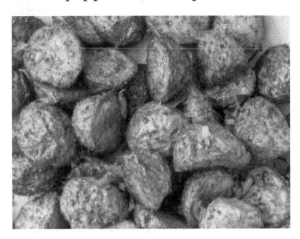

Method

1. Set the temperature of an air fryer to 160C.

2. Cut squash into two halves from length side and remove seeds. Again cut these halves into half inch slices.

3. Place a single layer of squash on buttered air fryer pot. Cook each side of squash for 5 minutes.

4. Mix butter into brown sugar and spread this mixture on the top of every squash. Cook for more 3 minutes. Dish out and serve immediately.

32. Air Fried Red Potatoes

Ingredients

- Baby potatoes - 2 pounds
- Olive oil - 2 tablespoons
- Fresh rosemary - 1 tablespoon
- Garlic - 2 cloves
- Salt - 1/2 teaspoon

Method

1. Set the temperature of an air fryer to 198C.

2. Cut potatoes into wedges. Coat them properly with minced garlic, rosemary, black pepper and salt.

3. Place coated potatoes on buttered air fryer pot. Cook potatoes for 5 minutes until golden brown and soft. Stir them at once. Dish out in a clean plate and serve immediately.

33. Air Fried Butter Cake

Ingredients

- Melted butter - 7 tablespoons
- White sugar - 1/4 cup & 2 tablespoons
- Plain flour - 1 & 2/3 cup
- Egg - 1
- Salt - 1 pinch
- Milk - 6 tablespoons
- Cooking oil - to spray

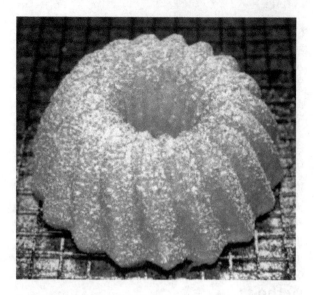

Method

1. Set the temperature of an air fryer to 180C and spray with cooking oil.

2. Beat white sugar, and butter together in a clean bowl until creamy and light. Then add egg and beautiful fluffy and smooth. Add salt and flour and stir. Then add milk and mix until batter is smooth. Shift batter to an preheated air fryer pot and level its surface by using spatula.

3. Place in an air fryer and set time of 15 minutes. Bake and check cake after 15 minutes by inserting toothpick in the cake. If toothpick comes out clean it means cake has fully baked.

4. Take out cake from air fryer and allow it to cool for 5-10 minutes. Serve immediately and enjoy.

34. Air Fried Jelly and Peanut Butter S'mores

Ingredients

- Chocolate topping peanut butter cup - 1
- Raspberry jam (seedless) - 1 teaspoon
- Marshmallow - 1 large
- Chocolate cracker squares – 2

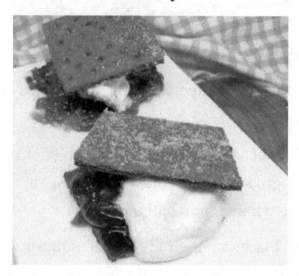

Method

1. Set the temperature of an air fryer to 200C.

2. Put peanut butter cup on one cracker square and topped with marshmallow and jelly. Carefully transfer it in the preheated air fryer.

3. Cook for 1 minute until marshmallow becomes soft and light brown. Remaining cracker squares is used for topping.

4. Shift this delicious in a clean plate and serve immediately.

35. Air Fried Sun-Dried Tomatoes

Ingredients

- Red grape tomatoes - 5 ounces
- Olive oil - 1/4 teaspoon
- Salt - to taste

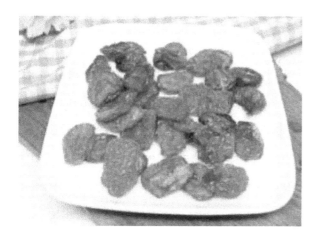

Method

1. Set the temperature of an air fryer to 115C.

2. Combine tomatoes halves, salt and olive oil evenly in a clean bowl. Shift tomatoes in an air fryer pot by placing skin side down.

3. Cook in air fryer for 45 minutes. Smash tomatoes by using spatula and cook for more 30 minutes. Repeat this step with the rest of tomatoes.

4. Shift this delicious dish in a clean plate and allow it to stand for 45 minutes to set. Serve this dish and enjoy.

36. Air Fried Sweet Potatoes Tots

Ingredients:

- Peeled Sweet Potatoes - 2 small (14oz.total)
- Garlic Powder - 1/8 tsp
- Potato Starch - 1 tbsp
- Kosher Salt, Divided - 11/4 tsp
- Unsalted Ketchup - 3/4 Cup
- Cooking Oil for spray

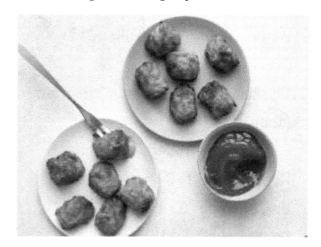

Method:

1. Take water in a medium pan and give a single boil over high flame. Then, add the sweet potatoes in the boiled water & cook for 15 minutes till potatoes becomes soft. Move the potatoes to a cooling plate for 15 minutes.

2. Rub potatoes using the wide hole's grater over a dish. Apply the potato starch, salt and garlic powder and toss gently. Make almost 24 shaped cylinders (1-inch) from the mixture.

3. Coat the air fryer pot gently with cooking oil. Put single layer of 1/2 of the tots in the pot and spray with cooking oil. Cook at 400 °F for about 12 to 14

minutes till lightly browned and flip tots midway. Remove from the pot and sprinkle with salt. Repeat with rest of the tots and salt left over. Serve with ketchup immediately.

37. Air Fried Banana Bread

Ingredients:

- White Whole Wheat Flour - 3/4 cup (3 oz.)
- Mashed Ripe Bananas - 2 medium or (about 3/4th cup)
- Cinnamon powder– 4 pinches
- Kosher Salt - 1/2 tsp
- Baking Soda - 1/4 tsp
- Large Eggs, Lightly Beaten - 2
- Regular Sugar - 1/2 cup
- Vanilla Essence - 1 tsp
- Vegetable Oil - 2 tbsp
- Roughly Chopped and toasted Walnuts - 2 table-spoons (3/4 oz.)
- Plain Non-Fat Yogurt - 1/3 cup
- Cooking Oil for Spray - as required

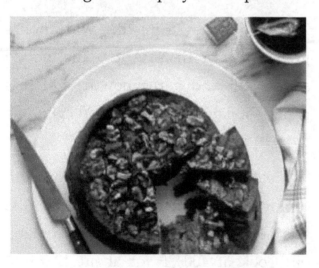

Method:

1. Cover the base of a 6-inches round cake baking pan with baking paper and lightly brush with melted butter. Beat the flour, baking soda, salt, and cinnamon together in a clean bowl and let it reserve.

2. Whisk the mashed bananas, eggs, sugar, cream, oil and vanilla together in a separate bowl. Stir the wet ingredients gently into the flour mixture until everything is blended. Pour the mixture in the prepared pan and sprinkle with the walnuts.

3. Set the temperature of an air fryer to 310 °F and put the pan in the air fryer. Cook until browned, about 30 to 35 minutes. Rotate the pan periodically until a wooden stick put in it and appears clean. Before flipping out & slicing, move the bread to a cooling rack for 15 minutes.

38. Air Fried Avocado Fries

Ingredients:

- Avocados --. 2 - Cut each into the 8 pieces
- All-purpose flour - 1/2 cup (about 21/8 oz.)
- Panko (Japanese Style Breadcrumbs) - 1/2 cup
- Large Eggs - 2

- Kosher Salt - 1/4 tsp
- Apple Cider - 1 tbsp
- Sriracha Chilli Sause - 1 tbsp
- Black pepper - 11/2 tsp
- Water - 1 tbsp
- Unsalted Ketchup - 1/2 cup
- Cooking spray

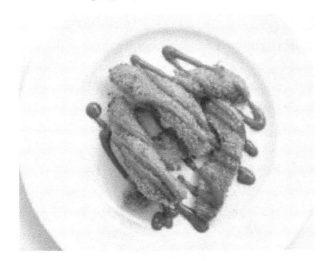

Method:

1. Mix flour and pepper collectively in a clean bowl. Whip eggs & water gently in another bowl. Take panko in a third bowl. Coat avocado slices in flour and remove extra flour by shaking. Then, dip the slices in the egg and remove any excess. Coat in panko by pushing to stick together. Spray well the avocado slices with cooking oil.

2. In the air fryer's basket, put avocado slices & fry at 400 ° F until it turns into golden for 7-8 minutes. Turn avocado wedges periodically while frying. Take out from an air fryer and use salt for sprinkling.

3. Mix the Sriracha, ketchup, vinegar, and mayonnaise together in a small bowl. Put two tablespoons of sauce on each plate with 4 avocado fries before serving.

39. "Strawberry Pop Tarts" in an Air Fryer

Ingredients:

- Quartered Strawberries - (about 13/4 cups equal to 8 ounces)
- White/Regular Sugar - 1/4 cup
- Refrigerated Piecrusts - 1/2(14.1-oz)
- Powdered Sugar - 1/2 cup (about 2-oz)
- Fresh Lemon Juice - 11/2 tsp
- Rainbow Candy Sprinkles - 1 tbsp(about 1/2 ounce)
- Cooking Spray

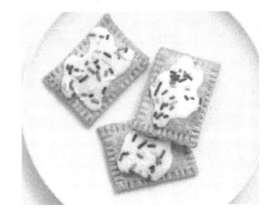

Method:

1. Mix strawberries & white sugar and stay for 15 minutes with periodically

stirring. Air fryer them for 10 minutes until glossy and reduced with constant stirring. Let it cool for 30 minutes.

2. Use the smooth floured surface to roll the pie crust and make 12-inches round shape. Cut the dough into 12 rectangles of (2 1/2- x 3-inch), re-rolling strips if necessary. Leaving a 1/2-inch boundary, add the spoon around 2 tea-spoons of strawberry mixture into the middle of 6 of dough rectangles. Brush the edges of the rectangles of the filled dough with water. Then, press the edges of rest dough rectangles with a fork to seal. Spray the tarts very well with cooking oil.

3. In an air fryer pot, put 3 tarts in a single layer and cook them at 350 ° F for 10 minutes till golden brown. With the rest of the tarts, repeat the process. Set aside for cooling for 30 minutes.

4. In a small cup, whip the powdered sugar & lemon juice together until it gets smooth. Glaze the spoon over the cooled tarts and sprinkle equally with candy.

40. Lighten up Empanadas in an Air Fryer

Ingredients:

- Lean Green Beef - 3 ounces
- Cremini Mushrooms - Chopped finely - 3 ounces
- White onion - Chopped finely - 1/4th cup
- Garlic – Chopped finely - 2 tsp.
- Pitted Green Olives - 6
- Olive Oil - 1 table-spoon
- Cumin - 1/4th tsp
- Cinnamon - 1/8th tsp
- Chopped tomatoes - 1/2 cup
- Paprika - 1/4 tea-spoon
- Large egg lightly Beaten - 1
- Square gyoza wrappers - 8

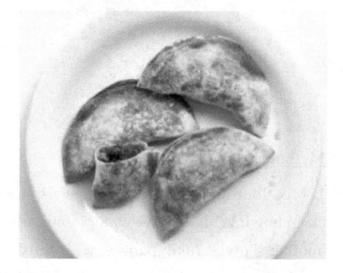

Method:

1. In a medium cooking pot, let heat oil on the medium/high temperature. Then, add beef & onion; for 3 minutes, cook them, mixing the crumble, until getting brown. Put the mushrooms; let them cook for 6 mins, till the mushrooms start to brown, stirring frequently. Add the paprika, olives, garlic, cinnamon, and cumin; cook for three minutes until the mushrooms are very tender and most of

the liquid has been released. Mix in the tomatoes and cook, turning periodically, for 1 minute. Put the filling in a bowl and let it cool for 5 minutes.

2. Arrange 4 wrappers of gyoza on a worktop. In each wrapper, put around 1 1/2 tablespoons of filling in the middle. Clean the edges of the egg wrappers; fold over the wrappers and pinch the edges to seal. Repeat with the remaining wrappers and filling process.

3. Place the 4 empanadas in one single layer in an air-fryer basket and cook for 7 minutes at 400 °F until browned well. Repeat with the empanadas that remain.

41. Air Fried Calzones

Ingredients:

- Spinach Leaves --> 3 ounces (about 3 cups)
- Shredded Chicken breast --> 2 ounces (about 1/3 cup)
- Fresh Whole Wheat Pizza Dough --> 6 ounces
- Shredded Mozzarella Cheese --> 11/2 ounces (about 6 tbsp)
- Low Sodium Marinara Sauce --> 1/3 cup

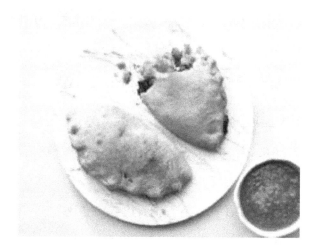

Method:

1. First of all, in a medium pan, let heat oil on medium/high temperature. Include onion & cook, continue mixing then well efficiently, for two min, till get soft. After that, add the spinach; then cover & cook it until softened. After that, take out the pan from the heat; mix the chicken & marinara sauce.

2. Divide the dough in to the four identical sections. Then, roll each section into a 6-inches circle on a gently floured surface. Place over half of each dough circular shape with one-fourth of the spinach mixture. Top with one-fourth of the cheese each. Fold the dough to make half-moons and over filling, tightening the edges to lock. Coat the calzones well with spray for cooking

3. In the basket of an air fryer, put the calzones and cook them at 325 ° F until the dough becomes nicely golden brown,

in 12 mins, changing the sides of the calzones after 8 mins.

42. Air Fried Mexican Style Corns

Ingredients:

- Unsalted Butter - 11/2 tbsp.
- Chopped Garlic -2 tsp
- Shucked Fresh Corns - 11/2 lb
- Fresh Chopped Cilantro - 2 tbsp.
- Lime zest - 1 tbsp.
- Lime Juice - 1 tsp
- Kosher Salt - 1/2 tsp
- Black Pepper - 1/2 tsp

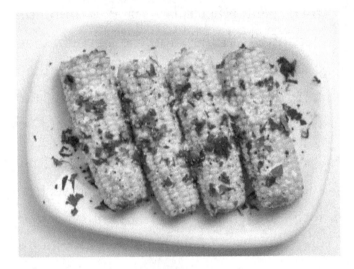

Method:

1. Coat the corn delicately with the cooking spray, and put the corn in the air fryer's basket in one single layer. Let it Cooking for 14 mins at 400 °F till tender then charred gently, changing the corn half the way via cooking.

2. In the meantime, whisk together all the garlic, lime juice, butter, & lime zest in the microwaveable pot. Let an air fryer on Fast, about 30 seconds, until the butter melts and the garlic is aromatic. Put the corn on the plate and drop the butter mixture on it. Using the salt, cilantro, and pepper to sprinkle. Instantly serve this delicious recipe.

43. Air Fryer Crunchy & Crispy Chocolate Bites

Ingredients:

- Frozen Shortcrust Pastry - Partially thawed -- 4
- Cinnamon for dusting -- as required
- Icing Sugar for dusting -- as required
- Mars Celebration Chocolates -- 24
- Whipped Cream - as required

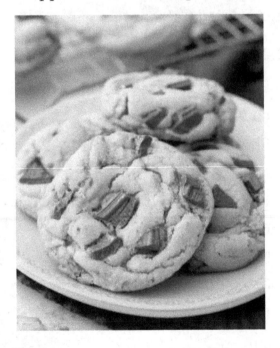

Method:

1. First of all, cut each pastry sheet into 6 equal rectangles. Brush the egg finely. In

the centre of each piece of the pastry, place one chocolate. Fold the pastry over to seal the chocolate. Trim the extra pastry, then press and lock the corners. Put it on a tray lined with baking sheet. Brush the tops with an egg. Use the mixture of cinnamon and sugar to sprinkle liberally.

2. In the air-fryer basket, put a layer of the baking paper, ensuring that the paper is 1 cm smaller than that of the basket to permit air to circulate well. Place the 6 pockets in basket, taking care that these pockets must not to overlap. Then, cook them for 8-9 mins at 190 ° C till they become golden and the pastry are prepared thoroughly. As the pockets cooked, transfer them into a dish. Repeat the process with the pockets that remain.

3. After taking out from the air fryer, dust the Icing sugar and at last with whipped cream. Serve them warm.

44. Doritos-Crumbled Chicken tenders in an Air fryer

Ingredients:

- Buttermilk -- 1 cup (about 250ml)
- Doritos Nacho Cheese Corn Chips -- 170g Packet
- Halved Crossways Chicken Tenderloins -- 500g
- Egg -- 1
- Plain Flour -- 50g
- Mild Salsa -- for serving

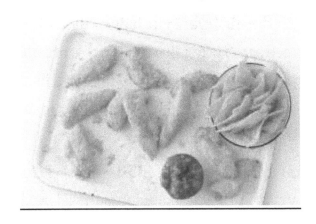

Method:

1.Take a ceramic bowl or glass and put the chicken in it. Then, c over the buttermilk with it. Wrap it and put it for 4 hours or may be overnight in the refrigerator to marinate.

2. Let Preheat an air fryer at 180C. Then, cover a Baking tray with grease-proof paper.

3. In a Chopper, add the corn chips then pulse them until the corn chips become coarsely chopped. Then, transfer the chopped chips to a dish. In a deep cup, put the egg and beat it. On another plate, put the flour.

4. Remove the unnecessary water from the chicken, and also discard the buttermilk. Then, dip the chicken in the flour mixture and wipe off the extra flour. After that, dip in the beaten egg and then into the chips of corn, press

it firmly to coat well. Transfer it to the tray that made ready to next step.

5. In the air fryer, put half of the chicken and then, fry for 8 to 10 mins until they are golden as well as cooked completely. Repeat the process with the chicken that remain.

Transfer the chicken in the serving dish. Enjoy this delicious recipe with salsa.

45. Air Fryer Ham & Cheese Croquettes

Ingredients:

- Chopped White Potatoes -- 1 kg
- Chopped Ham -- 100g
- Chopped Green Shallots -- 2
- Grated Cheddar Cheese -- 80g (about 1 cup)
- All-purpose flour -- 50g
- eggs -- 2
- Breadcrumbs -- 100g
- Lemon Slices -- for serving
- Tonkatsu Sause -- for serving

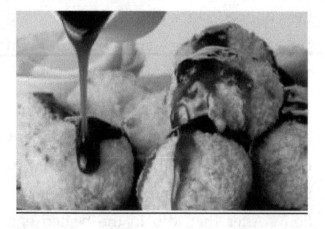

Method:

1. In a large-sized saucepan, put the potatoes. Cover with chill water. Carry it over high temperature to a boil. Boil till tender for 10 to 12 minutes. Drain thoroughly. Return over low heat to pan. Mix until it is smooth and has allowed to evaporate the certain water. Withdraw from the sun. Switch to a tub. Fully set aside to chill.

2. Then, add the shallot, Ham and cheese in the mashed potatoes also season with kosher salt. Mix it well. Take the 2 tablespoons of the mixture and make its balls. And repeat process for the rest of mixture.

3. Take the plain flour in a plate. Take another small bowl and beat the eggs. Take the third bowl and add the breadcrumbs in it. Toss the balls in the flour. Shake off the extra flour then in eggs and coat the breadcrumbs well. Make the balls ready for frying. Take all the coated balls in the fridge for about 15 minutes.

4. Preheat an air fryer at 200 ° C. Then, cook the croquettes for 8 to10 mints until they become nicely golden, in two rounds. Sprinkle the tonkatsu sauce and serve the croquettes with lemon slices.

46. Air Fryer Lemonade Scones

Ingredients:

- Self-raising flour -- 525g (about 3 1/2 cups)
- Thickened Cream -- 300ml
- Lemonade -- 185ml (about 3/4 cup)
- Caster Sugar -- 70g (1/3 cup)
- Vanilla Essence -- 1 tsp
- Milk -- for brushing
- Raspberry Jam -- for serving
- Whipped Cream -- for serving

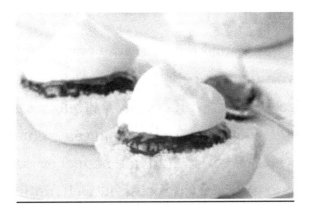

Method:

1. In a large-sized bowl, add the flour and sugar together. Mix it well. Add lemonade, vanilla and cream. In a big bowl, add the flour and sugar. Just make a well. Remove milk, vanilla and lemonade. Mix finely, by using a plain knife, till the dough comes at once.

2. Take out the dough on the flat surface and sprinkle the dry flour on the dough. Knead it gently for about 30 secs until the dough get smooth. On a floured surface, roll out the dough. Politely knead for thirty seconds, until it is just smooth. Form the dough into a round shape about 2.5 cm thick. Toss around 5.5 cm blade into the flour. Cut the scones out. Push the bits of remaining dough at once gently and repeat the process to make Sixteen scones.

3. In the air fryer bucket, put a layer of baking paper, ensuring that the paper is 1 cm shorter than the bucket to allow air to flow uniformly. Put 5 to 6 scones on paper in the bucket, even hitting them. Finely brush the surfaces with milk. Let cook them for about 15 mins at 160 ° C or when they tapped on the top, until become golden and empty-sounding. Move it safely to a wire or cooling rack. Repeat the same process with the rest of scones and milk two more times.

4. Serve the lemonade scones warm with raspberry jam & whipped cream.

47. Air Fryer Baked Potatoes

Ingredients:

- Baby Potatoes -- Halved shape -- 650g
- Fresh rosemary sprigs-- 2 large
- Sour Cream -- for serving
- Sweet Chilli Sauce -- for serving
- Salt -- for seasoning

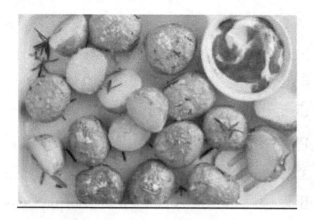

Method:

1. Firstly, at 180C, pre-heat the air fryer. In an air fryer, put the rosemary sprigs & baby potatoes. Use oil for spray and salt for seasoning. Then, cook them for fifteen min until become crispy and cooked completely, also turning partially.

2. Serve the baked potatoes sweet chilli Sause & sour cream to enhance its flavour.

48. Air Fryer Mozzarella Chips

Ingredients:

- All-purpose flour -- 1 tbsp
- Breadcrumbs -- 2/3 cup
- Garlic Powder -- 3 tbsp
- Lemon Juice -- 1/3 cup
- Avocado -- 1
- Basil Pesto -- 2 tbsp
- Plain Yogurt -- 1/4 cup
- Chopped Green Onion --1
- Cornflakes crumbs -- 1/4 cup
- Mozzarella block -- 550g

- Eggs – 2
- Olive Oil for spray

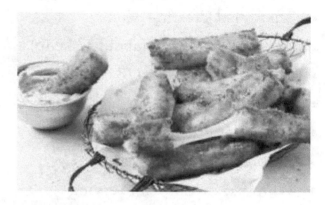

Method:

1. Start making Creamy and fluffy Avocado Dipped Sauce: In a small-sized food processor, put the yogurt, avocado, lemon juice, onion, and pesto. Also add the pepper & salt, blend properly. Process it well until it get mixed and smooth. Switch the batter to a bowl. Cover it. Place in the fridge, until It required.

2. Take a large-sized tray and place a baking sheet. In a large bowl, add the garlic powder & plain flour together. Also add the salt and season well. Take another medium bowl, whisk the eggs. Mix the breadcrumbs well in bowl.

3. Make the 2 cm thick wedges of mozzarella, then put them into the sticks. For coating, roll the cheese in the flour. Shake off the extra flour. Then, coat the sticks in the egg fusion, then in the breadcrumbs, operating in

rounds. Place the prepared plate on it. Freeze till solid, or even for around 1 hour.

4. Spray the oil on the mozzarella lightly. Wrap the air fryer bucket with baking sheet, leaving an edge of 1 cm to enable air to flow. Then, cook at 180C, for 4 to 4 1/2 mins until the sticks become crispy & golden. Serve warm with sauce to dip.

49. Air Fryer Fetta Nuggets

Ingredients:

- All-purpose flour -- 1 tbsp.
- Chilli flakes -- 1 tsp
- Onion powder -- 1 tsp
- Sesame Seeds -- 1/4 cup
- Fetta Cheese Cubes -- Cut in 2 cm 180g
- Fresh Chives -- for serving
- Breadcrumbs -- 1/4 cup

BARBECUE SAUSE:

- apple cider -- 11/2 tsp
- Chilli Flakes -- 1/2 tsp
- Barbecue Sause -- 1//4 cup

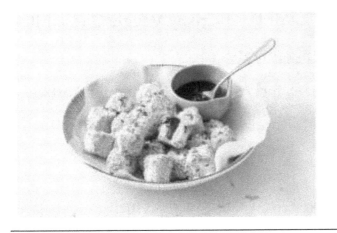

Method:

1. Mix the onion powder, flour and chilli flakes in a medium-sized bowl. Use pepper for seasoning. Take another bowl, and beat an egg. Take one more bowl and mix sesame seeds and breadcrumbs. Then, toss the fetta in the chilli flakes, onion powder & flour mixture. Dip the fetta in egg, and toss again in breadcrumbs fusion. Put them on a plate.

2. Pre- heat the air fryer at 180 °C. Put the cubes of fetta in a baking tray, in the basket of the air fryer. cook till fetta cubes become golden, or may be for 6 mins.

3. In the meantime, mix all the wet ingredients and create the Barbecue sauce.

4. Sprinkle the chives on the fetta and serve with Barbecue Sause.

50. Air Fryer Japanese Chicken Tender

Ingredients:

- McCormick Katsu Crumb for seasoning -- 25g
- Pickled Ginger -- 1 tbsp.
- Japanese-Style Mayonnaise -- 1/3 cup
- Chicken Tenderloins -- 500g
- Oil for spray

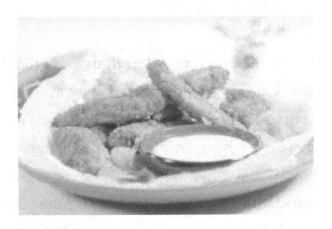

Method:

1. Put the chicken on tray in the form of single layer. Sprinkle the half seasoning on chicken. Then, turn chicken and sprinkle the seasoning again evenly. Use oil for spray on it.

2. Pre-heat at 180°C, an air fryer. Let the chicken cooking for about 12 - 14 mins until it becomes golden & cooked completely.

3. In the meantime, take a small-sized bowl, mix the mayonnaise and the remaining pickling sauce.

4. Serve the chicken with white sauce and put the ginger on the side, in a platter.

51. Whole-Wheat Pizzas in an Air Fryer

Ingredients:

- Low-sodium Marinara Sauce -- 1/4 cup
- Spinach leaves -- 1 cup
- Pita Breads -- 2

- Shredded Mozzarella Cheese -- 1/4 cup
- Parmigiano- Reggiano Cheese -- 1/4 ounces (about 1 tbsp.)
- Tomato slices -- 8
- Sliced Garlic Clove -- 1

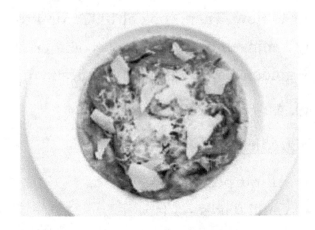

Method:

1. Spread the marinara sauce on 1 side of each pita bread uniformly. Cover the cheese spinach leaves, tomato slices and garlic, with half of each of these.

2. Put one pita bread in an air fryer pot, then cook it at 350°F till the cheese becomes melted and pita becomes crispy, 4 - 5 mins. Repeat the process with the pita leftover.

52. Air Fryer Crispy Veggie Quesadillas

Ingredients:

- 6 inches Whole Grain Flour Tortillas - - 4
- Full fat Cheddar Cheese -- 4 ounces (about 1 cup)
- Sliced Zucchini -- 1 cup

- Lime Zest -- 1 tbsp.
- Lime Juice -- 1 tsp.
- Fresh Cilantro -- 2 tbsp.
- Chopped Red Bell Pepper -- (about 1 cup)
- Cumin -- 1/4 tsp.
- Low-fat Yoghurt -- 2 ounces
- Refrigerated Pico de Gallo -- 1/2 cup
- Oil for spray

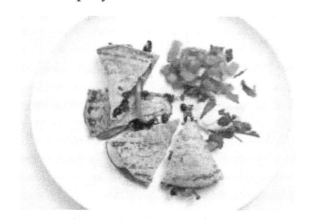

Method:

1. Put tortillas on the surface of the work. Sprinkle onto half of each tortilla with 2 tbsp. of grated cheese. Cover each tortilla with 1/4 cup of chopped red bell pepper, zucchini chunks & the black beans on the top of the cheese. Sprinkle finely with 1/2 cup of cheese left. Fold over the tortillas to create quesadillas form like half-moons. Coat the quesadillas slightly with a cooking spray, & lock them with match picks or toothpicks.

2. Lightly brush a bucket of air fryer with cooking oil spray. Place 2 quesadillas carefully in the basket. Cook at 400°F till the tortillas become golden brown & gently crispy. Melt the cheese & gradually tender the vegetables for ten mins, tossing the quesadillas partially throughout the cooking period. Repeat the process with leftover quesadillas.

3. Mix together lime zest, yogurt, cumin, & lime juice, in a small-sized bowl since the quesadillas getting prepare. Break each quesadilla in-to the pieces to serve and then sprinkle the coriander. With one tbsp. of cumin cream and two tablespoons of pico de gallo, and serve each.

53. Air Fried Curry Chickpeas

Ingredients:

- Drained & Rinsed Un-Salted Chickpeas -- 11/2 cups (15-oz.)
- Olive Oil -- 2 tbsp.
- Curry Powder -- 2 tsp.
- Coriander -- 1/4 tsp.
- Cumin -- 1/4 tsp.
- Cinnamon -- 1/4 tsp.
- Turmeric -- 1/2 tsp.
- Aleppo Pepper -- 1/2 tsp.
- Red Wine Vinegar -- 2 tbsp.
- Kosher Salt -- 1/4 tsp.
- Sliced Fresh Cilantro -- as required

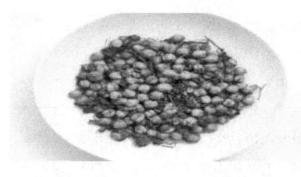 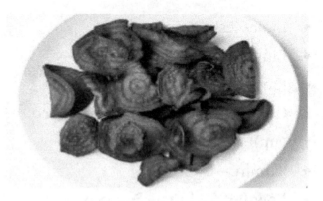

Method:

1. Break the chickpeas lightly in a medium-sized bowl with your hands (don't crush them); and then remove the skins of chickpea.

2. Add oil & vinegar to the chickpeas, and stir to coat. Then, add curry powder, turmeric, coriander, cumin, & cinnamon; mix gently to combine them.

3. In the air fryer bucket, put the chickpeas in one single layer & cook at 400°F temperature until becoming crispy, for about 15 min, stirring the chickpeas periodically throughout the cooking process.

4. Place the chickpeas in a dish. Sprinkle the salt, cilantro and Aleppo pepper on chickpeas; and cover it.

54. Air Fried Beet Chips

Ingredients:

- Canola Oil -- 1 tsp.
- Medium-sized Red Beets -- 3
- Black Pepper -- 1/4 tsp.
- Kosher Salt -- 3/4 tsp.

Method:

1. Cut and Peel the red beets. Make sure each beet cutted into 1/8-inch-thick slices. Take a large-sized bowl and toss the beets slices, pepper, salt and oil well.

2. Put half beets in air fryer bucket and then cook at the 320°F temperature about 25 - 30 mins or until they become crispy and dry. Flip the bucket about every 5 mins. Repeat the process for the beets that remain.

55. Double-Glazed Air Fried Cinnamon Biscuits

Ingredients:

- Cinnamon -- 1/4 tsp.
- Plain Flour -- 2/3 cup (about 27/8 oz.)
- Whole-Wheat Flour -- 2/3 cup (about22/3 oz.)
- Baking Powder -- 1 tsp.
- White Sugar -- 2 tbsp.
- Kosher Salt -- 1/4 tsp.
- Chill Salted Butter -- 4 tbsp.
- Powdered Sugar -- 2 cups (about 8-oz.)

- Water -- 3 tbsp.
- Whole Milk -- 1/3 cup
- Oil for spray -- as required

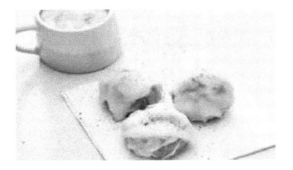

Method:

1. In a medium-sized bowl, stir together salt, plain flour, baking powder, white sugar cinnamon and butter. Use two knives or pastry cutter to cut mixture till butter becomes well mixed with the flour and the mixture seems to as coarse cornmeal. Add the milk, then mix well until the dough becomes a ball. Place the dough on a floury surface and knead for around 30 seconds until the dough becomes smooth. Break the dough into 16 identical parts. Roll each part carefully into a plain ball.

2. Coat the air fryer pot well with oil spray. Put 8 balls in the pot, by leaving the space between each one; spray with cooking oil. Cook them until get browned & puffed, for 10 - 12 mins at 350°F temperature. Take out the doughnut balls from the pot carefully and put them on a cooling rack having

foil for five mins. Repeat the process with the doughnut balls that remain.

3. In a medium pot, mix water and powdered sugar together until smooth. Then, spoon half of the glaze carefully over the doughnut balls. Cool for five mins and let it glaze once and enabling to drip off extra glaze.

56. Lemon Drizzle Cake in an Air Fryer

Ingredients:

- Grated Lemon rind -- 2 tsp.
- Cardamom -- 1 tsp.
- Softened Butter -- 150g
- Eggs -- 3
- Honey-flavoured Yoghurt -- 3/4 cup
- Self-raising flour -- 11/2 cups
- Caster Sugar -- 2/3 cup (150g)
- Lemon Zest -- for serving

LEMON ICING:

- Icing Sugar -- 1 cup
- Lemon Juice -- 11/2 tbsps.
- Softened Butter -- 10g

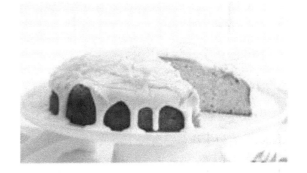

Method:

1. First, grease a 20 cm cake baking pan of round shape having butter paper. Take an electric beater and beat cardamom, sugar, lemon rind, and butter until the mixture becomes smooth & pale. Then, add the eggs one by one and beat well. Put the eggs in the flour and yoghurt. Fold by spatula and make the surface very smooth.

2. Pre-heat the air fryer at 180 C temperature. Put the pan in air fryer's pot. Bake it for about 35 mins. Check it by putting skewer in it that comes out clean without any sticky batter. Reserve it in the pan for 5 minutes to become cool before shifting it to a cooling rack.

3. Make the lemon glaze, add butter and icing sugar in a bowl. By adding lemon juice as required and form a smooth paste.

4. Put the cake on a plate to serve. Sprinkle the lemon zest and lemon icing to serve.

57. Air Fryer dukkah-Crumbed chicken

Ingredients:

- Chicken Thigh Fillets -- 8
- Herb or dukkah -- 45g packet
- Plain Flour -- 1/3 cup (about 50g)
- Kaleslaw kit -- 350g Packet
- Breadcrumbs -- 1 cup (about 80g)

- Eggs -- 2

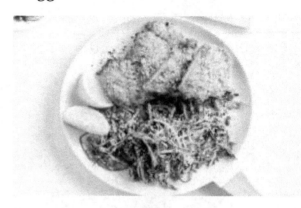

Method:

1. Put half of the chicken within 2 sheets of cling paper. Gently beat until it remains 2 cm thick by using a meat hammer or rolling pin. Repeat the process with the chicken that remains.

2. In a deep bowl, mix breadcrumbs and dukkah together. Beat an egg in medium bowl., Put the flour and all the seasoning on a tray. Coat chicken pieces one by one in the flour and shake off the extra. Dip chicken pieces into the egg, then in breadcrumbs for coating. Move them to a dish. Cover them with the plastic wrapper & leave it to marinate for 30 mins in the fridge.

3. Pre-heat air fryer at 200°C temperature. Use olive oil to spray the chicken pieces. Put half of the chicken in one single layer in the air fryer pot. Cook them for about 16 mins and turning partially until they become golden & get cooked completely. Move to a plate &

wrap them with foil to stay warm. Repeat the process with the chicken pieces that remains.

4. After that, place the kaleslaw kit in a serving bowl by following instructions mentioned in the packets.

5. Divide the prepared chicken & the kaleslaw between serving platters, and season it.

58. Air Fryer Vietnamese-style spring roll salad

Ingredients:

- Rice Noodles -- 340g
- Crushed Garlic -- 1 clove
- Grated Ginger -- 2 tsp.
- Pork Mince -- 250g
- Lemongrass paste -- 1 tsp
- Cutted into matchsticks the Peeled Carrots -- 2
- Sliced Spring onion -- 3
- Fish sauce -- 2 tsp.
- Spring roll pastries -- 10 sheets
- Coriander -- 1/2 cup
- Sliced Red Chilli - 1 long
- Vietnamese-style Salad -- for dressing
- Mint Leaves -- 1/2
- Bean Sprouts -- 1 cup

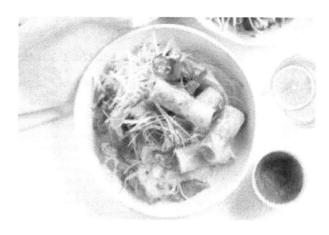

Method:

1. Take a large-sized saucepan and cook the noodles for about 4 mins until get soft. Take the cold water and discharge thoroughly. Cutting 1 cup of the boiled noodles into the short lengths, with the leftover noodles reserved.

2. Take a large-sized bowl, add the mince, lemongrass, ginger, garlic, half carrot, spring onion, and fish sauce together and mix them well.

3. On a clean surface, put one pastry paper. Add two tablespoons across 1 side of the mince fusion diagonally. With just a little spray, brush its opposite side. Fold and roll on the sides to completely cover the mince filling. Repeat the process with the sheets of pastry and fill the thin layer of mince mixture, that remain.

4. Pre-heat at 200°C, an air fryer. Use olive oil, spray on the spring rolls. Put in

the bucket of air fryer and cook the spring rolls for fifteen mins until cooked completely. Change the sides half-way during cooking.

5. After that, equally split reserved noodles in the serving bowls. Place coriander, bean sprouts, mint and the remaining spring onion and carrots at the top of the serving bowl.

6. Then, break the spring rolls in the half and place them over the mixture of noodles. Sprinkle the chili and serve with Vietnamese-style salad dressing according to your taste.

59. Air Fryer Pizza Pockets

Ingredients:

- Olive oil - 2 tsp.
- Sliced Mushrooms - 6 (about 100g)
- Chopped Leg Ham - 50g
- Crumbled Fetta - 80g
- White Wraps - 4
- Basil Leaves - 1/4 cup
- Baby Spinach - 120g
- Tomato Paste - 1/3 cup
- Chopped Red Capsicum - 1/2
- Dried Oregano - 1/2 tsp
- Olive oil - for spray
- Green Salad - for serving

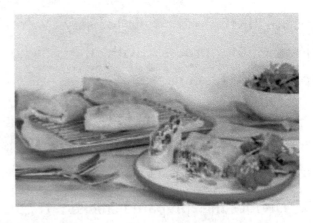

Method:

1. Heat oil on medium temperature in an air fryer. Cook capsicum for about five minutes until it starts to soften. Add mushrooms and cook them for another five mins until mushrooms become golden and evaporating any water left in the pan. Move mushrooms to another bowl. Leave them to cool for 10 mins.

2. Take a heatproof bowl and put spinach in it. Cover it with boiling water. Wait for 1 min until slightly wilted. Drain water and leave it to cool for about 10 mins.

3. Excessive spinach moisture is squeezed and applied to the capsicum mixture. Add the oregano, basil, ham and fetta. Season it with both salt & pepper. Mix it well to combine properly.

4. Put one wrapper on the smooth surface. Add 1 tbsp of tomato paste to the middle of the wrap. Cover it with a

combination of 1-quarter of the capsicum. Roll up the wrap to completely enclose the filling, give it as the shape of parcel and folding the sides. To build four parcels, repeat the procedure with the remaining wraps, mixture of capsicum & tomato paste. Use oil spray on the tops.

5. Pre-heat the air fryer at 180 C temperature. Cook the parcels for 6 - 8 mins until they become golden & crispy, take out them and move to 2 more batches. Serve along with the salad.

60. Air Fryer Popcorn Fetta with Maple Hot Sauce

Ingredients:

- Marinated Fetta cubes - 265g
- Cajun for seasoning - 2 tsp.
- Breadcrumbs - 2/3 cups
- Corn flour - 2 tbsp.
- Egg - 1
- Chopped Fresh Coriander - 1 tbsp.
- Coriander leaves - for serving

Maple hot sauce:

- Maple syrup - 2 tbsp.
- Sriracha - 1 tbsps.

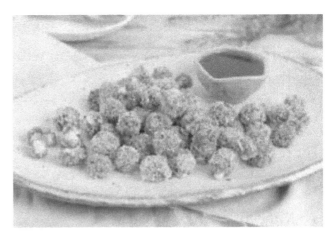

Method:

1. Drain the fetta, then reserve 1 tbsp of oil making sauce.

2. Take a bowl, mix the cornflour and the Cajun seasoning together. Beat the egg in another bowl. Take one more bowl and combine the breadcrumbs & cilantro in it. Season it with salt & pepper. Work in batches, coat the fetta in cornflour mixture, then dip in the egg. After that, toss them in breadcrumb mixture for coating. Place them on the plate and freeze them for one hour.

3. Take a saucepan, add Sriracha, reserved oil and maple syrup together and put on medium low heat. Stir it for 3 - 4 minutes continuously until sauce get start to thicken. Then, remove the maple sauce from heat.

4. Pre-heat the air fryer at 180C. Place the cubes of fetta in a single layer in the air fryer's pot. Cook them for 3 - 4 mins until just staring softened, and fettas

become golden. Sprinkled with extra coriander leaves and serve them with the maple hot sauce.

61. Air fryer Steak Fajitas

Ingredients:

- Chopped tomatoes - 2 large
- Minced Jalapeno pepper - 1
- Cumin - 2 tsp.
- Lime juice - 1/4 cup
- Fresh minced Cilantro - 3 tbsp.
- Diced Red Onion - 1/2 cup
- 8-inches long Whole-wheat tortillas - 6
- Large onion - 1 sliced
- Salt - 3/4 tsp divided
- Beef steak - 1

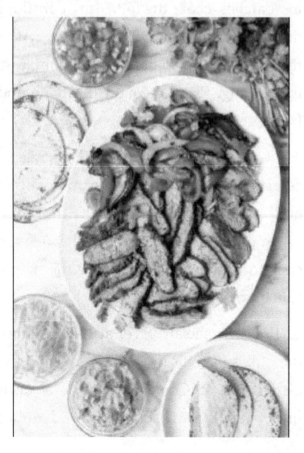

Method:

1. Mix first 5 ingredients in a clean bowl then stir in cumin and salt. Let it stand till before you serve.

2. Pre-heat the air fryer at 400 degrees. Sprinkle the cumin and salt with the steak that remain. Place them on buttered air-fryer pot and cook the steak until the meat reaches the appropriate thickness (a thermometer should read 135 ° for medium-rare; 140 °; moderate, 145 °), for 6 to 8 mins per side. Remove from the air fryer and leave for five min to stand.

3. Then, put the onion in the air-fryer pot. Cook it until get crispy-tender, stirring once for 2 - 3 mins. Thinly slice the steak and serve with onion & salsa in the tortillas. Serve it with avocado & lime slices if needed.

62. Air-Fryer Fajita-Stuffed Chicken

Ingredients:

- Boneless Chicken breast - 4
- Finely Sliced Onion - 1 small
- Finely Sliced Green pepper - 1/2 medium-sized
- Olive oil - 1 tbsp.
- Salt - 1/2 tsp.
- Chilli Powder - 1 tbsp.
- Cheddar Cheese - 4 ounces

- Cumin - 1 tsp.
- Salsa or jalapeno slices - optional

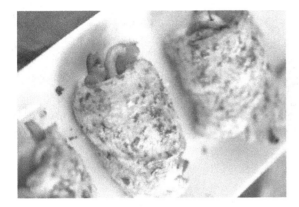

Method:

1. Pre-heat the air fryer at the 375 degrees. In the widest part of every chicken breast, cut a gap horizontally. Fill it with green pepper and onion. Combine olive oil and the seasonings in a clean bowl and apply over the chicken.

2. Place the chicken on a greased dish in the form of batches in an air-fryer pot. Cook it for 6 minutes. Stuff the chicken with cheese slices and secure the chicken pieces with toothpicks. Cook at 165° until for 6 to 8 minutes. Take off the toothpicks. Serve the delicious chicken with toppings of your choosing, if wanted.

63. Nashvilla Hot Chicken in an Air Fryer

Ingredients:

- Chicken Tenderloins - 2 pounds
- Plain flour - 1 cup
- Hot pepper Sauce - 2 tbsp.
- Egg - 1 large
- Salt - 1 tsp.
- Pepper - 1/2 tsp.
- Buttermilk - 1/2 cup
- Cayenne Pepper - 2 tbsp.
- Chilli powder - 1 tsp.
- Pickle Juice - 2 tbsp.
- Garlic Powder - 1/2 tsp.
- Paprika - 1 tsp.
- Brown Sugar - 2 tbsp.
- Olive oil - 1/2 cup
- Cooling oil for spray

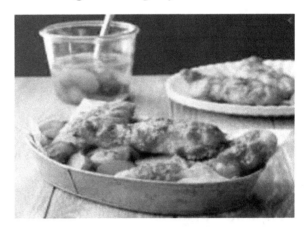

Method:

1. Combine pickle juice, hot sauce and salt in a clean bowl and coat the chicken on its both sides. Put it in the fridge, cover it, for a minimum 1 hour. Throwing away some marinade.

2. Pre-heat the air fryer at 375 degrees. Mix the flour, the remaining salt and the pepper in another bowl. Whisk together the buttermilk, eggs, pickle juice and hot

sauce well. For coating the both sides, dip the chicken in plain flour; drip off the excess. Dip chicken in egg mixture and then again dip in flour mixture.

3. Arrange the single layer of chicken on a greased air-fryer pot and spray with cooking oil. Cook for 5 to 6 minutes until it becomes golden brown. Turn and spray well. Again, cook it until golden brown, for more 5-6 minutes.

4. Mix oil, brown sugar, cayenne pepper and seasonings together. Then, pour on the hot chicken and toss to cover. Serve the hot chicken with pickles.

64. Southern-style Chicken

Ingredients:

- Crushed Crackers - 2 cups (about 50)
- Fresh minced parsley - 1 tbsp.
- Paprika - 1 tsp.
- Pepper - 1/2 tsp.
- Garlic salt - 1 tsp.
- Fryer Chicken - 1
- Cumin - 1/4 tsp.
- Egg - 1
- Cooking Oil for spray

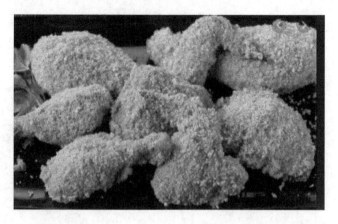

Method:

1. Set the temperature of an air fryer at 375 degrees. Mix the first 7 ingredients in a deep bowl. Beat an egg in deep bowl. Soak the chicken in egg, then pat in the cracker mixture for proper coat. Place the chicken in a single layer on the greased air-fryer pot and spray with cooking oil.

2. Cook it for 10 minutes. Change the sides of chicken and squirt with cooking oil spray. Cook until the chicken becomes golden brown & juices seem to be clear, for 10 - 20 minutes longer.

65. Chicken Parmesan in an Air Fryer

Ingredients:

- Breadcrumbs - 1/2 cup
- Pepper - 1/4 tsp.
- Pasta Sauce - 1 cup
- Boneless Chicken breast - 4
- Mozzarella Cheese - 1 cup
- Parmesan Cheese - 1/3 cup
- Large Eggs - 2

- Fresh basil - Optional

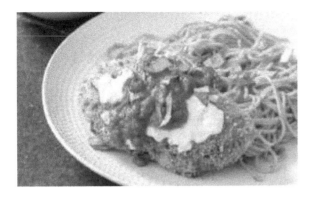

Method:

1. Set the temperature of an air-fryer at 375 degrees. In a deep bowl, beat the eggs gently. Combine the breadcrumbs, pepper and parmesan cheese in another bowl. Dip the chicken in beaten egg and coat the chicken parmesan with breadcrumbs mixture.

2. In an air-fryer pot, put the chicken in single layer. Cook the chicken for 10 to 12 mins with changing the sides partially. Cover the chicken with cheese and sauce. Cook it for 3 to 4 minutes until cheese has melted. Then, sprinkle with basil leaves and serve.

66. Lemon Chicken Thigh in an Air Fryer

Ingredients:

- Bone-in Chicken thighs- 4
- Pepper - 1/8 tsp.
- Salt - 1/8 tsp.
- Pasta Sauce - 1 cup
- Lemon Juice - 1 tbsp.

- Lemon Zest - 1 tsp.
- Minced Garlic - 3 cloves
- Butter - 1/4 cup
- Dried or Fresh Rosemary - 1 tsp.
- Dried or Fresh Thyme - 1/4 tsp.

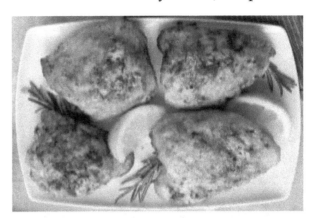

Method:

1. Pre-heat the air fryer at 400 degrees. Combine the butter, thyme, rosemary, garlic, lemon juice & zest in a clean bowl. Spread a mixture on each of the thigh's skin. Use salt and pepper to sprinkle.

2. Place the chicken, then side up the skin, in a greased air-fryer pot. Cook for 20 mins and flip once. Switch the chicken again (side up the skin) and cook it for about 5 mins until the thermometer will read 170 degrees to 175 degrees. Then, place in the serving plate and serve it.

67. Salmon with Maple-Dijon Glaze in air fryer

Ingredients:

- Salmon Fillets - 4 (about ounces)
- Salt - 1/4 tsp.
- Pepper - 1/4 tsp.
- Butter - 3 tbsp.
- Mustard - 1 tbsp.
- Lemon Juice - 1 medium-sized
- Garlic clove - 1 minced
- Olive oil

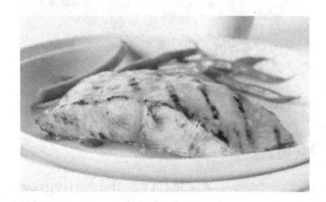

Method:

1. Pre-heat the air fryer at 400 degrees. Melt butter in a medium-sized pan on medium temperature. Put the mustard, minced garlic, maple syrup & lemon juice. Lower the heat and cook for 2 - 3 minutes before the mixture thickens significantly. Take off from the heat and set aside for few mins.

2. Brush the salmon with olive oil and also sprinkle the salt and pepper on it.

3. In an air fryer bucket, put the fish in a single baking sheet. Cook for 5 to 7 mins until fish is browned and easy to flake rapidly with help of fork. Sprinkle before to serve the salmon with sauce.

68. Air Fryer Roasted Beans

Ingredients:

- Fresh Sliced Mushrooms - 1/2 pounds
- Green Beans cut into 2-inch wedges - 1 pound
- Italian Seasoning - 1 tsp.
- Pepper - 1/8 tsp.
- Salt - 1/4 tsp.
- Red onion - 1 small
- Olive oil - 2 tbsp.

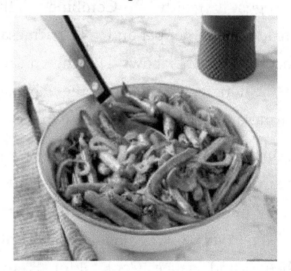

Method:

1. Pre-heat the air fryer at 375 degrees. Merge all of the ingredients in the large-sized bowl by tossing.

2. Assemble the vegetables on the greased air-fryer pot. Cook for 8 -10 minutes until become tender. Redistribute by tossing and cook for 8-10 minutes until they get browned.

69. Air Fried Radishes

Ingredients:

- Quartered Radishes - (about 6 cups)
- Fresh Oregano - 1 tbsp.
- Dried Oregano - 1 tbsp.
- Pepper - 1/8 tsp.
- Salt - 1/4 tsp.
- Olive Oil - 3 tbsp.

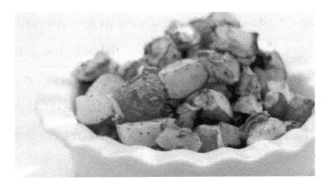

Method:

1. Set the temperature of an air fryer to 375 degrees. Mix the rest of the ingredients with radishes. In an air-fryer pot, put the radishes on greased dish.

2. Cook them for 12-15 minutes until they become crispy & tender with periodically stirring. Take out from the air fryer and serve the radishes in a clean dish.

70. Air Fried Catfish Nuggets

Ingredients

- Catfish fillets (1 inch) - 1 pound
- Seasoned fish fry coating - 3/4 cup
- Cooking oil - to spray

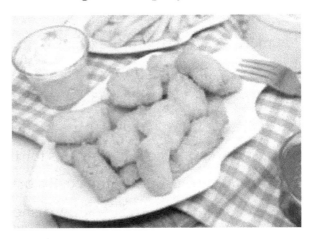

Method

1. Set the temperature of an air fryer to 200C.

2. Coat catfish pieces with seasoned coating mix by proper mixing from all sides.

3. Place nuggets evenly in an oiled air fryer pot. Spray both sides of nuggets with cooking oil. You can work in batches if the size of your air fryer is small.

4. Air fry nuggets for 5-8 minutes. Change sides of nuggets with the help of tongs and cook for more 5 minutes. Shift these delicious nuggets in a clean plate and serve immediately.

CONCLUSION:

This manual served you the easiest, quick, healthy and delicious foods that are made in an air fryer. It is also very necessary to cook food easily and timely without getting so much tired. We've discussed all the 70 easy, short, quick, delicious and healthy foods and dishes. These recipes can be made within few minutes. This manual provides the handiest or helpful cooking recipes for the busy people who are performing their routine tasks. Instead of ordering the costly or unhealthy food from hotels, you will be able to make the easy, tasty and healthy dishes with minimum cost. By reading this the most informative handbook, you can learn, experience or make lots of recipes in an air with great taste because cooking food traditionally on the stove is quite difficult for the professional persons. With the help of an air fryer, you can make various dishes for a single person as well as the entire family timely and effortlessly. We conclude that this cook book will maintain your health and it would also be the source of enjoying dishes without doing great effort in less and budget.

The Healthy Air Fryer Cookbook with Pictures

By Mark Machino

Table of Contents:

Introduction

An air fryer is a little kitchen appliance which imitates the outcomes of deep frying foods with the excess grease. As opposed to submerging food in order to fry it, the more food is put within the fryer together with a rather tiny quantity of oil. The food is subsequently "fried" having just hot air cooking. Food is cooked fast Because of the high heat and, because of the small quantity of oil onto the exterior of the meals, the outside will be emptied, like it was fried!

So, here we have discussed 70 best and healthy recipes for you that you can try at home and enjoy cooking using an air fryer.

Chapter 1: Air fryer Basics and 20 Recipes

Type of air fryer:

There're some air fryers that are over $300 and the one I used was less than a hundred. I didn't want you to splurge on the expensive one immediately because I was like what if I don't even use this thing? I want you to know that I'm going to use it first so I bought this for less than $100. This one is perfectly fine. It's big, it cooks a lot and it works just as good if not better than the more expensive models.

I'm going to bring you many air fryer recipes that are super easy. Even though it takes up quite a bit of counter space, it does a good job getting things crispy and delicious. Let's start with four recipes i.e. Bacon, Brussels sprouts, chicken wings and chicken breasts. So, let's get started.

1. Air fryer Bacon Recipe

I'm going to use four slices of bacon and I'm going to cut them in half on the cutting board.

So, here's the air fryer that I have:

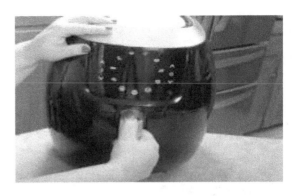

It is a 5.7 quart which is a pretty large air fryer. You take out the drawer and then we're going to lay the bacon inside of the air fryer, as it all fits. You want it to be a single layer so that they get evenly cooked. We're going to put this back in so we set the temperature for 350 degrees and they will cook for about nine minutes. We will also check them a couple of times just to make sure they're not getting too overdone. That's all there is to it, so our air fryer bacon is already and let's pull it out.

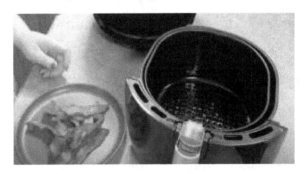

If you wanted it a little crispy, you could leave it in for probably just one more minute but I like it like this.

2. Air Fryer Apple Pie Chips

Let us be honest: If you are craving super-crispy, crunchy apple chips, then baking them in the oven is not good for you. The air fryer, on the other hand, is best.

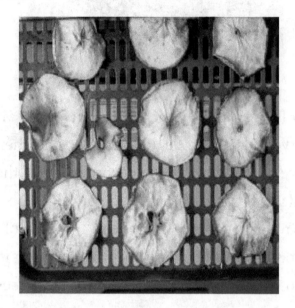

You'll begin by slicing an apple (any variety will probably work, although a red apple generates extra-pretty processors), and in case you've got a mandolin, utilize it as the thinner the slice, the crispier the processor. Toss the pieces with cinnamon and nutmeg, put an even coating into a preheated air fryer, coat with cooking spray, and stir fry until golden. You will have a tasty snack in under 10 minutes. For maximum crunchiness, let cool completely before eating.

Ingredients

- Moderate red apple
- 1/4 tsp ground nutmeg
- 1/2 tsp ground cinnamon

- Cooking spray

Instructions

❑ Thinly slice the apple into 1/8-inch-thick slices using a knife or rather on a mandoline.

❑ Toss the apple slices with 1/2 teaspoon ground cinnamon along with 1/4 teaspoon ground nutmeg.

❑ Preheat in an air fryer into 375°F and place for 17 minutes. Coat the fryer basket with cooking spray. Put just one layer of apple pieces into a basket and then spray with cooking spray.

❑ Air fry until golden-brown, rotating the trays halfway through to keep the apples at level, about 7 minutes total.

❑ Allow the chips to cool entirely too crisp.

❑ Repeat with the air fryer for the remaining apple pieces.

3. **Air-fryer Chicken Wings**

We will get started on the chicken wings.

Ingredients:

- 12 Chicken wings
- Salt
- Pepper

Method:

I'm going to put them in the air fryer basket and then I'm going to season them with salt and pepper. I've got these all in a single layer and they're kind of snug in there which is fine because they're going to shrink as they cook.

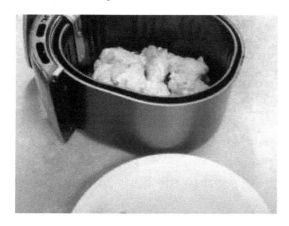

I put in about 12 chicken wings fit in my air fryer basket and now we're going to cook them for 25 minutes at 380 degrees. What that's going to do is it really get them cooked and then we're going to bump up the temperature and we will get them crispy. The first cook on our wings is done and now we are going to put it back in the air fryer at 400 degrees for about three to five minutes to get them nice and crispy. With this recipe and most air fryer recipes, whenever you're cooking things for longer than I would say five minutes, you may want to pull the basket out and shake what's inside. It is to make sure that it gets evenly cooked and I like to do that about every five minutes. Our wings are done. Look at how good they look in there nice and crispy.

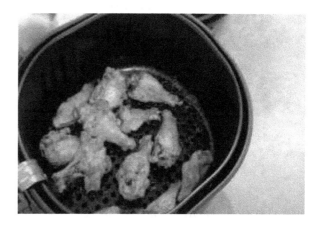

This took about three minutes as I didn't have to do the full five minutes for these.

4. **Air Fryer Mini Breakfast Burritos**

All these air-fried miniature burritos are fantastic to get a catch's go breakfast or perhaps to get a midday snack. Leave the serrano Chile pepper for a spicy version.

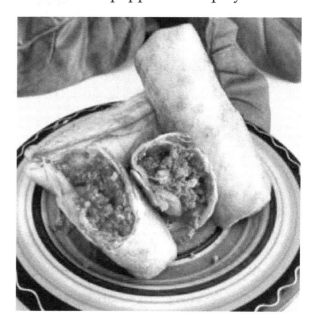

Ingredients

- 1 tablespoon bacon grease

- 1/4 cup Mexican-style chorizo
- 2 tbsp. sliced onion
- 1 serrano pepper, chopped
- salt and ground black pepper to taste
- 4 (8 inch) flour tortillas
- 1/2 cup diced potatoes
- 2 large eggs
- avocado oil cooking spray

Instructions

- ❖ Cook chorizo in an air fryer over medium-high heat, stirring often, until sausage operates into a dark crimson, 6 to 8 minutes.

- ❖ Melt bacon grease in precisely the exact way over medium-high warmth.

- ❖ Add onion and serrano pepper and continue stirring and cooking until berries are fork-tender, onion is translucent, and serrano pepper is tender in 2 to 6 minutes.

- ❖ Add eggs and chorizo; stir fry till cooked and fully integrated into curry mixture in about 5 minutes. Season with pepper and salt.

- ❖ Meanwhile, heat tortillas directly onto the grates of a gasoline stove until pliable and soft.

- ❖ Put 1/3 cup chorizo mixture down the middle of each tortilla.

- ❖ Fold top and bottom of tortillas over the filling, then roll into a burrito form. Mist with cooking spray and put in the basket of a fryer.

- ❖ Flip each burrito above, peppermint with cooking spray, and fry until lightly browned, 2 to 4 minutes longer.

5. **Herb Chicken Breast**

Now let's get to the herb chicken breast.

Ingredients

- Salt
- Pepper
- Chicken Breast
- Smoked Paprika
- Butter

Method:

We've got two chicken breasts. We've got butter, Italian seasoning salt, pepper and smoked paprika. We're going to mix all of that into the butter to give it a quick mix. Now we've got our two chicken breasts here and we're going to spread the mixture over each chicken breast to give it a nice flavorful crust.

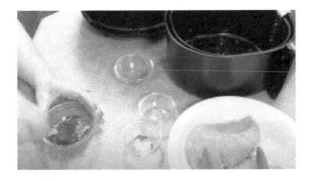

Put these in the air fryer with some tongs. We're ready to cook these in the air fryer.

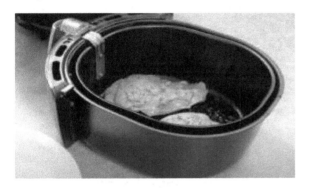

Cook them at 370 degrees for about 10 to 15 minutes and then check it with a meat thermometer to make sure that they're perfectly cooked. Because we don't want them to be overcooked, then they'll be dry and we definitely don't want them to be undercooked.

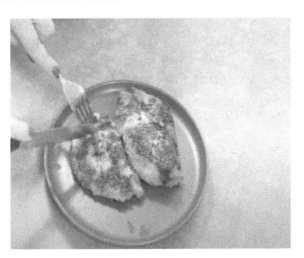

Okay, we pulled our chicken out of the air fryer. We had one chicken breast that was smaller so it came out a little bit earlier and now we have this one that's ready and its right at 165. So, we know that our chickens are not going to be dry. Let's cut into one of these. Those are perfectly cooked and juicy

6. Three Cheese Omelet

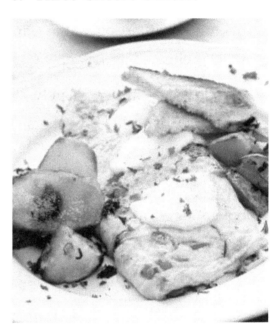

Ingredients

- 3 Tbsp. heavy whipping cream
- ½ tsp salt
- 4 eggs
- ¼ cup cheddar cheese, grated
- ¼ cup provolone cheese
- ¼ tsp ground black pepper
- ¼ cup feta cheese

Method:

❖ Preheat your air fryer to 350 degrees F and line a baking pan using parchment paper. Be sure the pan will fit on your fryer-normally a seven inch round pan will do the job flawlessly.

❖ In a small bowl, whisk together the eggs, cream, pepper and salt

❖ Pour the mixture into the prepared baking pan then place the pan on your preheated air fryer.

❖ Cook for approximately ten minutes or till the eggs are completely set.

❖ Sprinkle the cheeses round the boiled eggs and then return the pan into the air fryer for one more moment to melt the cheese.

7. Patty Pan Frittata

I had a gorgeous patty pan squash sitting on my counter tops and was wondering exactly what to do with this was fresh and yummy for my loved ones. I had not made breakfast however so a summer squash frittata appeared in order! Comparable to zucchini, patty pan squash leant itself well to my fundamental frittata recipe. Serve with your favorite brunch sides or independently. You could also cool and serve cold within 24 hours.

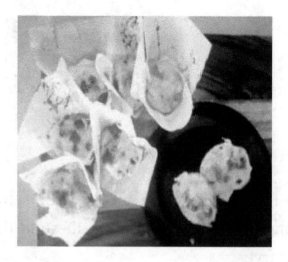

Ingredients

- 1 patty pan squash
- 1 tbsp. unsalted butter
- 4 large eggs
- 1/4 cup crumbled goat cheese
- 1/4 cup grated Parmesan cheese
- salt and ground black pepper to taste
- 1/4 cup
- 2 medium scallions, chopped, green and white parts split
- 1 tsp garlic, minced
- 1 small tomato, seeded and diced
- 1 tsp hot sauce, or to flavor

Instructions

❖ Press 5-inch squares of parchment paper to 8 cups of a muffin tin, creasing where essential.

❖ Heat butter over moderate heat; stir fry into patty pan, scallion whites, salt, garlic, and pepper. Transfer into a bowl and set aside.

❖ Add sausage in the identical way and cook until heated through, about 3 minutes. Add sausage into patty pan mix.

❖ Fold in goat milk, Parmesan cheese, and tomato. Add hot sauce and season with pepper and salt. Twist in patty pan-sausage mix. Put frittata mixture to the prepared muffin cups, filling to the peak of every cup and then overfilling only when the parchment paper may encourage the mix.

❖ Put muffin tin in addition to a cookie sheet in the middle of the toaster.

8. Bacon and Cheese Frittata

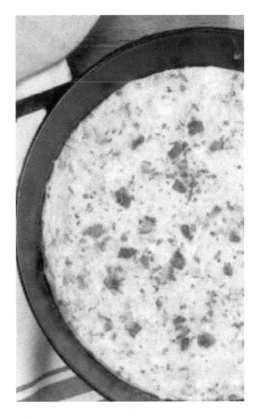

Ingredients

- ½ cup cheddar cheese, grated
- 4 eggs
- ½ cup chopped, cooked bacon
- ½ tsp salt
- 3 Tbsp. heavy whipping cream
- ¼ tsp ground black pepper

Method:

❖ Preheat your air fryer to 350 degrees F and line a baking pan using parchment paper. Be sure the pan will fit on your fryer-normally a seven inch round pan will do the job flawlessly.

❖ In a small bowl, whisk together the eggs, cream, pepper and salt

❖ Stir in the cheese and bacon into the bowl.

❖ Pour the mixture into the prepared baking pan then place the pan on your preheated air fryer.

❖ Cook for approximately 15 minutes or till the eggs are completely set.

9. Meat Lovers Omelet

Ingredients:

- ¼ cup cheddar cheese, grated

- ¼ cup cooked, crumbled bacon

- ½ tsp salt

- 4 eggs

- ¼ cup cooked, crumbled sausage

- 3 Tbsp. heavy whipping cream

- ¼ tsp ground black pepper

Method:

❏ Preheat your air fryer to 350 degrees F and line a baking pan using parchment paper. Be sure the pan will fit on your fryer-normally a seven inch round pan will do the job flawlessly.

❏ In a small bowl whisk together the eggs, cream, pepper and salt.

❏ Pour the mixture into the prepared baking pan then place the pan on your preheated air fryer.

❏ Cook for approximately ten minutes or till the eggs are completely set.

❏ Sprinkle the cheeses round the boiled eggs and then return the pan into the fryer for another two minutes to melt the cheese.

10. Crispy Brussels sprouts

Next on our list is air fryer crispy Brussels sprouts.

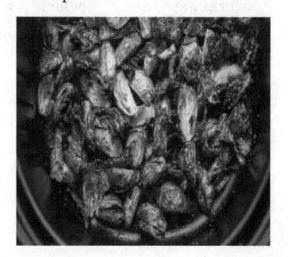

Ingredients:

- Brussels sprouts

- Salt

- Pepper

Method:

Let's get started with these Brussels sprouts. Use fresh Brussels sprouts and we could also use frozen ones. I've got a bag of frozen Brussels sprouts and actually they're still broke. I'm going to season them with some salt and some pepper.

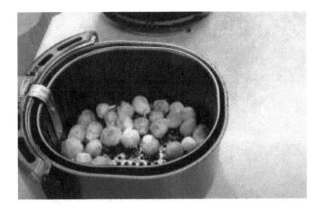

Shake them up and now I'm going to cook them at 400 or I'm going to start with 10 minutes. Let's see how it goes. I think you're going to be surprised because they're crispy. Can you believe that? I think these are better than fresh ones.

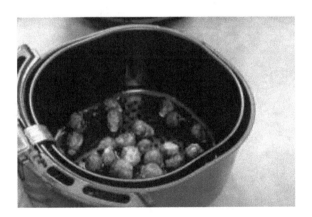

Use frozen if you want to make air fryer Brussels sprouts because the fresh ones take forever to get soft on the inside. You got to cut them into quarters, you've got to trim the leaves off these. They're

frozen. I just threw them in the air fryer for 15minutes and they're good to go.

Now what I'm going to show you are actually dessert ideas that you can cook in your air fryer. They come in different sizes and one and a half liter is quite common too, so just check when you buy your own if you do that.

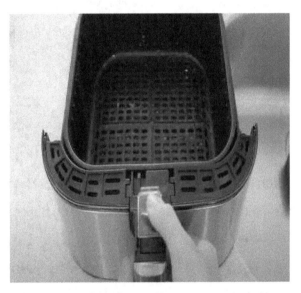

It is a bigger liter air fryer because I promise you, you're going to want to cook everything in this. What I love about this style of air fryer is that it's so simple on the front. You will see that you have got different settings but if you want to cook chips, prawns, fish, steak and muffins as well, it's really easy to adjust the temperature up and down. Also the time up and down as well. Then once you put your tray back in, all you need to do is select your setting and press the play button and the air fryer does everything else for you. It is also really really easy to clean. All you need to do is remove your tray from your air fryer, press the button on at the handle and detach your basket from the tray.

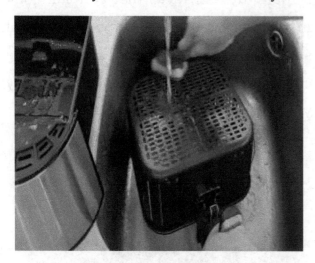

I then use a handheld scrubbing brush which dispenses washing-up liquid and I just go over my basket and my outer tray as well which is where all the fats from your food drip. I just go in with some warm water and my washing up liquid washes it all away. It's got a really nice TEFL coating so everything just wipes off. It's nonstick, then I just leave it on the side, let it dry and then pop it back in my air fryer. At once it is dry, so with all that said I'm just going to jump straight on into the recipes.

11. Hard Boiled Eggs

Ingredients:

- 4 eggs

Method:

➢ Preheat your air fryer to 250 degrees F.

➢ Place a wire rack in the fryer and set the eggs in addition to the rack.

➢ Cook for 17 minutes then remove the eggs and put them into an

➢ Ice water bath to cool and then stop the cooking procedure.

➢ Peel the eggs and love!

1. Spinach Parmesan Baked Eggs

Ingredients:

- 1 Tbsp. frozen, chopped spinach, thawed

- 1 Tbsp. grated parmesan cheese

- 2 eggs

- 1 Tbsp. heavy cream

- ¼ tsp salt

- 1/8 tsp ground black pepper

Method:

❑ Preheat your air fryer to 330 degrees F.

❑ Spray a silicone muffin cup or a little ramekin with cooking spray.

❑ In a small bowl, whisk together all of the components

❑ Pour the eggs into the ready ramekin and bake for 2 minutes.

❏ Enjoy directly from the skillet!

12. Fried hushpuppies.

Inside my home, stuffing is consistently the very popular Thanksgiving dish on the table. Because of this, we create double the amount we all actually need just so we can eat leftovers for a week! And while remaining stuffing alone is yummy, turning it into hushpuppies? Now that is only pure wizardry. Here is the way to use your air fryer to produce near-instant two-ingredient fried hushpuppies.

Ingredients:

- large egg
- cold stuffing
- Cooking spray

Directions:

★ Put 1 large egg in a large bowl and gently beat. Add 3 cups leftover stuffing and stir till blended.

★ Preheat in an air fryer into 355°F and place it for 12 minutes. Put one layer of hushpuppies on the racks and then spray the tops with cooking spray.

★ Repeat with the remaining mixture.

13. Keto Breakfast Pizza

An egg, sausage, and pork rind "crust" holds sauce, cheese, and other savory toppings within this keto-friendly breakfast pizza recipe.

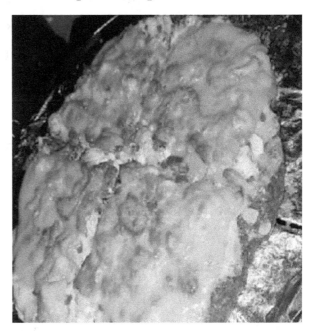

Ingredients

- 3 large eggs, split
- 2 tbsp. Italian seasoning
- 1 cup ready country-style sauce
- 10 tbsp. bacon pieces
- 1 pound bulk breakfast sausage
- cooking spray
- 1/3 cup crushed pork rinds
- 2 tbsp. chopped yellow onion
- 2 tbsp. diced jalapeno pepper
- 1 cup shredded Cheddar cheese

Instructions

★ Grease a rimmed pizza sheet.

★ Spread mixture out on the pizza sheet at a big, thin circle.

★ Meanwhile, spray a large air fryer with cooking spray and heat over medium-high heat. Whisk remaining eggs together in a bowl and then pour into it.

★ Place an oven rack about 6 inches from the heat source and then turn on the oven's broiler.

★ Spread sausage evenly over the beef "crust", sprinkle scrambled eggs. Sprinkle with bacon pieces, onion, and jalapeno.

★ Broil pizza in the preheated oven till cheese is melted, bubbling, and lightly browned, 3 to 5 minutes. Let cool and cut into fourths prior to serving.

14. Mozzarella stick

Ready for the simplest mozzarella stick recipe? These air fryer mozzarella sticks are created completely from pantry and refrigerator staples (cheese sticks and breadcrumbs), which means that you can dig to the crispy-coated, nostalgic bite anytime you would like.

INGREDIENTS:

➢ 1 (12-ounce) bundle mayonnaise

➢ 1 large egg

➢ 1/2 tsp garlic powder

➢ all-purpose flour

➢ 1/2 tsp onion powder

Method:

★ Before frying pan, set the halved cheese sticks onto a rimmed baking sheet lined with parchment paper. Freeze for half an hour. Meanwhile, construct the breading and get outside the air fryer.

★ Whisk the egg and lettuce together in a skillet. Put the flour, breadcrumbs, onion, and garlic powder in a large bowl and whisk to mix.

★ Working in batches of 6, then roll the suspended cheese sticks at the mayo-egg mix to coat, and then in the flour mixture.

★ Pour the coated cheese sticks into the parchment-lined baking sheet. Pour the baking sheet into the freezer for 10 minutes.

★ Heat the fryer to 370°F. Fry 6 the mozzarella sticks for 5 minutes -- it's important not to overcrowd the fryer.

★ Repeat with the rest of the sticks and serve hot with the marinara for dipping.

15. Raspberry Muffins

Ingredients:

- ¼ cup whole milk

- 1 egg

- 1 Tbsp. powdered stevia

- ¼ tsp salt

- ¼ tsp ground cinnamon

- 1 ½ tsp baking powder

- 1 cup almond flour

- ½ cup frozen or fresh raspberries

Steps:

I. Preheat your air fryer to 350 degrees F.

II. In a large bowl, stir together the almond milk, stevia, salt, cinnamon, and baking powder.

III. Add the milk and eggs and then stir well.

IV. Split the muffin batter involving each muffin cup, filling roughly 3/4 of this way complete.

V. Set the muffins to the fryer basket and cook for 14 minutes or till a toothpick comes out when inserted to the middle.

VI. Eliminate from the fryer and let cool.

16. Sausage Tray Bake

I have just chopped up some new potatoes and then I've got some chipolata sausages so I'm going to make a tray bake.

Ingredients:

- Potatoes

- Chipolata Sausage

- corvette

- Onion

- Garlic

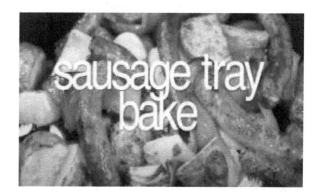

Method:

I would put potato and chipotle sausage into the air fryer for about 20 minutes at first before I add in my other veggies.

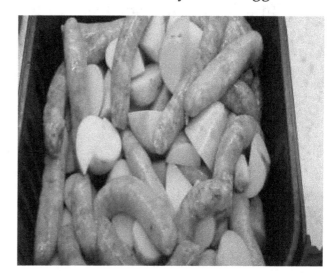

Once these have been in for 20 minutes or so, I will then add in two papers of corvette, an onion and some garlic to go in as well. Cook them for a further 10 minutes and then dinner should be ready.

17. Strawberry Muffins

Ingredients:

- ¼ cup whole milk
- 1 ½ tsp baking powder
- ½ cup chopped strawberries
- 1 egg
- ¼ tsp salt
- ¼ tsp ground cinnamon
- 1 cup almond flour
- 1 Tbsp. powdered stevia

Steps:

1. Preheat your air fryer to 350 degrees F.

2. In a large bowl, stir together the almond milk, stevia, salt, cinnamon, and baking powder.

3. Add the milk and eggs and then stir well.

4. Fold in the berries.

5. Split the muffin batter involving each muffin cup, filling roughly 3/4 of this way complete.

6. Set the muffins to the fryer basket and cook for 14 minutes or till a toothpick comes out when inserted to the middle.

7. Eliminate from the fryer and let cool.

18. Bacon and Eggs for a single

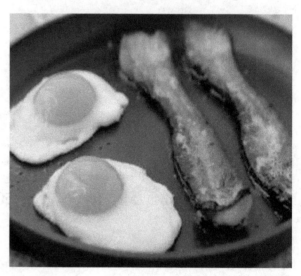

Ingredients:

- 1 Tbsp. heavy cream
- two Tbsp. cooked, crumbled bacon
- 1/4 tsp salt
- 2 eggs
- 1/8 tsp ground black pepper

Directions

❏ Preheat your air fryer to 330 degrees F.

❏ Spray a silicone muffin cup or a little ramekin with cooking spray.

❏ In a small bowl, whisk together all of the components

❏ Pour the eggs into the ready ramekin and bake for 2 minutes.

❏ Enjoy directly from the skillet!

19. Mini Sausage Pancake Skewers with Spicy Syrup

These small savory skewers are fantastic for breakfast or a fantastic addition to your brunch buffet. The hot maple syrup garnish kicks up the flavor and adds some zest to sandwiches and sausage.

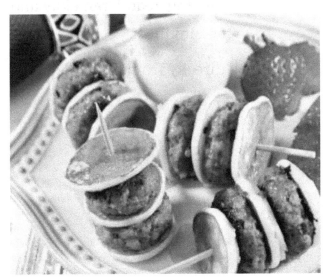

Ingredients

Syrup:

- 4 tbsp. unsalted butter

- 1/2 tsp salt

- 1/2 cup maple syrup

- 1 tsp red pepper flakes, or to taste

Pancake

- 1 cup buttermilk

- 2 tbsp. unsalted butter, melted

- 1 cup all-purpose flour

- 1 large egg

- 1 tbsp. olive oil

- 1 lb. ounce standard pork sausage (like Jimmy Dean®)

- 13 4-inch bamboo skewers

- 2 tablespoons sour cream

- 1/2 tbsp. brown sugar

- 1/4 tsp baking powder

- 1/4 tsp salt

- 2 tsp maple syrup

Instructions

❏ Bring to a boil and cook for 3 to 4 minutes.

❏ Meanwhile, prepare pancakes: whisk flour, sugar, baking powder, and salt in a huge bowl. Whisk buttermilk, egg, sour cream, melted butter and maple syrup together in another bowl. Pour the wet ingredients into the flour mixture. Stir lightly until just blended but slightly lumpy; don't overmix. Let sit for 10 minutes.

❏ Heat in an air fryer over moderate heat. Drop teaspoonfuls of batter onto them to make 1-inch diameter sandwiches.

❏ Cook for approximately 1 to 2 minutes, then reverse, and keep cooking until golden brown, about 1 minute. Transfer cooked pancakes into a plate and repeat with remaining batter.

❏ Heat olive oil at precisely the exact same fryer over moderate heat. Form table-spoonfuls of sausage to 1-inch patties, exactly the exact same size as the miniature pancakes.

❏ Cook until patties are cooked through, about 3 minutes each side. Transfer to a newspaper towel-lined plate.

❏ Blend 3 pancakes and two sausage patties onto each skewer, beginning and end with a pancake.

❏ Repeat to create staying skewers. Serve drizzled with hot syrup.

20. Avocado Baked Eggs

Ingredients:

- 1 Tbsp. heavy cream
- ¼ tsp salt
- ¼ avocado, diced
- 1 Tbsp. grated cheddar cheese
- 2 eggs
- 1/8 tsp ground black pepper

Method:

❏ Preheat your air fryer to 330 degrees F.

❏ Spray a silicone muffin cup or a little ramekin with cooking spray.

❏ In a small bowl, whisk together the eggs, cream, cheddar cheese, salt, and pepper.

❏ Stir in the avocado and pour the eggs into the ready ramekin and bake for 2 minutes.

❏ Enjoy directly from the skillet!

Chapter 2: Air Fryer 50 more Recipes for You!

21. Sausage and Cheese Omelet

Ingredients:

- ¼ cup cheddar cheese, grated
- ½ cup cooked, crumbled sausage
- 4 eggs
- 3 Tbsp. heavy whipping cream
- ½ tsp salt
- ¼ tsp ground black pepper

Method

01. Preheat your air fryer to 320 degrees F and line a baking pan using parchment paper. Be sure the pan will fit on your fryer-normally a seven inch round pan will do the job flawlessly.

02. In a small bowl, whisk together the eggs, cream, pepper and salt.

03. Pour the mixture into the prepared baking pan then place the pan on your preheated air fryer.

04. Cook for approximately ten minutes or till the eggs are completely set.

05. Sprinkle the cheeses round the boiled eggs and then return the pan into the fryer for another two minutes to melt the cheese.

22. Pita bread Pizza

I am making some pita bread pizzas now.

Ingredients:

- Bread
- Tomato puree
- Passat

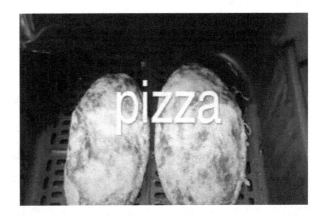

Method:

I usually would make these in the oven and I would put them in there for about 10 to 15 minutes. I'm just going to put some ketchup on top of the pizza bread base.

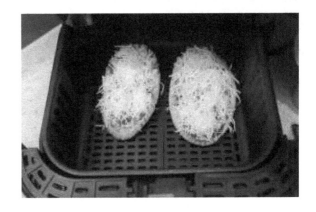

Or you can put tomato puree on there or some pasta whatever you've got. Then I'm just going to put some cheese on really nice and simple. I'm going to pop them on the pizza setting in the air fryer so that's eight minutes when I do my pizzas in the oven the base isn't really nice and crispy. So, I am really pleased with how they've turned out in the air fryer. Pizzas are done, crispy delicious, ready to eat.

23. Air Fryer Hanukkah Latkes

If you have never needed a latke, it is about time we change this. Traditionally served throughout Hanukkah, these crispy fritters -- frequently made with grated potatoes, lettuce, onion, and matzo meal -- are kind of impossible to not love.

Traditionally latkes are fried in oil (or poultry schmaltz!)) , however I wanted to see if I could create them using the popular air fryer. Since the fryer is a high-heat convection oven, the large fan speed and focused warmth yields a crispy potato pancake that is also soft at the middle.

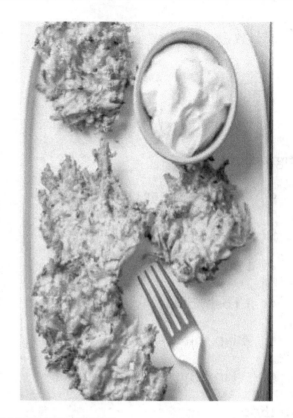

INGREDIENTS

- 1 1/2 Pounds Russet potatoes (2 to 3 tbsp.)

- ½ medium yellow onion

- 1/2 tsp freshly ground black pepper

- Cooking spray

- Two large eggs

- matzo meal

- 2 tsp kosher salt

Description:

❖ Peel 1 1/2 lbs. russet potatoes. Grate the potatoes and 1/2 yellow onion onto the large holes of a box grater. Put with a clean kitchen towel, then pull up the sides of the towel to make a package, and squeeze out excess moisture.

❖ Transfer the curry mixture into a large bowl. Add two large eggs, 1/4 cup matzo meal, two tsp kosher salt, and 1/2 tsp black pepper, and stir to blend.

❖ Preheat the Air Fryer into 375°F and place it for 16 minutes. Coat the air fryer racks together with cooking spray.

❖ Dip the latke mix in 2-tablespoon dollops to the fryer, flattening the shirts to make a patty.

❖ Air fry, rotating the trays halfway through, for 2 minutes total. Repeat with the rest of the latke mix.

24. Salmon Fillet

Now, I'm going to cook some salmon in it.

Ingredients:

- Salmon

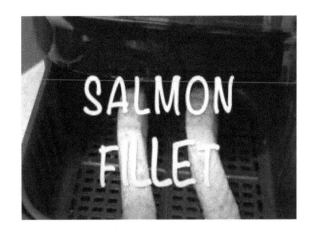

Method:

I put my salmon in, with nothing on top of it, just a salmon filet. I pop it in on the fish sitting for ten minutes and when it comes out it has got the crispy skin ever. The salmon was in for ten minutes and I wanted to show you how crispy the skin is.

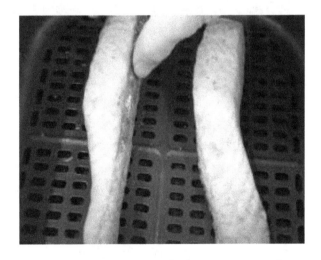

I'm someone who loves eating salmon skin and that is just perfectly done right.

25. Air Fryer Mini Calzones

Among the greatest approaches to utilize an air fryer is a miniature oven that will not heat up your entire kitchen for party snacks. It's possible to turn out batch after batch of wings, mozzarella sticks, and also, yes, miniature calzones which are hot, crispy, and superbly nostalgic by one air fryer.

These mini calzones utilize ready pizza dough to produce delicious pockets full of gooey cheese, piquant tomato sauce, and hot pepperoni that are fantastic for celebrations, after-school snacks, or even for satisfying your craving to get your dessert rolls of your childhood.

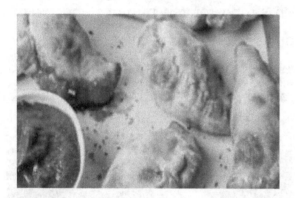

Ingredients:

- All-purpose flour, for rolling the dough out

- Pizza sauce, and more for dipping

- Thinly sliced pepperoni

- miniature pepperoni, chopped

Directions:

- ❖ Utilize a 3-inch round cutter or a large glass to cut 8 to 10 rounds of bread.

- ❖ Transfer the rounds into some parchment paper-lined baking

sheet. Gather up the dough scraps, then reroll and replicate cutting rounds out until you've got 16.

- ❖ Top each round with two tsp of sauce, 1 tablespoon of cheese, and one tsp of pepperoni.

- ❖ Working with a single dough around at a time, fold in half an hour, then pinch the edges together to seal. When every calzone is sealed, then use a fork to crimp the borders shut to additional seal.

- ❖ Heat the air fryer into 375°F. Working in batches of 4, air fry the calzones until golden brown and crispy, about 8 minutes. Serve with extra pizza sauce for dipping, if desired.

26. Fajitas

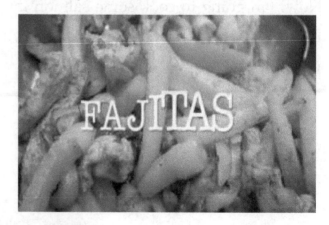

Ingredients:

- Turkey Strips

- Yellow Pepper

- Onion

- Orange Pepper

Method:

It's a night that we are going to be having for heaters. So, here, I've chopped up yellow and orange pepper and also half an onion. I have got some turkey strips.

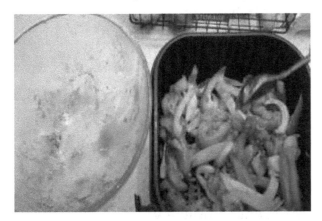

I'll pass it over heat as it makes barbecue flavor onto all of this. So, I'm just going to pop these all into the air fryer together because I think they'll actually cook through at a very similar rate. Then I am going to pop them on the chicken setting and let the air fryer get cooking alright. This is the fajita mix in ten minutes.

I put on the chicken setting which is actually 20 minutes but I was just checking it.

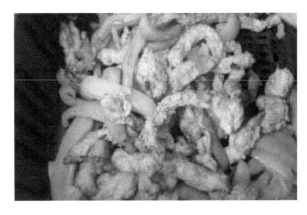

I cut a piece of the turkey and it's perfect all the way through, I cut it like one of the biggest pieces up as well. So, it's absolutely perfect so all this needs is ten minutes in the air fryer and it's done right.

27. Pot Sweet Potato Chips

Replace the humble sweet potato to a freshly-fried bite, and it is sure to be yummy. Sweet potato chips, sweet potato tater tots -- you name it, we will take it. The comparison between the sweetness of the curry and the saltiness of this bite is really impossible to not love.

These air fryer sweet potato chips provide everything you adore about these deep-fried snacks. That is the great thing about the air fryer that it requires less oil, after all -- you have to bypass the hassle and clutter of heating a massive pot of oil to the stove -- but the "fried" cure comes out evenly as yummy. And unlike a store-bought bag of chips, you have to personalize the seasonings. Here, we are using dried herbs and a pinch of cayenne for an earthy, somewhat spicy beverage.

Ingredients:

- medium sweet potato
- 1 tbsp. canola oil
- 1/2 tsp freshly ground black pepper
- 1/4 tsp paprika
- 1 tsp kosher salt
- 3/4 tsp dried thyme leaves
- Cooking spray

Directions:

- ❏ Wash 1 sweet potato and dry nicely. Thinly slice 1/8-inch thick using a knife or rather on a mandolin. Set in a bowl, then cover with cool water, and then soak at room temperature for 20 minutes to remove the excess starch.

- ❏ Drain the pieces and pat very dry with towels. Put into a large bowl, then add 1 tbsp. canola oil, 1 tsp kosher salt, 3/4 tsp dried thyme leaves, 1/2 tsp black pepper, 1/4 tsp paprika, and a pinch cayenne pepper if using, and toss to blend.

- ❏ Gently coat in an air fryer rotisserie basket with cooking spray.

- ❏ Air fry in batches: put one layer of sweet potato pieces from the rotisserie basket. Put the rotisserie basket at the fryer and press on.

- ❏ Preheat the fryer into 340°F and place for 22 minutes, until the sweet potatoes are golden brown and the edges are crispy, 19 to 22 minutes.

- ❏ Transfer the chips into a newspaper towel-lined plate to cool completely

- ❏ They will crisp as they cool. Repeat with the remaining sweet potato pieces.

28. **Easy Baked Eggs**

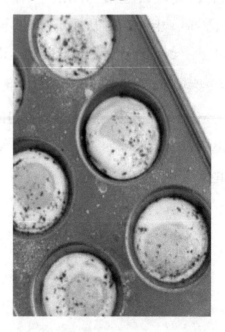

Ingredients:

- 1 Tbsp. heavy cream
- ¼ tsp salt
- 2 eggs
- 1/8 tsp ground black pepper

Method:

➢ Preheat your fryer to 330 degrees F.

➢ Spray a silicone muffin cup or a little ramekin with cooking spray.

➢ In a small bowl, whisk together all of the components

➢ Pour the eggs into the ready ramekin and bake for 6 minutes.

➢ Enjoy directly from the skillet!

29. Air Fryer Buttermilk Fried Chicken

I went to school in the South, so I have had my fair share of crispy, succulent, finger-licking fried chicken. As you might imagine, I had been skeptical about creating a much healthier version from the air fryer.

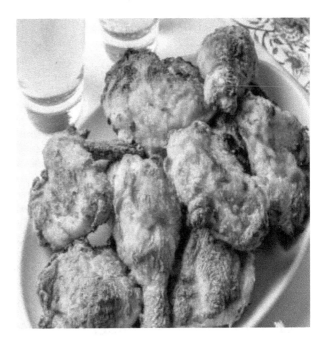

The second I pulled out my first batch, but my worries disappeared. The epidermis was crispy, the coat was cracker-crisp (as it ought to be), and also, above all, the chicken itself was tender and succulent -- the indication of a perfect piece of fried chicken.

Air fryer fried chicken is lighter, quicker, than and not as cluttered as deep-fried chicken. Here is the way to get it done.

Ingredients

- 1 tsp Freshly ground black pepper, divided
- Buttermilk
- 1 tsp Cayenne pepper
- 1 tbsp. Garlic powder
- 2 tbsp. paprika
- 1 tbsp. onion powder

- 1 tsp kosher salt, divided
- all-purpose flour
- 1 tbsp. ground mustard
- Cooking spray

Directions

❏ Put all ingredients into a large bowl and season with 1 teaspoon of the kosher salt and 1/2 tsp of honey.

❏ Add 2 cups buttermilk and simmer for 1 hour in the fridge. Meanwhile, whisk the remaining 1 tbsp. kosher salt, staying 1/2 tsp black pepper, 2 cups all-purpose flour, 1 tbsp. garlic powder, 2 tbsp. paprika, 1 teaspoon cayenne pepper, 1 tbsp. onion powder, plus one tbsp. ground mustard together into a huge bowl.

❏ Preheat an air fryer into 390ºF. Coat the fryer racks together with cooking spray. Remove the chicken in the buttermilk, allowing any excess to drip off. Dredge in the flour mixture, shaking off any excess. Put one layer of chicken in the basket, with distance between the bits. Air fry, turning the chicken hallway through, until an instant-read thermometer registers 165ºF from the thickest part

❏ Cook for 18 to 20 minutes, then complete.

30. **Keto Chocolate Chip Muffins**

Ingredients:

- ¼ tsp salt
- 1 Tbsp. powdered stevia
- ¼ cup whole milk
- 1 egg
- 1 cup almond flour
- 1 ½ tsp baking powder
- ½ cup mini dark chocolate chips (sugar free)

Method:

❖ Preheat your air fryer to 350 degrees F.

❖ In a large bowl, stir together the almond milk, stevia, salt, cinnamon, and baking powder.

❖ Add the milk and eggs and then stir well.

❖ Split the muffin batter involving each muffin cup, filling around 3/4 of this way complete.

❖ Set the muffins to the air fryer basket and cook for 14 minutes or till a toothpick comes out when put to the middle.

❖ Eliminate from the fryer and let cool.

31. Crispy Chickpeas

What, I've got in here are some chickpeas.

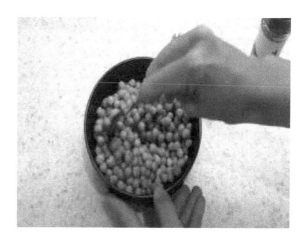

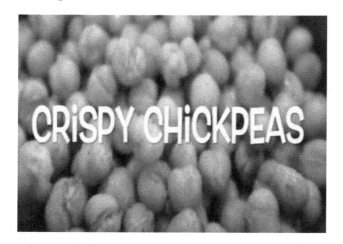

Ingredients:

- Chickpeas

- Olive oil

- Per-peril salt

Method:

I've drained and washed chickpeas and then what I'm going to do is add on some olive oil and then also the periphery salt. The reason I put some olive oil on is because it just helps the pair of results stick to the chickpeas.

Then I'm just going to mix everything in together and pop them into the air fryer for about 15 minutes. On the chip setting these are great little snacks to make like pre dinner snacks. Instead of having crisps or if you're watching a movie, instead of having popcorn these are good little things. Also, if you are having a salad they're really nice to go in your salad as well.

32. Keto Blueberry Muffins

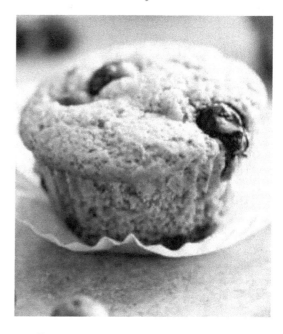

Ingredients:

- 1 egg

- ¼ tsp salt

- 1 cup almond flour

- 1 Tbsp. powdered stevia

- 1 ½ tsp baking powder

- ¼ cup whole milk

- ¼ tsp ground cinnamon

- ½ cup frozen or fresh blueberries

Steps:

1) Preheat your air fryer to 350 degrees F.

2) In a large bowl, stir together the almond milk, stevia, salt, cinnamon, and baking powder.

3) Add the milk and eggs and then stir well.

4) Split the muffin batter involving each muffin cup, filling roughly 3/4 of this way complete.

5) Set the muffins to the air fryer basket and cook for 14 minutes or till a toothpick comes out when put to the middle.

6) Eliminate from the fryer and let cool.

33. **Air Fryer Donuts**

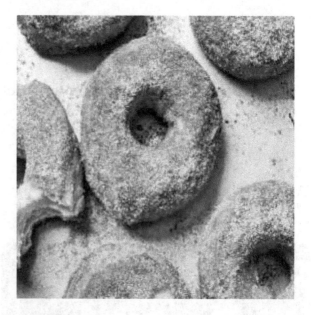

Ingredients

- ground cinnamon

- granulated sugar

- Flaky large snacks,

- Jojoba oil spray or coconut oil spray

Instructions

★ Combine sugar and cinnamon in a shallow bowl; place aside.

★ Remove the cookies from the tin, separate them and set them onto the baking sheet.

★ Utilize a 1-inch round biscuit cutter (or similarly-sized jar cap) to cut holes from the middle of each biscuit.

★ Lightly coat an air fryer basket using coconut or olive oil spray (don't use nonstick cooking spray like Pam, which may damage the coating onto the basket)

★ Put 3 to 4 donuts in one layer in the air fryer (that they shouldn't be touching). Close to the air fryer and place to 350°F. Transfer donuts into the baking sheet.

★ Repeat with the rest of the biscuits. You can also cook the donut holes they will take approximately 3 minutes total

★ Brush both sides of this hot donut with melted butter, put in the cinnamon sugar, and then turn to coat both sides.

34. Sausage and Spinach Omelet

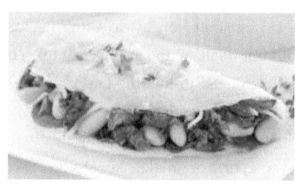

Ingredients:

½ cup baby spinach

4 eggs

¼ cup cheddar cheese, grated

½ cup cooked, crumbled sausage

3 Tbsp. heavy whipping cream

½ tsp salt

¼ tsp ground black pepper

Directions

I.   Preheat the air fryer at around 330 F.

II.   In a small bowl, whisk together the eggs, cream, pepper and salt.

III. Fold in the cooked sausage and sausage.

IV.   Pour the mixture into the prepared baking pan then place the pan on your

V.   Cook for approximately ten minutes or till the eggs are completely set.

VI.   Sprinkle the cheeses round the boiled eggs and then return the pan into the fryer

VII. Fryer for another two minutes to melt the cheese.

35. Air Fryer Potato Wedges

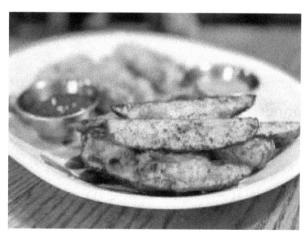

Perfectly crisp and seasoned potato wedges directly from your air fryer. It will not get any simpler than this!

Ingredients

- → 2 medium Russet potatoes, cut into wedges
- → 1/2 tsp sea salt
- → 1 1/2 tsp olive oil
- → 1/2 tsp chili powder
- → ⅛ teaspoon ground black pepper
- → 1/2 tsp paprika
- → 1/2 tsp parsley flakes

Instructions

- ❖ Place potato wedges in a large bowl.
- ❖ Put 8 wedges at the jar of the air fryer and cook for 10 minutes.
- ❖ Flip wedges with tongs and cook for another five minutes.

36. **Chocolate Chip Cookies in Air fryer**

They are my day pick-me-up, my after-dinner treat, also, sometimes, a part of my breakfast. I keep either frozen cookies or baked biscuits in my freezer -- true my friends know and have come to appreciate when they come around for dinner or even a glass of wine.

The kind of chocolate chip cookie I enjoy all, depends upon my mood. Sometimes I need them super doughy, and sometimes challenging and crisp. If you're searching for one someplace in between -- gooey on the inside and crunchy on the outside -- I have discovered the foolproof way of you. It entails cooking them on your air fryer.

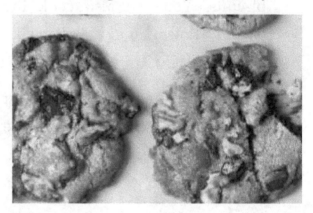

When using your fryer to create biscuits, be certain that you always line its base with foil to aid with simple cleanup. You will also need to line the basket or racks using parchment paper. Buy paper which has holes in it, cut some slits to the newspaper, or make sure you leave space around it which will allow for even cooking and flow of the air. With these suggestions, you're on your way to cookie victory!

Ingredients:

- Granulated sugar
- vanilla extract
- dark brown sugar

- 1 tsp kosher salt

- 2 large eggs

- 3/4 cup chopped walnuts

- 1 tsp baking soda

- Flaky sea salt, for garnish (optional)

- all-purpose flour

- Cooking spray

INSTRUCTIONS

❖ Put 2 sticks unsalted butter in the bowl of a stand mixer, fitted with the paddle attachment and also let it sit till softened. Insert 3/4 cup granulated sugar and 3/4 cup packed dark brown sugar and beat it on medium speed till blended and fluffy within 3 to 4 minutes. Add 1 tablespoon lemon extract, 2 big eggs, and 1 tsp kosher salt, and beat until just blended. After that, add 1 tea-spoon baking soda plus 2 1/3 cups all-purpose flour in increments, mixing until just blended.

❖ Add 2 cups chocolate balls and 3/4 cup chopped peppers and stir with a rubber spatula until just blended.

❖ Preheat in an air fryer, at 350°F and set to 5 minutes. Line the fryer racks with parchment paper, make sure you leave space on all sides for air to leak.

❖ Reduce 2-tablespoon scoops of this dough on the racks, setting them 1-inch apart. Gently flatten each spade marginally to earn a cookie form.

❖ Sprinkle with flaky sea salt, if using. Bake until golden brown, about 5 minutes. Remove the racks out of the fryer and let it cool for 3 to 5 minutes to place. Repeat with the remaining dough.

37. Crispy Coated Veggies

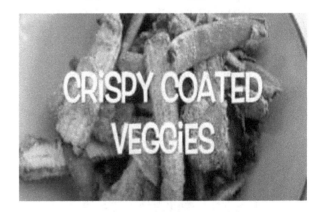

Ingredients:

- Vegetables

- Egg

- Paprika

- Salt & Pepper

Method:

I'm making some crispy coating of vegetables in this bowl. I have got one egg beaten up. This is actually almond flour but you can use normal flour and then I popped in some paprika. I've also put in some salt and pepper here too. Then I'm going to dip my veggies into my egg and then I'll put them into the flour mixture, then into the air fryer for probably about eight minutes.

38. Ranch Pork Chops in Air fryer

Ingredients

- 4 boneless, center-cut pork chops, 1-inch thick

- aluminum foil

- cooking spray

- 2 Tsp dry ranch salad dressing mix

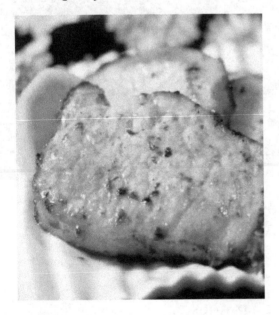

Directions

★ Put pork chops on a plate and then gently spray both sides with cooking spray. Sprinkle both sides with ranch seasoning mixture and let them sit at room temperature for 10 minutes.

★ Spray the basket of an air fryer with cooking spray and preheat at 390 degrees F (200 degrees C).

★ Place chops in the preheated air fryer, working in batches if needed, to guarantee the fryer isn't overcrowded.

★ Flip chops and cook for 5 minutes longer. Let rest on a foil-covered plate for 5 minutes prior to serving.

39. Quesadillas

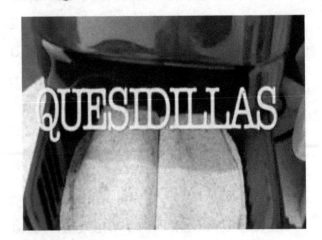

Ingredients:

- Refried Beans

- Cheese

- Peppers

- Chicken

Method:

I'm going to be using the El Paso refried beans in the tin. I will spread that onto the wrap and then I'm just going to sprinkle some cheese on top.

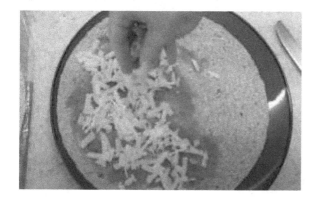

This is a really basic wrap so usually when we have routes we'll add some like peppers in here as well and loads of other bits like chicken. I just wanted to show you how well they cook in the air fryer. You pop them in on the pizza setting and in 8 to10 minutes they are done. Really crispy and ready to eat.

40. Pecan Crusted Pork Chops at the Air Fryer

The air-fryer makes simple work of those yummy pork chops. The chops make good leftovers too, since the pecan crust does not get soggy!

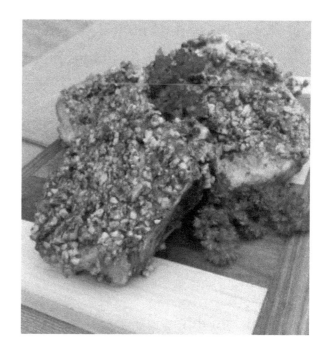

Ingredients:

- Egg

- Pork

- Pecans

- Simmer

Instructions

➢ Add egg and simmer until all ingredients are well blended. Place pecans onto a plate.

➢ Dip each pork dip in the egg mix, then put onto the plate together with the pecans

➢ Press pecans firmly onto either side until coated. Spray the chops on both sides with cooking spray and set from the fryer basket.

➢ Cook at the fryer for 6 minutes. Turn chops closely with tongs, and fry until pork is no longer pink in the middle, about 6 minutes more.

41. Crispy Chicken Thighs

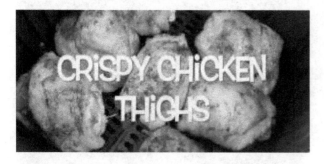

Ingredients

- Chicken thighs

- Pepper

- Olive oil

- Paprika

- Salt

Method:

I've got some chicken thighs. These have got bone-in and skinned on so what I've done is just put some olive oil on top of them with some paprika and some salt and pepper. Then I just rubbed everything into the chicken skin so I'm going to pop these into my air fryer. Press the chicken button and let the air fryer just do its thing.

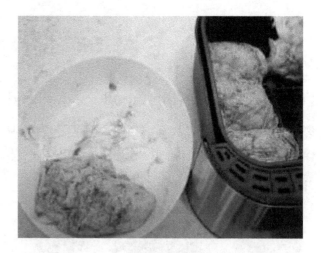

This skin is super crispy that is perfectly done and it's been in there for 20 minutes. I just wanted to show you all the fat that came out of that chicken so here are all the oils that came off.

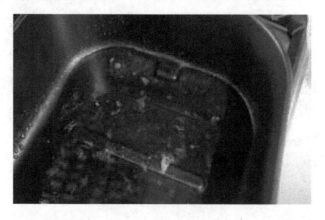

So those are what your chicken would be sitting in but instead it's all just tripped underneath the air fryer.

42. Bacon-Wrapped Scallops with Sirach Mayo

This yummy appetizer is ready quickly and easily in the air fryer and served with a hot Sirach mayo skillet. I use the smaller bay scallops because of this. If you're using jumbo scallops, it'll require a longer cooking time and more bits of bacon.

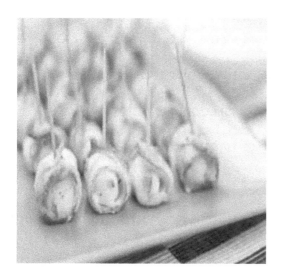

Ingredients

- 1/2 cup mayonnaise

- 1 pinch coarse salt

- 2 tbsp. Sirach sauce

- 1 pound bay scallops (about 36 small scallops)

- 1 pinch freshly cracked black pepper

- 12 slices bacon, cut into thirds

- 1 serving olive oil cooking spray

Instructions

★ Mix mayonnaise and Sirach sauce together in a little bowl.

★ Preheat the air fryer to 390 degrees F (200 degrees C).

★ Season with pepper and salt. Wrap each scallop with 1/3 piece of bacon and fasten with a toothpick.

★ Spray the air fryer basket with cooking spray. Put bacon-wrapped scallops from the basket in one layer; divide into two batches if needed.

★ Cook at the air fryer for 7 minutes. Check for doneness; scallops should be wheat and opaque ought to be crispy. Cook 1 to 2 minutes more, if needed, checking every moment. Remove scallops carefully with tongs and put on a newspaper towel-lined plate to absorb extra oil out of the bacon.

43. Homemade Chips

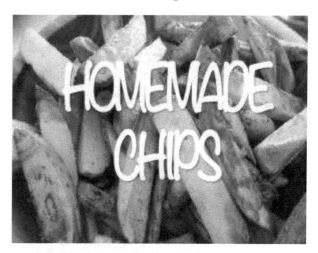

Ingredients

- Chip

- Olive oil

- Paprika

- Salt

Method:

Now I'm going to do some chips. I've just cut up some potatoes into chip shapes and then I am going to put some olive oil on top. Some paprika and some salt and the main reason I'm putting olive oil on top is basically for the paprika and the salt to stick to the surface of the chips. I'll just pop these in and then I'll put them onto the chip setting and let them cook away for about 18 minutes. I will be staring these halfway through because I'm doing quite a few chips as well. I will probably have to put these on for another 10 minutes after the 18 minutes is done.

44. Easy Air Fryer Pork Chops

Boneless pork chops cooked to perfection with the help of an air fryer. This recipe is super easy and you could not ask for a more tender and succulent chop.

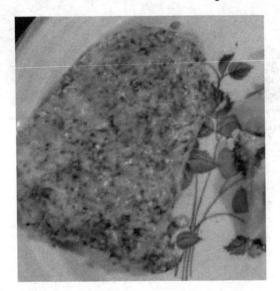

Ingredients

- 1/2 cup grated Parmesan cheese
- 1 tsp kosher salt
- 4 (5 oz.) center-cut pork chops
- 2 tbsp. extra virgin olive oil
- 1 tsp dried parsley
- 1 tsp paprika
- 1 tsp garlic powder
- 1/2 teaspoon ground black pepper

Instructions

- ❏ Preheat the fryer to 390 degrees F.

- ❏ Combine Parmesan cheese, paprika, garlic powder, salt, parsley, and pepper in a level shallow dish; combine well.

- ❏ Stir every pork chop with olive oil. Dredge both sides of each dip from the Parmesan mixture and put on a plate.

- ❏ Put 2 chops from the basket of the fryer and cook for 10 minutes; turning halfway through cook time.

45. Corn on the Cob

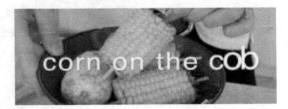

Ingredients:

- Corn

- Butter

- Salt

Method:

We're going to do some corn on the cob. What I'm going to do is just pop them into my air fryer but not put anything on top of them. I'm going to put them in on the prawn settings.

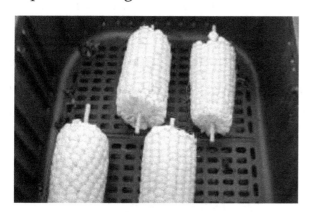

It's just eight minutes, after ten minutes like I said, I will then add some butter on top and a little bit of salt. They're ready to eat.

46. Air Fryer Broiled Grapefruit

This hot and warm grapefruit with a buttery candy topping is the best accompaniment for your Sunday brunch and makes a lovely snack or dessert. I love to add a pinch of sea salt in the end to actually bring out the tastes.

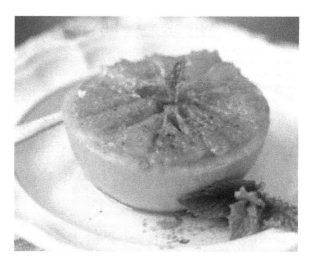

Ingredients

- 1 red grapefruit, refrigerated

- aluminum foil

- 1 tbsp. brown sugar

- 1/2 teaspoon ground cinnamon

- 1 tbsp. softened butter

- 2 tsp sugar

Instructions

➢ Cut grapefruit in half crosswise and slice off a thin sliver away from the base of every half, when the fruit is not sitting at level. Use a sharp paring knife to cut around the outer edge of this grapefruit and involve every section to generate the fruit easier to consume after cooking.

➢ Combine softened butter 1 tbsp. brown sugar in a small bowl. Spread mix over each grapefruit in half. Sprinkle with remaining brown sugar levels.

➤ Cut aluminum foil into two 5-inch squares and put each grapefruit half one square; fold the edges up to catch any juices. Place in the air fryer basket.

➤ Broil in the fryer until the sugar mixture is bubbling, 6 to 7 minutes.

47. Kale Crisps

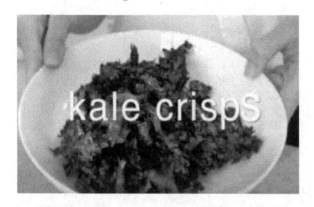

Ingredients:

- Kale

- Olive oil

- Salt

Method:

I'm going to make some kale crisps now. So, the first thing we're going to do list, get my kale and chop off the thick stocky bits. Once I've chopped that out, I will then just dice my kale up into kind of chunks and then I'll pop them into a bowl. Put some olive oil on top and some salts give everything a mix around.

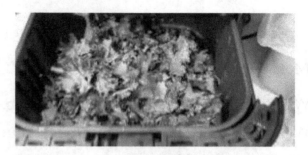

I'll pop them into my air fryer and on the prong setting. The reason I put them on the prong setting is because that's just a quick eight minute setting and that's the perfect amount of time that these kale crisps take to cook. When they come out, they are super nice and crunchy and they taste delicious.

48. Air Fryer Brown Sugar and Pecan Roasted Apples

A sweet and nutty topping made with brown sugar and pecans adds amazing flavor to apples since they cook to tender perfection at the air fryer.

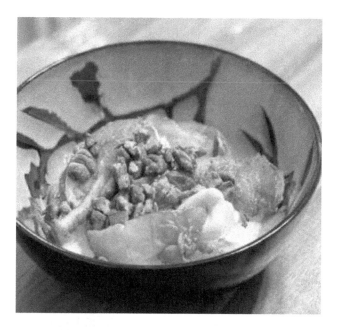

Ingredients

- 1/4 tsp apple pie spice

- 2 tbsp. coarsely chopped pecans

- 1 tbsp. brown sugar

- 1 tbsp. butter, melted

- 1 tsp all-purpose flour

- 2 medium apples, cored and cut into wedges

Instructions

→ Preheat the air fryer to 350 degrees F

→ Put apple wedges in a skillet drizzle with butter and toss to coat. Arrange apples in one layer in the air fryer basket and then sprinkle with pecan mixture.

→ Cook in the preheated air fryer until apples are tender, 10 to 15 minutes.

49. Sausage Rolls

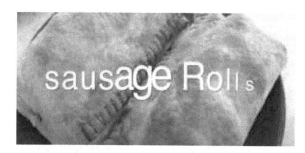

Ingredients:

- Sausage

- Puff pastry

- Cheese

- Chutney

- Milk

Methods:

Today we're going to make some really easy sausage rolls. So, I've just got some puff pastry and some sausages. What I'll do is I'll cut the puff pastry into four pieces. I'll then lay a sausage into each one of the pieces along with some grated cheese.

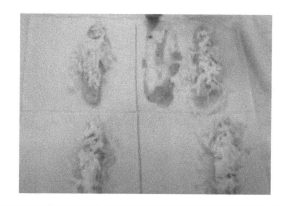

I like to have some chutney in the house as well. I'll just fold over the pastry and then secure it with a fork at the edges. So, it doesn't open up. I then just also get a bit of milk as well or you can use a beaten egg and just brush it over the top so it goes nice and golden brown. I'll pop it into my air fryer on the chip setting because they do need a good18 minutes in there to make sure the sausages are nice and cooked.

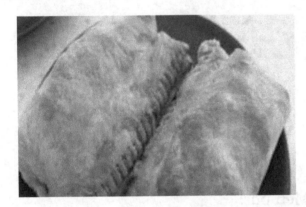

After the 18 minutes they're ready to eat.

50. Air Fryer French Fries

It will not get more classic than French fries; the normally accepted technique is fairly, dare I say, air tight, but I really do have one additional trick in shop! Last, dip them in honey mustard, hot ketchup, garlic aioli, or all 3 blended together, such as I did

Ingredients

- 1 lb. russet potatoes, peeled
- 1/2 tsp kosher salt
- 2 tsp vegetable oil
- 1 pinch cayenne pepper

Instructions

- ❖ Slice segments into sticks too around 3/8 inch-wide.
- ❖ Cover potatoes with water and let boil for 5 minutes to discharge excess starches.
- ❖ Drain and cover with boiling water with several inches (or put in a bowl of boiling water). Let sit for 10 minutes.
- ❖ Drain potatoes and move onto several paper towels. Transfer to a mixing bowl drizzle with oil, season with cayenne, and toss to coat.
- ❖ Stack potatoes in a dual layer in the fryer basket. Slide out basket and throw fries; keep frying until golden brown, about 10 minutes longer. Toss chips with salt in a mixing bowl.

51. Cheese on Toast

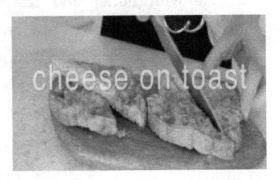

Ingredients:

- Bread

- Garlic butter

- cayenne pepper

Method:

I'm going to show you how to make a really quick and easy cheese on toast. How I make my cheese on toast is I get the bread and I put garlic butter on each side of the bread.

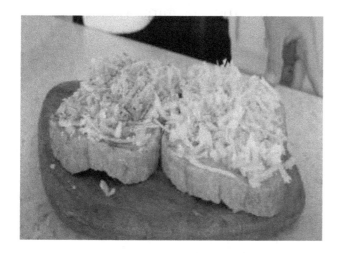

For me this is a very important step. I then grate quite a generous amount of cheese and then sprinkle it over the top. I will also add a little dash of cayenne pepper on top. Pop into my air fryer on the pizza button so that is for eight minutes at 160 degrees. Once the time is up, it comes out perfect every single time with a real nice crunchy piece of toast.

52. Tomato Pork Chops

It is a rather quick and easy recipe.

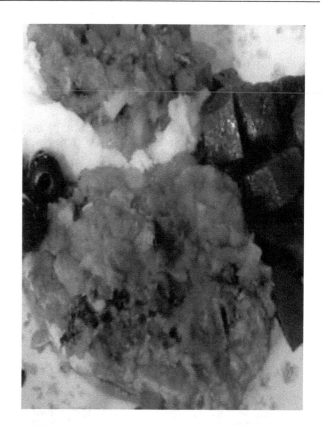

Ingredients

- 1 bell pepper - sliced, your color option

- 1 (15 oz.) can tomato sauce

- garlic powder to flavor

- 4 pork chops

- 1 tsp, sliced

- pepper and salt to taste

Directions

❖ Dredge the pork chops in flour, add to the pan and brown well on both sides.

❖ Add the onion and bell pepper, stir and cook for 5 minutes in the air fryer, or until nearly tender. Return pork chops to skillet and pour into the sauce. Permit the sauce to begin bubbling and reduce heat.

❖ Simmer for half an hour and season with garlic powder, pepper and salt to taste.

53. Veggie Egg Bread

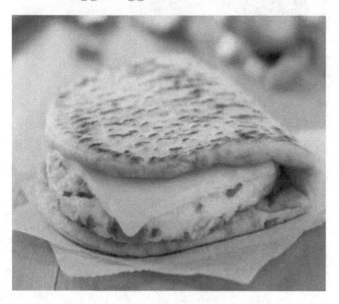

Ingredients:

- 1 tsp salt
- ½ pound cream cheese
- 10 eggs
- 4 cups grated zucchini
- 1 cup grated cheddar cheese
- ½ cup chopped tomatoes
- ½ tsp ground black pepper
- ½ cup sliced mushrooms, cooked
- ½ cup almond flour
- 2 tsp baking powder

Directions

❖ Be sure the pan will fit on your air fryer- normally a seven inch round pan will do the job flawlessly.

❖ Stir together the almond milk, pepper, salt and baking powder.

❖ In another bowl, beat the cream cheese until its smooth and nice afterward insert the eggs. Beat until well blended.

❖ Add the zucchini into the cream cheese mixture and stir until incorporated.

❖ Add the dry mix to the cream cheese jar and then stir well.

❖ Pour into the prepared pan and then cook at the fryer for 45 minutes

54. Easy Muffins

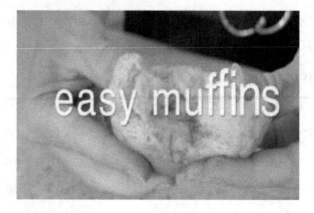

Ingredients:

- Sugar
- Butter

- Flour

- Eggs

- Milk

- Salt

Method:

We're going to make cupcakes. I have got a hundred grams of sugar, 250 grams of butter, 250 grams of flour, 4 eggs, a splash of milk and a dash of salt. We're just going to whisk this all up. I have got some of these cupcake holders. They're silicon ones. I'm going to add it to those and then we'll put them into the air fryer on the cupcake setting and let them cook away.

55. Almond Flour Pancake

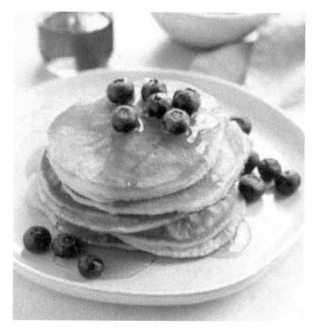

Ingredients:

- 1 teaspoon vanilla extract

- 1 1/4 cup almond milk

- two Tbsp. granulated erythritol

- 1 teaspoon baking powder

- 2 eggs

- 1/2 cup whole milk

- 2 Tbsp. butter, melted

- 1/8 tsp salt

Directions

❖ Be sure the pan will fit on your air fryer- normally a seven inch round pan will do the job flawlessly.

❖ Put the eggs, butter, milk and vanilla extract in a blender and puree for around thirty minutes.

❖ Add the remaining ingredients into the blender and puree until smooth.

❖ Pour the pancake batter to the prepared pan and set from the fryer.

❖ Cook for 2 minutes or until the pancake is puffed and the top is gold brown.

❖ Slice and serve with keto sugar free!

56. Zucchini and Bacon Egg Bread

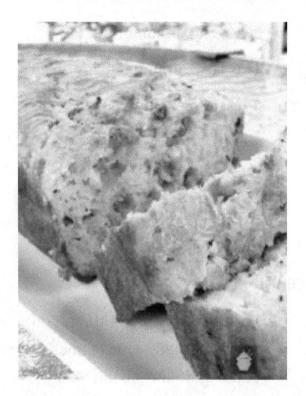

Ingredients:

- ½ cup almond flour

- 1 tsp salt

- ½ pound cream cheese

- 10 eggs

- 2 tsp baking powder

- ½ tsp ground black pepper

- 1 pound bacon cooked and crumbled

- 4 cups grated zucchini

- 1 cup grated cheddar cheese

Directions

- ❖ Be sure the pan will fit on your air fryer- normally a seven inch round pan will do the job flawlessly.

- ❖ Stir together the almond milk, pepper, salt and baking powder.

- ❖ In another bowl, beat the cream cheese until its smooth and nice afterward insert the eggs. Beat until well blended.

- ❖ Add the zucchini into the cream cheese mixture and stir until incorporated.

- ❖ Add the dry mix to the cream cheese jar and then stir well.

- ❖ Pour into the prepared pan and then cook at the fryer for 45 minutes

57. Raspberry Almond Pancake

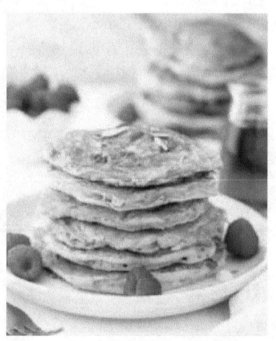

Ingredients:

- 1/2 cup whole milk

- 2 Tbsp. butter, melted

- 1 teaspoon almond extract

- 2 eggs

- two Tbsp. granulated erythritol

- 1 teaspoon baking powder

- 1/8 tsp salt

- 1 1/4 cup almond milk

- 1/4 cup frozen or fresh desserts

Directions

I. Preheat your air fryer to 420 degrees F and line a baking pan using parchment paper. Be sure the pan will fit on your air fryer- normally a seven inch round pan will do the job flawlessly.

II. Put the eggs, butter, milk and almond extract in a blender and puree for around thirty minutes.

III. Add the remaining ingredients into the blender and puree until smooth.

IV. Pour the pancake batter to the pan and stir in the raspberries

V. Lightly.

VI. Put in the fryer.

VII. Slice and serve with keto sugar free!

58. **Maple Brussel Sprout Chips**

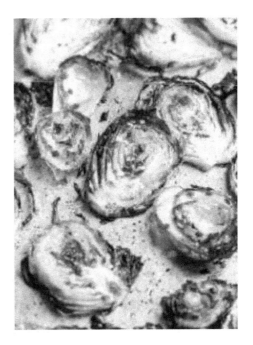

Ingredients:

- 2 Tbsp. olive oil

- 1 tsp sea salt

- 1 Pound Brussel Sprouts, ends removed

- 1 tsp maple extract

Method:

➢ Preheat your air fryer to 2400 degrees F and line the fryer tray with parchment paper.

➢ Peel the Brussels sprouts leaf at a time, putting the leaves in a massive bowl as you pare them.

➢ Toss the leaves using the olive oil, maple extract and salt then disperse onto the prepared tray.

➤ Bake for 15 minutes at the fryer, tossing halfway through to cook evenly.

➤ Serve warm or wrap in an airtight container after chilled.

59. Sweet and Tangy Apple Pork Chops

That is a recipe that I made using the thought that apples and pork go beautifully together! The seasonings provide the pork a pleasant and slightly spicy flavor. The apple cider increases the sweetness, while still bringing an exceptional tartness, since it's absorbed into the meat. Serve with applesauce, if wanted. Hope you like it!

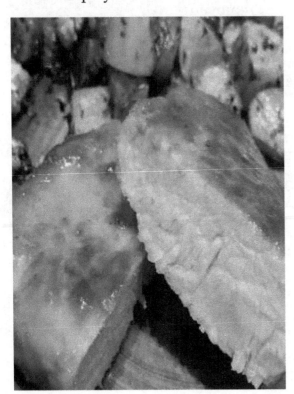

Ingredients:

- 3 tbsp. brown sugar
- 1/2 tsp garlic powder
- 2 tbsp. honey mustard
- 1 tsp mustard powder
- 1/2 teaspoon ground cumin
- 1 lb. pork chops
- 2 tbsp. butter
- 1/2 tsp cayenne pepper (Optional)
- 3/4 cup apple cider

Instructions

❑ Mix brown sugar, honey mustard, mustard powder, cumin, cayenne pepper, and garlic powder together in a small bowl. Rub pork chops and let sit on a plate for flavors to split into pork chops, about 10 minutes.

❑ Melt butter in a large skillet over moderate heat; include apple cider. Organize coated pork chops from the skillet;

❑ Cook until pork chops are browned, 5 to 7 minutes each side.

60. Maple Brussel Sprout Chips

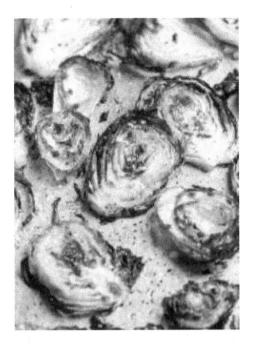

Ingredients:

- 2 Tbsp. olive oil

- 1 tsp sea salt

- 1 Pound Brussel Sprouts, ends removed

- 1 tsp maple extract

Method:

- ➢ Preheat your air fryer to 2400 degrees F and line the fryer tray with parchment paper.

- ➢ Peel the Brussels sprouts leaf at a time, putting the leaves in a massive bowl as you pare them.

- ➢ Toss the leaves using the olive oil, maple extract and salt then disperse onto the prepared tray.

- ➢ Bake for 15 minutes at the fryer, tossing halfway through to cook evenly.

- ➢ Serve warm or wrap in an airtight container after chilled.

61. Blueberry Pancake

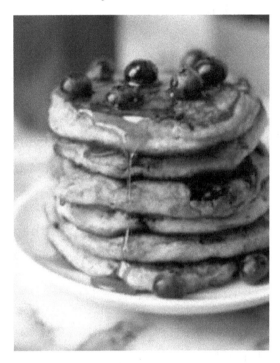

Ingredients:

- 2 Tbsp. butter, melted

- 1 teaspoon vanilla extract

- 1 1/4 cup almond milk

- 2 eggs

- 1 teaspoon baking powder

- 1/8 tsp salt

- 1/4 cup frozen or fresh blueberries

- 1/2 cup whole milk

- Two Tbsp. granulated erythritol

Directions

1. Preheat your air fryer to 400 degrees F and line a baking pan using parchment paper. Be sure the pan will fit on your fryer- normally a seven inch round pan will do the job flawlessly.

2. Put the eggs, butter, milk and vanilla extract in a blender and puree for around thirty minutes.

3. Add the remaining ingredients into the blender and puree until smooth.

4. Pour the pancake batter to the pan and stir in the blueberries

5. Put in the fryer.

6. Slice and serve with keto sugar free!

62. Chocolate Croissants

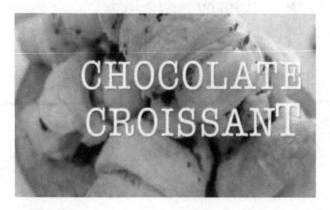

Ingredients

- Puff pastry

- Flake chocolate

Method:

I wanted to show you how to make some chocolate croissants in your air fryer as well. So, what I have got here is one roll of puff pastry and then to go on top to make it chocolatey, I have got some flake chocolate. What I'm going to do is roll out my puff pastry and then I'm going to crumble some flake chocolates all over the pastry.

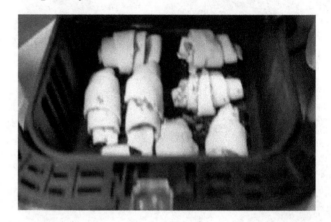

I'm then going to cut my pastry into eight. I'm going to cut them into fours and then I'll cut each four diagonally and then I'll roll them up into a croissant shape. Pop them into my air fryer, cook them on the muffin button which is a twelve minutes setting and then when they come out they are really really nice, chocolatey and delicious.

63. Strawberry Pancake

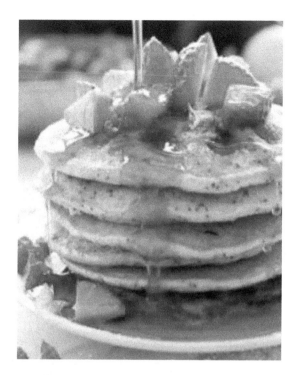

Ingredients:

- 1 teaspoon baking powder

- 1/8 tsp salt

- 1/4 cup fresh chopped tomatoes

- 2 eggs

- 1 teaspoon vanilla extract

- 1 1/4 cup almond milk

Directions

I.   Pre-heat the air fryer for around 15 minutes.

II. Put the eggs, butter, milk and vanilla extract in a blender and simmer for about half an hour.

III. Add the remaining ingredients into the blender and puree until smooth.

IV. Pour the pancake batter to the pan and stir in the berries gently.

V.   Put in the fryer.

VI. Slice and serve with keto sugar free!

64. Cheesy Zucchini Bake

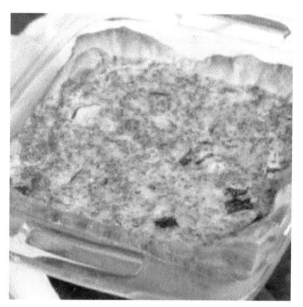

Ingredients:

- 2 tsp baking powder

- ½ tsp ground black pepper

- 1 tsp salt

- ½ cup almond flour

- 4 cups grated zucchini

- ½ pound cream cheese

- 10 eggs

- 1 cup grated cheddar cheese

Method:

1.   Be sure the pan will fit on your air fryer- normally a seven inch round

pan will do the job flawlessly. If it's possible to fit a bigger pan, then do so!

2. Stir together the almond milk, pepper, salt and baking powder.

3. In another bowl beat the cream cheese until its smooth and nice afterward insert the eggs. Beat until well blended.

4. Add the zucchini into the cream cheese mixture and stir until incorporated.

5. Add the dry mix to the cream cheese jar and then stir well.

6. Pour into the prepared pan and then cook at the fryer for 45 minutes.

65. Basil-Garlic Grilled Pork Chops

I had been tired of the exact same old agendas, and opted to try out something new... WOW! These chops are excellent!! They're fantastic for casual entertaining or family dinner. Together with the fresh basil and grated garlic, the taste is quite refreshing! Everybody will adore these!

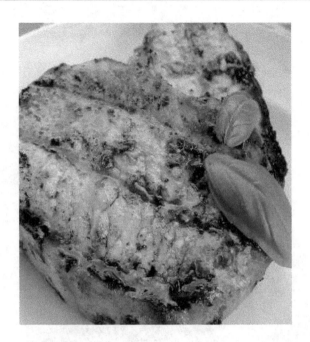

Ingredients

- 4 (8 ounce) pork chops
- 4 cloves garlic, minced
- ¼ cup chopped fresh basil
- 1 lime, juiced
- salt and black pepper to taste

Instructions

❖ Toss the pork chops with all the carrot juice in a bowl until evenly coated. Toss with ginger and garlic. Season the chops to taste with pepper and salt. Set aside to marinate for half an hour.

❖ Cook the pork chops on the fryer till no longer pink at the middle, 5 to 10 minutes each side.

66. Full English breakfast

Full English breakfast is one that my family really really likes. We have lived in England for a while so my kids really look forward to Saturday morning so that we make full English breakfast. However today I'm going to be showing you a special way to make it stress free.

I'm going to be starting off with the hash browns.

Ingredients:

- Potatoes
- Cheese
- Egg
- Salt
- Pepper
- Chili Flakes
- Sausage

Method:

So, the hash brownies are going to be composed of potatoes. I'm going to be using two, then I'm also going to be using cheese. This is shredded cheese and this is like the equivalent of one and a half cups of cheese. We are also going to be using one egg, this is one raw egg and some all-purpose flour, and this is the equivalent of two huge teaspoons of flour. We will be using some pepper along with chili flakes and finally of

course some salt to taste. Right, so these are the ingredients that I'm going to be using for the hash browns.

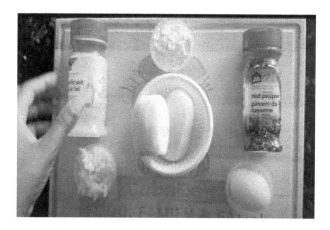

Before we start off with hash browns let's move on to all the other ingredients or condiments that are going to make up the English breakfast so part of the traditional ones we also use would be the eggs so this will make up we're going to make sunny side up eggs I'm going to be using some tomatoes some sausage, so this is not this is not the same way you have a traditional English breakfast.

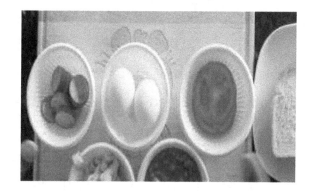

This isn't the same kind of way the sausage is or the way to slice but this is fine. Then we're going to be including baked beans right. So, this is a shop bought and actually there's still one more ingredient I'm going to be using: bacon. This is raw thinly sliced bacon and we have two slices of bread right. So, that's all the components or the condiments are going to go into the full English breakfast.

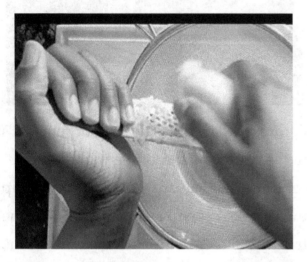

Let's start off straight away with the hash browns because all these other things are pretty much ready to go. Let's start with the preparation of the hash browns. So the first thing I'm going to be doing to grate the potatoes. With grated you can use any size. I want to use the really thin size because I want it more or less almost if it's already mashed or boiled. Because I'm going to be putting it in an array, I want it to take as little time as possible in order to get the potatoes done. If you've had English breakfast before let me know what you include or what you remove. I know people have different types of English breakfast at different

times. Yeah, I know there's the black pudding, if you're a traditional English person you probably like black pudding instead.

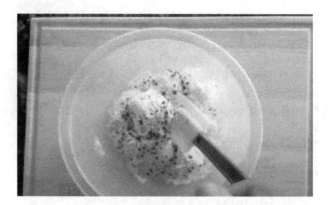

We're done with the grating of the potatoes and I've rinsed it out in sense that I've put some water in. I'm giving it a good squeeze to make sure all the water is gone. This helps to remove the majority of the starch in the potatoes. So it's completely up to you, if you want to skip this process in the sense that you want to rinse out some of the water from the potatoes. Okay so that done, the next thing we're going to move on to the mixing. I'm going to put in my flour. This is two teaspoons but it seems like I'm going to use only one. Then I remember eggs, had a full raw egg for my potato to make the hash browns. I also have some cheese, add some salt to taste and some chili flakes. I like something hot and spicy and yeah that's why I add that. So, I give this a really good mix for hash browns, people usually sometimes add butter so it's completely up to you what you want to include in your own hash browns. I'm just keeping my own soft shots sweet and simple. You can add or subtract as much as you want.

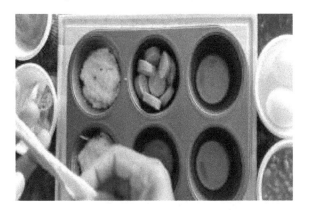

I'm going to give my tray a spray just to oil it, because what I'm going to do guys, this is something different. I'm going to start off with the hash browns. I'm putting everything and it's going to come out like a cup sort of like a cupcake, because my cans are a bit deep. I'm going to spread it into two sections right because I want it to cook all the way through so the potatoes are going to come out, sort of like a cupcake or potato cups. I'm also going to give this another spray right now, this is different.

I'm going to put in oops my sausages right, to line them all in here. As I'm using the air fryer for everything stress less so hopefully this should work for a bachelor or spencer or a small family or just making breakfast for somebody for

just one person in the family. This works pretty good. I'm going to put them in first so the next thing that is going to be included in the air fryer all three of them are going in now is the bacon. I'm going to put the bacon this way, alternatively, I could have chopped up the bacon and put them in one of these sections. Maybe I would actually just do that so that you have a look-see at its rest of the bacon. I'm just going to cut this one in here.

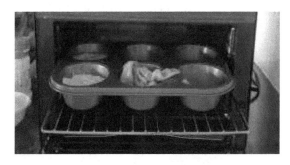

Throw it into the extra bit there again, I'm not going to be bothered about these bacon, because you know they're going to come up with their own oil. It's going to go into the air fryer oven. Put it in the air fryer oven and let it fry just turning the timer to one hour. It's an air fryer oven and the specific degree setting should be up on your screen and yeah so once this is ready again, like I said it's halfway into the cooking of the sausages of the hash browns and the bacon.

I'm now going to include the baked beans and the eggs because those ones will actually take less time compared to what you've got in the oven. I've had these in the air fryer and I can see that my bacon is coming out nicely.

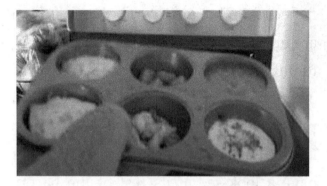

You see that so it depends on you if this is how you like your bacons this is the point in which you take them out. So, I'm just going to chuck the monotone section of the cupcake bits. What I'm going to do is to put the ones that are under done on the top and the ones that are already getting as crisp, I'm going to put them at the bottom. Now I'm just trying to get my stuff together. I'm scooping out all the sausages tone section so that I have two sections free for me to put my eggs and my baked beans. I'm going to have the egg sunny side up, I'm not going to spray the container again because all the bacon oil is in the egg, is in the cupcake holder. I'm just going to break two eggs and putting two into one section and then add some salt and some chili flakes. Our egg begins to cool, then I'm also going to put in the baked beans right in the final section. We are all good to go so

I just want to show you guys what it looks like.

We've got the eggs we've got the baked beans we've got everything in the section in the containers. I'm going to have the the tomatoes, I'm just going to line them on top here and yeah voila. I know for some people it's a lot of work but this is really stress less. The only bit where you have lots of work to do is with the grating of the potatoes and that's pretty much it. We're going to allow these now to cook all the way through by the time the egg is done and the baked paint is ready, the entire dish should be ready. We're about 30 minutes into the entire thing and it's looking really really good. I just want to bring this and mix up the sausages a bit, yeah and put this back because you need a couple of minutes to go. You can see the egg, you can see the bacon everything is looking wonderful. I'm going to move this all the way back because I want to put my tomatoes just to give it a little bit of somehow grilled max and then my bread right just to heat it up.

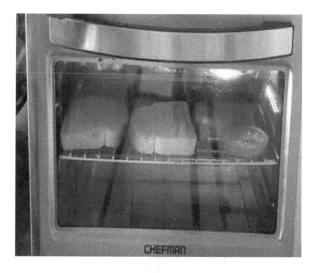

Let it give me somewhat like a mini toast. I'm going to shut this down now its done 30 minutes and it's done right. I'm not looking to get toasted bread but I just want this really warm. It's not toasted but it's warm and really crispy. I'm going to get the bread out of the way and the same thing with the tomatoes. So they're just warm so that when the breakfast is being eaten it's really nice and warm and fuzzy. Let's get onto plating it okay we are all ready, can you see that looks really good so and this is every single thing in one place right. So, our potatoes looks properly cooked a bit hot, our hash browns potatoes looks good and you can see our sausages. It did really really well cooked properly right and the same thing with the bacon so you can see all crispy or crunchy. I was able to achieve breakfast.

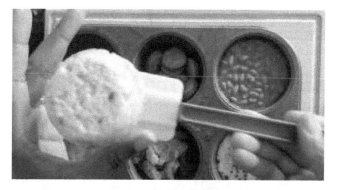

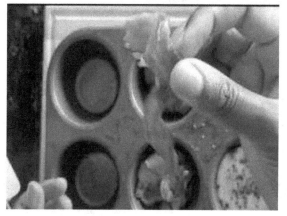

It took me about 30 minutes to make the entire dish so you can see my eggs yummy yummy yummy. I'm just going to dish this out and yeah so you can see the entire dish all presented for you. This is our English breakfast right you have the bread, we've got the bacon, I'm going to put in the sausages. This is a wonderful breakfast. All I really did was just to check it up at various times and baked beans is ready. This could actually is pretty decent meal and I think can it's perfect for more than one person. We have got egg there's not mushroom, there is no black pudding but this is completely fine the way it is right. So, this is what our full English breakfast looks like on some days and I've got the eggs, I've got the bacon, I still have some bacon there in the tray because I did make a lot so, still have some eggs.

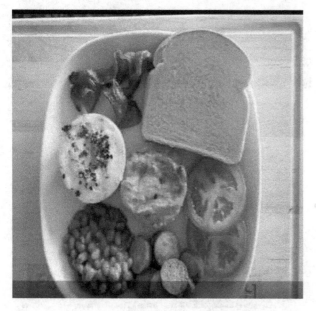

I have got some bacon some bread, yeah with a glass of milk or a cup of coffee you're good to go.

67. Garlic Brussel Sprout Chips

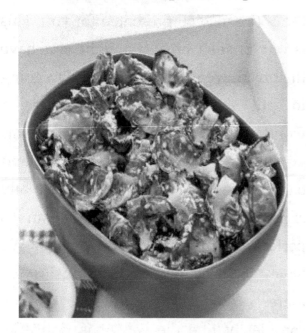

Ingredients:

- 1 tsp sea salt
- 1 Pound Brussel Sprouts, ends removed
- 2 Tbsp. olive oil
- 1 tsp garlic powder

Method:

- ❖ Preheat your air fryer to 2400 degrees F and line the fryer tray with parchment paper.
- ❖ Peel the Brussels sprouts leaf at a time, putting the leaves in a massive bowl as you pare them.
- ❖ Toss the leaves together with olive oil, garlic powder and salt then disperse onto the prepared tray.
- ❖ Bake for 15 minutes at the fryer, tossing halfway through to cook evenly.

68. Home and Asparagus

Ingredients:

- 1/4 teaspoon ground black pepper
- 1/4 tsp salt
- 1 lb. asparagus spears

Directions

- ❑ Preheat your air fryer to 400 degrees F and line your fryer tray using a
- ❑ Set the cod filets onto the parchment and sprinkle with the

pepper and salt and rub the spices to the fish.

❏ Top the fish with the remaining components then wrap the parchment paper around the fish filets, surrounding them entirely.

❏ Put the tray in the fryer and bake for 20 minutes.

69. Herbed Parmesan Crackers

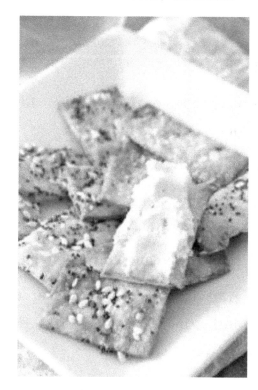

Ingredients:

- 2 Tbsp. Italian seasoning
- ½ cup chia seeds
- 1 ½ cups sunflower seeds
- 1 egg
- 2 Tbsp. butter, melted
- Salt

- ½ tsp garlic powder
- ½ tsp baking powder
- ¾ cup parmesan cheese, grated

Method:

❏ Set the sunflower seeds and chia seeds in a food processor until finely mixed to a powder. Put into a large bowl.

❏ Add the cheese, Italian seasoning, garlic powder and baking powder to the bowl and combine well.

❏ Add the melted butter and egg and stir till a wonderful dough forms.

❏ Put the dough onto a sheet of parchment and then put the following slice of parchment on top.

❏ Roll the dough into a thin sheet around 1/8 inch thick.

❏ Remove the top piece of parchment and lift the dough with the underside parchment and set onto a sheet tray which can fit in the air fryer.

❏ Score the cracker dough to your desired shape and bake for 40-45cminutes.

❏ Break the crackers aside and enjoy!

70. Salmon and Asparagus

Ingredients:

- ¼ tsp ground black pepper
- 1 ¾ pound salmon fillets
- ¼ tsp salt
- 1 pound asparagus spears
- 1 Tbsp. lemon juice
- 1 Tbsp. fresh chopped parsley
- 3 Tbsp. olive oil

Method

→ Preheat your air fryer to 400 degrees F and line your fryer tray using a long piece of parchment paper.

→ Set the salmon filets onto the parchment and sprinkle with the salt and pepper and rub the spices to the fish.

→ Top the fish with the rest of the ingredients then wrap the parchment paper around the fish filets, surrounding them completely.

→ Put the tray in the fryer and bake for 20 minutes.

71. Super Seed Parmesan Crackers

Ingredients:

- ½ tsp baking powder
- 1 egg
- 2 Tbsp. butter, melted
- 1 cups sunflower seeds
- ¾ cup parmesan cheese, grated
- 2 Tbsp. Italian seasoning
- ½ cup chia seeds
- ½ cup hulled hemp seeds
- ½ tsp garlic powder
- Salt

Method:

★ Preheat your air fryer to 300 degrees F.

★ Put into a large bowl.

★ Add the cheese, Italian seasoning, garlic powder and baking powder to the bowl and combine well.

★ Add the melted butter and egg and stir till a wonderful dough forms.

★ Put the dough onto a sheet of parchment and then put the following slice of parchment on top.

★ Roll the dough into a thin sheet around 1/8 inch thick.

★ Remove the top piece of parchment and lift the dough with the underside parchment and set onto a sheet tray which will fit from the air fryer.

★ Score the cracker dough to your desired shape and bake for 40-45 minutes.

★ Break the crackers aside and enjoy!

Conclusion

We have included 70 best recipes for you in this book. So, just try it out and then give us feedback with images of cooking.

Breville Smart Air Fryer Oven Cookbook

BY

Mark
Machino

Table of Contents

Introduction

A convenient way to prepare tasty, nutritious meals is the Breville Air Fryer Cooker. The system uses powerful warm air to flow around and cook foods, instead of cooking in a hot and oil fat meal. Which makes it easier to be crispy on the surface of the food to ensure sure the inner layers are cooked thru. The Breville Air Fryer Oven helps us to cook several dishes and almost everything. The Breville Air Fryer Oven may be used for frying beef, seafood, herbs, berries, poultry, and a broad selection of desserts. All your meals, ranging from appetizers to main meals and desserts, can be packed. Homemade or even tasty desserts and cakes are even permitted in the Breville Air Fryer Oven. Benefits of the Breville Air Fryer Oven:- Cleaner, oil-free foods- By inner filters of air, it removes cooking odors- Allows cleaning simpler free of oil- Air Fryers can bake, barbecue, roast more choices- A better cooking process opposed to frying with exposed warm oil- seems to have the potential to put and quit than other versions and provides a digital time.

To cook and crisp food that people put in a basket within the unit, air fryers use rotating warm air and oil. People might want to suggest introducing the fryer to their kitchen equipment collection. It is a relatively modern appliance that helps make healthy versions of the fried foods you love, from French fries to chicken nuggets, and is common. "Robin Plotkin, a licensed dietitian and culinary nutritionist located in Dallas, says, "The appeal is that it is a modern way to be 'healthier.' "This is a pleasant new way to achieve the objectives they are seeking to attain without getting depressed, particularly for people adopting low-carb diets."

The air fryer operates and lies on the countertop like a conventional oven. To cook and crisp the food in the basket inside, it uses swirling hot air and some oil. Without adding some gasoline, you can do it, or you can put a bit, which Plotkin says usually enhances the taste. "If people don't consume the food, diet doesn't matter, because people just want the food to taste good, and that's where I'd suggest you need some oil to appreciate the meal," she says. Either way, lowering the amount of oil consumed can decrease fat and calorie consumption. Instead of cooking meat, the Cleveland Clinic reports that air frying can help you reduce your calorie consumption by 80 - 85%. Jane Pelcher,

RDN, a Mountain View, California-based recipe creation and fitness writer, claims it is one of the finest kitchen appliances. "It's simple to use and in far less than halves the time that it takes in the oven, I can air-fried my rice," she says. According to the Cleveland Clinic, the consequence is food that is crispy on the outside and juicy on the ground. Keeping things safe is about the meals you produce. "It depends on what you placed in there, whether the air fryer is safe or not," Pelcher says. Quite certainly, frozen ready - to - cook fish sticks, chips, and wings is thoroughly fried in advance, but warming them high in an air fryer would not make them good. The nutritious way to go is to roast new tomatoes and broccoli, air fried raw proteins, and produce fries from scratch.

A better option to deep frying is the air fryer, although that does not render it the healthful form of cooking anywhere. The Cleveland Clinic warns that air frying can cause people to believe it's fine to eat fried food as often as they should. "If you consume this kind of meal over and over again, it would not be as good for you as you initially meant it to be," says Plotkin. "Eat it from time to time, play with it, prepare with that as well, and make it part of your toolbox for food."

Like those from brands such as Cuisinart, Philips, and NuWave, many air fryers are on the market. 6 They vary from around $60 to $360 in volume. For individuals living in tiny spaces with no oven or stove, such as college students living in dorms, Pelcher says they can be fantastic. The quantity of counter room you have is one factor you will want to remember since they come in multiple sizes. When picking the best air fryer, also remember life. e.g., a tiny one, whether you would like to support a family, maybe challenging, Plotkin says. According to the Cleveland Clinic, most people will cook around 2 - 3 lbs. at a time. Conclude, Plotkin claims that hers is quick and clear to scrub. Pelcher says there is typically a flexible basket bottom for the higher-end fryers that helps wash and extract food from each inch of the air fryer basket. Many lacking a flexible base are often more challenging to scrub, but the key should be to soak it for a prolonged amount of time in hot soapy water.

In recent years, air fryer is becoming a common addition to kitchen utensils and does not indicate slowing or stopping. Whether you still spotted one below

Christmas tree, bought either from a sale on Cyber Monday, or treated yourself to your party, then you are in fortune. This air fryer can give you the capacity or cook tasty meals by producing a crispy coating with minimal or oil free meal. It will free up your place to a completely different era of recipes, and you will get a grasp of how to operate an air fryer. While you can believe that the air fryer is restricted to fried classics such as Fries or chicken nuggets, a broad range of dishes can be made. Whip up some freshly made mini apple pies, challenge your beloved Italian restaurant's eggplant Parmesan, or even replicate equal foods such as fried pickles.

If people want to make a crunchy meal, it is time for the air fryer to heat up and start cooking. In each group, we have combined up 5-6 of our favorite meals, so you have got a baseline to start your air frying adventure. These meals will expose to the strengths of the appliance, and you will soon be able to play with a large variety of air-fried foods.

With these unforgettable air fryer meals in the air fryer, launch the day off. These Breakfast Frittata or Scotch Eggs could hit the flavor if savory is what crave early in the morning. But if the taste is sweeter, stay with the Sugar Doughnuts or Simple French Toast Sticks. Many of these meals include components that can be cooked in the afternoon unless you are in a hurry around breakfast time.

When bad weather helps prevent from cooking outdoors, Steak is perfect. Both and Breaded Pork Chops and Crumbled Chicken are made in the oven quicker than frying. Plus, every time they fall out wet and delicate. If you want to surf more than turf, the famous seafood recipes are Coconut Shrimp and Salmon. Parmesan Eggplant is a guaranteed crowd-pleaser for a full vegetarian Air Fryer oven.

When cooking dinner, save the stovetop room by tossing a side meal into the air fryer. Ratatouille Italian-Style and Green Beans (spicy) both are recipes that, if overcooked, will quickly turn soggy, suggesting they are ideal for the air fryer. With this process, making Baked Potatoes guarantees a crispy, fluffy coating of skin, but every time, French fries do not have all the fun. If you are trying to make picky eater-friendly veggies, frying Roasted Cauliflower and Okra makes crunchy and tasty vegetables in the air fryer. Corn in the air fryer on the Cob offers it the perfect feel, although the grilled flavor can be added with a splashing of paprika.

If someone is preparing treats for a Movie evening or looking for appetizers or snacks to serve at a picnic, the latest take-to for finger foods would be the air fryer. French Fries are the main food that most people attempt in an air fryer, and with valid reason: with a little oil usually used; hence, get crunchy and golden fries. Cheese and Sausage Filled Chicken Wings or small Peppers are also sophisticated enough to function as hors d'oeuvres, but still low-key enough as to serve at your next tailgate. Because people are hoping to bend fast food cravings, it's sure to please cooking up a bowl of Onion Rings, Mozzarella Sticks, or Fried Pickles.

And sweets, when it happens to an air fryer, work out delicious. Take typically deep-fried meals such as Beignets, or Fried chocolate bars or Apple pies to get crispy outside and tender indoors for a turn in the air fryer. For a moister product, producing baked products, such as Butter and Banana Cake, Roasted bananas served with a splashing of cinnamon or confectioner's sugar is a perfect way to finish your meal if you want to serve a nutritious dessert.

Chapter 1: Health Benefits of Air and Deeply Fried Meals

Air frying is, on certain standards, easier than frying in grease. It decreases calories by 60 to 90% and has a ton of fat. This form of cooking may also minimize any of the other adverse consequences of oil processing when you fried potatoes or other starchy foods, the reaction that occurs creates the organic acrylamide, which literature ties to higher cancer risks. One research reveals that acrylamide volume in fried potatoes is decreased by 89 percent by air frying. Any air-frying stuff might not be good. Air frying of fish improved the quantity of a material labeled 'cholesterol oxidation products' (COPs) in one report. COPs develop as, during frying, the cholesterol in fish or meat breaks down. Studies relate these compounds to cardiovascular disease, cancer, artery hardening and other diseases.

The study reveals that one way to reduce the number of COPs when you air-fried fish is to incorporate chives, parsley, or a combination of the two. Analysis reveals that these herbs function in air-fried foods as antioxidants. It also suggests that air frying curbs the saturated omega-3 fats in trout. These "healthy fats" help reduce blood pressure and increase the amounts of "healthy" HDL cholesterol, protecting the core.

The batter consumes the oil that is used to prepare it when fried the rice. This makes fried foods on the outside their happy crunch while holding the inward soft. Frying often adds a deep, dark coloring to foods that are appealing to the eyes. You can get a crunch with air frying, but it doesn't produce the same look or sound of the mouth like oil frying. One research contrasting oil frying with air frying showed that the two approaches contributed to foods with varying textures and sensory properties, but with a similar color and moisture content.

1.1 Statistics of Deeply Fried Foods

Generally, deep-fried foods are rich in calories than foods cooked with other types of frying. For instance, about 30 percent more fat is contained in a chicken breast that has been frying than an equivalent amount of roasted chicken. Some manufacturers say that fried foods' saturated fat can be decreased by up to 75% using an air fryer. It is due to air fryers need considerably reduced fat than conventional deep fryers. Although many recipes need up to 3 cups of oil for deeply fried dishes, just around 1 tablespoon of air-fried food is required. This indicates that deep fryers require up to 49 times much more oil than air fryers, and although the product consumes not all of the oil, the total fat content of the meal will be decreased when utilizing an air fryer.

1.2 Comparison of Deeply Fried and Air Fried Meals

One research contrasted the properties of deeply fried & air-fried fries said that a finished product of considerably reduced fat but a higher color and water absorption rate resulted from air-frying. As a larger consumption of fatty acids from vegetable oils has also been linked with a higher risk of conditions such as heart failure and arthritis, this may have a direct influence on your wellbeing. Not only are deeply fried meals rich in calories, but they are often higher in fat, which causes weight gain. Dietary fat produces almost twice as much energy per serving as other essential nutrients such as carbohydrates and protein, weighing in at 8.9 calories throughout. Since air-fried meals are low in saturated fat than deeply fried items, it can be a convenient way to reduce calories and facilitate weight reduction by converting to an electric oven.

Frying meals may produce toxic compounds such as acrylamide and become rich in calories and fats. Acrylamide is a substance produced during higher heating and cooking procedures such as frying in carbohydrate-rich meals. Acrylamide is listed as a 'probable carcinogen,' as per the International Organization for Testing on Cancer, indicating that certain research suggests that acrylamide could be related to cancer growth. Rather than using a deep fryer, wind frying food can help reduce acrylamide content in fried foods. It's important to note, though, that other hazardous substances can also be produced during the air-frying process.

Chapter 2: Breakfast & Main Dishes

1. Ninja Foodi Low-Carb Breakfast Casserole

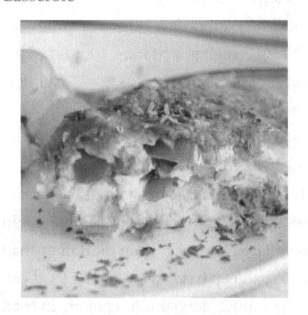

Ingredients

- ❖ Ground Sausage 1 LB
- ❖ Shredded Cheese 1/2 Cup
- ❖ Green Bell Pepper 1 Diced
- ❖ Eggs 8 Whole
- ❖ Diced White Onion 1/4 Cup
- ❖ Garlic Salt 1/2 Tsp
- ❖ Fennel Seed 1 Tsp

Steps

1. Add the pepper and onion and steam till the vegetables are soft and the sausage is fried, along with the ground sausage.

2. Spray it with non-stick cooking spray using the Air Fryer pan.

3. Position the bottom part with the ground sausage mixture.

4. Marinade equally with cheese.

5. Over the cheese and bacon, place the pounded eggs equally.

6. Similarly, sprinkle fennel seed and garlic salt to the chickens.

7. In the Ninja Foodi, put the rack in the low spot and put the pan on top.

8. Set at 390 degrees for 15 minutes on Air Crisp.

9. If you use an air fryer, put the dish directly in the air fryer's basket and cook at 390 degrees for 15 minutes.

10. Remove carefully and serve.

2. Air Fryer Breakfast Sausage

Ingredients

- ❖ Pork 1 lb.
- ❖ Fennel seeds 2 tsp
- ❖ Turkey 1 lb. ground
- ❖ Paprika 1 tsp
- ❖ Rubbed sage 2 tsp
- ❖ Sea salt 1 tsp

- ❖ Maple syrup 1 tbsp

- ❖ Dried thyme 1 tsp

- ❖ Garlic powder 2 tsp

Steps

1. Start by combining in a wide bowl the pork and turkey together. Mix the remaining ingredients in a shallow bowl: sage, fennel, ground garlic, paprika, thyme, and cinnamon. Add spices into the meat and keep combining until the spices are thoroughly added.

2. Spoon into balls and flatten into patties (about 2-3 tbsp of meat).

3. At 370 degrees, set the temperature and heat for 10 minutes. Remove and repeat for the leftover sausage from the air fryer.

3. Air Fryer Avocado Boats

Ingredients

- ❖ Avocados 2

- ❖ Plum tomatoes 2

- ❖ Lime juice 1 tbsp

- ❖ Red onion ¼ cup

- ❖ Black pepper ¼ tsp

- ❖ Jalapeno 1 tbsp

- ❖ Fresh sliced cilantro 2 tbsp

- ❖ Eggs 4 medium

- ❖ Salt ½ teaspoon

Steps

1. Squeeze the avocado pulp out from the skin with a spoon, leaving the shell intact. Dice the avocado and put it in a medium dish. Combine the peppers, onion, lime juice, cilantro, salt, and jalapeno, if needed. Cover and refrigerate the combination of avocado until fit for usage.

2. Heat the air fryer to 350 degrees Fahrenheit.

3. Put them on a foil ring to make sure the avocado shells wouldn't rock when frying. Simply wrap two 3-inch-wide strips of aluminum foil into rope shaped to build them, and form each into a 3-inch circle. In an air fryer bowl, put every avocado shell on a foil frame. Break 1 egg into each avocado shell and fried for 5 to 7 minutes or until the doneness is needed.

4. Remove from the basket; cover with salsa with avocado and eat.

4. Air Fryer Breakfast Stuffed Peppers

Ingredients

- ❖ Bell pepper 1

- ❖ Olive oil 1 tsp

❖ Salt 1 pinch

❖ Eggs 4

Steps

1. Lengthwise, split bell peppers in half and discard the seeds and base, keeping the sides as bowls intact.

2. Rub a little of olive oil only on the raw edges using your finger.

3. Crack 2 eggs into each half of the bell pepper. Sprinkle with the spices you desire.

4. Set them within your Ninja Foody on a trivet.

5. Close the cover (the one attached to your Ninja Foody machine) on the air fryer.

6. Switch on the computer, click the air crisper button for 13 minutes at 390 degrees.

7. Add the bell pepper and less brown egg on the exterior, add just one egg to the pepper and set the air fryer for 15 minutes to 330 degrees. (for consistency over hard eggs)

5. Air Fryer Breakfast Pockets

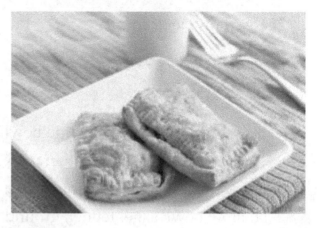

Ingredients

❖ Pastry sheets 1 box

❖ Sausage crumbles ½ cup

❖ Cheddar cheese ½ cup

❖ Bacon ½ cup

❖ Eggs 5

Steps

1. Eggs should be cooked like regular scrambled eggs. If needed, add meat to the egg mixture as you cook.

2. On a cutting board, lay out puff pastry sheets and slice out rectangles with a cookie blade, make sure they are all standardized enough to come together well.

3. On half of the pastry rectangles, Spoon chose a mixture of beef, milk, and cheese.

4. Cover the mixture with a pastry rectangle and press the sides together with a fork to cover.

5. Put breakfast pockets in an air-fryer basket and cook at 370 degrees for 8-10 minutes.

6. Monitor closely and test for ideal every 2-3 minutes.

6. Air Fryer Bacon and Egg Breakfast Biscuit Bombs

Ingredients

- ❖ Eggs 2
- ❖ Biscuit bombs
- ❖ Bacon 4 pieces
- ❖ Butter 1 tablespoon
- ❖ Pillsbury 1 can
- ❖ Pepper 1 teaspoon
- ❖ Egg 1
- ❖ Water 1 tablespoon
- ❖ Cheddar cheese 2 oz

Steps

1. Break the cooking parchment paper into two 8-inch rounds. Set one round at the bottom of the basket of the air fryer. Spray with spray for frying.

2. Cook the bacon over medium-high heat in a 10-inch nonstick skillet until crisp. Put on a paper towel, extract from the sauce. Wipe the pan gently with a paper towel. To the skillet, add butter; melt over medium heat. Add 2 pounded eggs and pepper to the skillet; boil until the eggs are thickened, stirring regularly, yet still moist. Remove from the heat; add bacon and swirl. Cool for five minutes.

3. Meanwhile, divide the dough into five biscuits; divide each biscuit into two layers. Push into a 4-inch round each. Spoon 1 into the middle of each circular heaping tablespoonful of the egg mixture. Cover it with one of the cheese bits. Fold the sides carefully up and over the filling, press to seal. Beat most of the egg and water in a shallow cup. Rub the biscuits with egg wash on both ends.

4. Put 5 of the biscuit bombs on the parchment in the air fryer bowl, seam side down. With cooking water, water all sides of the second round of parchment. Cover the second parchment round biscuit bombs in the bowl, then cover it with the leftover 5 biscuit bombs.

5. Set to 325 degrees F; cook for 8 minutes. Remove the circular parchment; use tongs to carefully transform the biscuits and position them in a single layer in the basket. Cook 5 minutes longer or (at least 165 ° F) before cooked through.

7. Air Fryer Breakfast Potatoes

Ingredients

- ❖ Potatoes 1 1/2 pounds
- ❖ Onion ¼ sliced
- ❖ Garlic cloves 2
- ❖ Green bell pepper 1
- ❖ Olive oil 1 Tablespoon
- ❖ Paprika 1/2 teaspoon
- ❖ Pepper 1/4 teaspoon
- ❖ Salt 1/2 teaspoon

Steps

1. Clean the potatoes and bell pepper.

2. Dice the potatoes and boil them for 30 minutes in water. Pat dry after 30 minutes.

3. Chop the mushrooms, cabbage, and bell pepper. Garlic is minced.

4. In a bowl, put all the ingredients and combine them. Put it into an air-fryer.

5. Cook in an air fryer for 10 minutes at 390-400 degrees. Move the bowl and cook for another 10 minutes, then lift the bowl again and cook for another 5 minutes, for a total of 25 minutes.

6. Only serve.

8. Breakfast Egg Rolls

Ingredients

- ❖ Salt and pepper
- ❖ Milk 2 T
- ❖ Eggs 2
- ❖ Cheddar cheese ½ cup
- ❖ Olive oil 1 tablespoon
- ❖ Egg rolls 6
- ❖ Sausage patties 2
- ❖ Water

Steps

1. Cook the sausage in a small skillet or replace it according to the packet. Remove and cut into bite-sized bits from the skillet.

2. Combine the chickens, sugar, and a touch of salt and pepper. Over medium / low flame adds a

teaspoon of oil or a little butter to a plate. Pour in the egg mixture and fry, stirring regularly to render scrambled eggs for a few minutes. Stir the sausage in. Only put back.

3. Put the egg roll wrapper on a working surface to create a diamond formation with points. Position roughly 1 T of the cheese on the bottom third of the wrapper. Comb with a blend of chickens.

4. Water the finger or pastry brush and rub all the egg roll wrapper's sides, allowing it to close.

5. Fold the egg roll up and over the filling at the bottom stage, attempting to keep it as close as you can. Then, fold the sides together to make an envelope-looking form. Last, tie the whole wrapping around the top. Put the seam side down and begin the remaining rolls to assemble.

6. Heat the fryer for 5 minutes to 400 F.

7. Rub rolls with grease or spray them. Placed the hot oven bowl in place. Set for 8 minutes to 400 F.

8. Flip over the egg rolls after 5 minutes. For a further 3 minutes, return the egg rolls to the air fryer.

9. Air Fryer Sausage Breakfast Casserole

Ingredients

- ❖ Onion ¼ cup
- ❖ Red Bell pepper 1
- ❖ Green Bell pepper 1
- ❖ Breakfast sausage 1 lb.
- ❖ Hash Browns 1 lb.
- ❖ Eggs 4
- ❖ Yellow Bell pepper 1

Steps

1. Foil fills the air fryer's basket.

2. Cover the uncooked sausage with it.

3. Put the peppers and onions uniformly on top.

4. Cook for 10 minutes at 355 *.

5. Open an air fryer and, if necessary, blend the casserole a little.

6. In a bowl, crack every egg, then pour it right in the middle of the casserole.

7. Cook for another 10 minutes on 355 *.

8. To try, mix with salt and pepper.

10. Air Fryer Egg in Hole

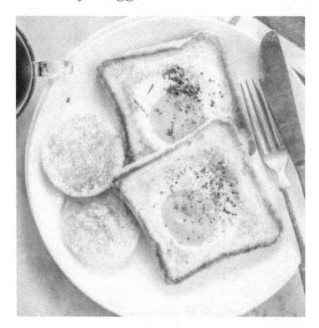

Ingredients

- ❖ Egg 1
- ❖ Salt and pepper
- ❖ Toast piece 1

Steps

1. Spray the safe pan of the air fryer with nonstick oil spray.

2. Put a slice of bread in a healthy pan inside the air fryer.

3. Create a spot, then slice the bread with a cup.

4. Into the hole, crack the egg.

5. Fry for 6 minutes at 330 degrees, then use a large spoon and rotate the egg and fry for another 4 minutes.

11. Air Fryer Baked Egg Cups with Spinach & Cheese

Ingredients

- ❖ Milk 1 tablespoon
- ❖ Cheese 1-2 teaspoons
- ❖ Egg 1 large
- ❖ Frozen spinach 1 tablespoon
- ❖ Cooking spray
- ❖ Salt and black pepper

Steps

1. Spray with oil spray inside the silicone muffin cups.

2. In a muffin cup, incorporate the cream, potato, spinach, and cheese.

3. Gently combine the egg whites with the liquids without separating the yolk and salt and pepper to taste.

4. For around 6-12 minutes, Air Fried at 330 ° F (single egg cups typically take about 5 minutes-several or doubled cups require as many as 12.

5. It may take a bit longer to cook in a ceramic ramekin. Cook for less time if you like runny yolks. After 5 minutes, regularly check the eggs to make sure the egg is of your desired texture.

12. Air Fryer French Toast Sticks

Ingredients

- ❖ Butter 2 tablespoon
- ❖ Salt 1 pinch
- ❖ Eggs 2
- ❖ Bread pieces 4
- ❖ Cinnamon 1 pinch
- ❖ Ground cloves 1 pinch
- ❖ Nutmeg 1 pinch
- ❖ Icing sugar 1 teaspoon

Steps

1. Heat the air fryer at 180 degrees centigrade.

2. Two eggs, a sprinkle of salt, a few hard-cinnamon shakes, and tiny pinches of both nutmeg and ground cloves are softly pounded together in a cup.

3. Butter all sides of the pieces of bread and break them into segments.

4. In the egg mixture, dredge-strip and place it in an air fryer.

5. After 2 minutes of frying, stop the air fryer, remove the pan, make sure you put the pan on a heat-safe surface and sprinkle the bread with cooking spray.

6. Flip and spray the second side till you have adequately sprayed the strips, as well.

7. Return the pan to the fryer and cook for another 4 minutes, testing after a few minutes to ensure that they are uniformly fried and not burnt.

8. Remove from the air fryer until the egg is fried, and the bread is golden brown and eat immediately.

9. Sprinkle with icing sugar for garnishing and serving, finish with ice cream, drizzle with maple syrup, or represent a little dipping cup of syrup.

13. Air Fryer Apple Fritters

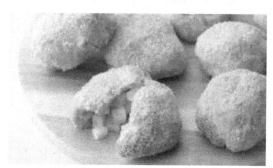

Ingredients

- ❖ Cooking spray
- ❖ Flour 1-1/2 cups
- ❖ Sugar 1/4 cup
- ❖ Baking powder 2 teaspoons
- ❖ Cinnamon 1-1/2 teaspoons

- ❖ Salt 1/2 teaspoon

- ❖ 2% Milk 2/3 cup

- ❖ Eggs 2 large

- ❖ 1 tablespoon lemon juice

- ❖ Honey Crisp apples 2 medium sliced

- ❖ Butter 1/4 cup

- ❖ Confectioners' sugar 1 cup

- ❖ 2% Milk 1 tablespoon

- ❖ Vanilla extract 1-1/2 teaspoons

Steps

1. Heat an air-fryer at 410 degrees.

2. Integrate the sugar, starch, baking powder, salt, and cinnamon in a wide dish. Transfer the milk, eggs, lemon juice and 1 teaspoon of vanilla extract leftover; whisk until it is moistened. Fold the apples in.

3. Drop 1/4 cup 2-in dough into batches. Detached from the air-fryer bowl. Spritz with spray for frying. Cook for 5-6 minutes till it is lightly browned. Switch the fritters over; proceed to fried for 1-2 minutes till lightly browned.

4. Melt butter over medium-high heat in a shallow saucepan. Cook gently for 5 minutes, before the butter and foam begins to tan. Remove from heat; mildly cold. Add browned butter with confectioner's sugar, milk and 1/2 teaspoon vanilla extract: whisk until smooth. Drizzle before serving over the fritters.

14. Air Fryer French Toast Sticks

Ingredients

- ❖ Bread pieces 4

- ❖ Eggs 2

- ❖ Salt and cinnamon 1 pinch

- ❖ Nutmeg 1 pinch

- ❖ Icing sugar 1 teaspoon

- ❖ Butter 2 tablespoon

Steps

1. Heat the air fryer at 180 degrees centigrade.

2. Two eggs, a sprinkle of salt, a few hard-cinnamon shakes, and tiny pinches of both nutmeg and ground cloves are softly pounded together in a cup.

3. Butter all sides of the pieces of bread and break them into segments.

4. In the egg mixture, dredge-strip and place it in an air fryer.

5. After 2 minutes of frying, stop the Air Fryer, remove the oil, make sure you put the oil on a heat-safe surface and sprinkle the bread with cooking spray.

6. Flip and spray the second side till you have adequately sprayed the strips, as well.

7. Return the pan to the fryer and cook for another 4 minutes, testing after a few minutes to ensure that they are uniformly fried and not burnt.

8. Take from the Air Fryer till the egg is fried, and the bread is lightly browned and eat immediately.

9. Sprinkle with icing sugar for garnishing and serving, finish with ice cream, drizzle with maple syrup, or represent a little dipping cup of syrup.

15. Air Fryer Breakfast Toad-in-the-Hole Tarts

Ingredients

❖ Frozen puff pastry 1 sheet
❖ Sliced cooked ham 4 tablespoons
❖ Cheddar cheese 4 tablespoons
❖ Sliced fresh chives 1 tablespoon
❖ Large Eggs 4

Steps

1. Heat up to 400 degrees F for the air fryer.

2. On a flat surface, spread the pastry sheet and break it into 4 squares.

3. In the air-fryer bowl, put 2 pastry squares and cook for 6 to 8 minutes.

4. Remove the air fryer from the bowl. To form an oval shape, use a metal tablespoon to press every square gently. In each hole, put 1 tbsp of Cheddar cheese and 1 tbsp of ham and pour 1 egg on top.

5. Move the basket back to the air fryer. Cook until necessary, around 6 more minutes. Take the tart out of the basket and let it cool for 5 minutes. With the leftover squares of pastry, cheese, ham, and eggs, repeat.

6. Tarts with chives to garnish.

16. Air Fryer Churros

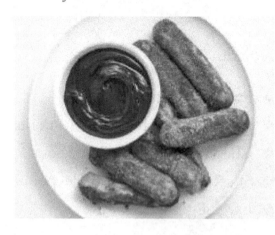

Ingredients

- ❖ Butter ¼ cup
- ❖ Salt 1 pinch
- ❖ Milk ½ cup
- ❖ Eggs 2 large
- ❖ Flour ½ cup
- ❖ Ground cinnamon ½ teaspoon
- ❖ White sugar ¼ cup

Steps

1. Melt butter on medium-high heat in a saucepan. Sprinkle with milk and apply salt. Lower the flame to low and carry it to a boil, stirring vigorously with a wooden spoon. Add flour easily all at a time. Keep stirring until it fits along with the pastry.

2. Turn off the heat and leave for 5 to 7 minutes to cool down. Mix the wooden spoon with the eggs before the pastry is blended. Spoon the dough into a pastry bag with a big star tip attached. Pipe the dough into strips directly into the basket of the air fryer.

3. Air fried the churros for 5 minutes at 340 degrees F.

4. Meanwhile, in a small bowl, combine the sugar and cinnamon and pour over a shallow plate.

5. Take the fried churros from the air fryer and roll them in the mixture of cinnamon-sugar.

17. Air Fryer Hard Boiled Eggs

Ingredients

- ❖ Eggs 4

Steps

1. To 250F / 120C, heat the air fryer.

2. In the air fryer bowl, put the wire rack and position the eggs on top.

3. For 16 minutes, cook.

4. To interrupt the frying method, extract the air fryer's eggs and quickly immerse them in ice water.

5. Peel and serve until cooled.

18. Air Fryer Omelette

Ingredients

- ❖ Salt 1 pinch
- ❖ Milk ¼ cup
- ❖ Eggs 2
- ❖ Shredded cheese ¼ cup
- ❖ Breakfast seasoning Garden herb 1 teaspoon
- ❖ Fresh meat and veggies

Steps

1. Mix the eggs and milk in a shallow bowl until well mixed.

2. Add the egg mixture with a sprinkle of salt.

3. Apply the egg mixture to vegetables.

4. Pour a well-greased 6"x3" pan into the egg mixture.

5. Place the pan in the air fryer's basket.

6. Cook for 8-10 minutes at 350 ° Fahrenheit.

7. Sprinkle the breakfast seasoning on the eggs and sprinkle the cheese over the surface midway during preparation.

8. Soften the omelet from the pan's sides with a thin spatula and pass it to a tray.

19. Air Fryer McDonald's Copycat Egg McMuffin

Ingredients

- ❖ Eggs 2
- ❖ Muffins 2
- ❖ Bacon 2 slices
- ❖ Cheese 2 slices

Steps

1. Heat the air fryer at 400 degrees.

2. Put foil on the rack.

3. Sprinkle the cooking oil spray.

4. Break one egg in every jar cover.

5. Put bacon on the rack.

6. Heat up to 5 mins and rotate the bacon.

7. Cook further for another 5 mins.

8. Take off the eggs.

9. Put sliced muffin in the air fryer and bake for 5 mins till light brown.

10. Place a piece of cheese on the muffin, bacon, and egg.

20. Air Fryer Breakfast Pizza

Ingredients

- ❖ Crescent Dough
- ❖ Eggs 3 scrambled
- ❖ Crumbled sausage
- ❖ Pepper 1/2 minced
- ❖ Cheddar cheese 1/2 cup
- ❖ Mozzarella cheese 1/2 cup

Steps

1. Sprinkle oil on the pan.

2. Spread out the dough in the lower layer of a pan.

3. Put the air fryer for 5 mins at 350 degrees till the upper layer is lightly browned.

4. Take off the air fryer.

5. Cover it with sausage, cheese, peppers, and eggs.

6. Put air fryer for extra 5-10 mins.

21. Air Fryer Cherry and Cream Cheese Danish

Ingredients

- ❖ Icing
- ❖ Pillsbury Crescent Rolls Dough
- ❖ Cream Cheese 8 oz
- ❖ Cherry Pie Filling 16 oz

Steps

1. Heat the air fryer at 350 degrees.

2. Wrapped out the crescent dough.

3. Wrap the very upper layer for one time. Packed the edges to make a circle and fill every roll with cream cheese.

4. Put an air fryer on a rack.

5. Heat up to 390 degrees for 10 mins.

6. The upper layer will become lightly browned.

7. Put foil on the top of the tray and heat again for extra 10 mins.

8. Take it off and drizzle with icing.

22. Air-Fryer Southern Bacon, Egg, and Cheese Breakfast Sandwich

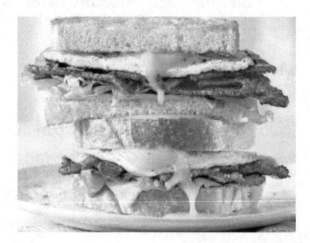

Ingredients

- ❖ Bread slices 2
- ❖ Eggs 2
- ❖ Bacon 3 to 4 pieces
- ❖ Mayonnaise 1 tablespoon
- ❖ Butter ½-1 tablespoon

Steps

1. At high temperatures, put 3 to 4 slices of bacon in an air-fryer, around 375-390 degrees.

2. Cook the bacon for around 3 minutes or set aside for your preferred crispiness.

3. Set aside with a medium-hot skillet, butter, and a slightly toasted slice of bread.

4. Fry two eggs in a skillet and form the sandwich bread to order.

5. To cook on both sides, flip the egg halfway.

6. Put one slice of cheese on top before moving the fried egg to the toasted crust.

7. Next, on top of a scrambled egg with cheese, incorporate air-fried, crispy bacon.

8. To complete the sandwich, put the other slice of cheese on top of the bacon, then position the other slice of toasted bread.

9. Finally, for around one to two minutes, place the breakfast sandwich in the air-fryer to toast your sandwich and make it good, sweet, and crispy.

10. Take from the freezer.

23. Air-Fried Breakfast Bombs

Ingredients

- ❖ Bacon slices 3
- ❖ Eggs 3 large
- ❖ Fresh chives 1 tablespoon
- ❖ Cream cheese 1 ounce
- ❖ Cooking oil spray
- ❖ Wheat pizza dough 4 ounces

Steps

1. Cook the bacon in a small skillet for around 10 minutes, mild to crisp. Bring the bacon out of the pan, crumble. Add the eggs to the bacon drippings in the pan; cook, constantly stirring, around 1 minute, until almost firm but still loose. Put the eggs in a bowl; add the cream cheese, the chives, and the crumbled bacon.

2. Cut the dough into four identical pieces. Wrap each piece into a 5-inch circle on a lightly floured. Place a quarter of the egg mixture in the center of each circle of dough. Clean the dough's outer edge with water; tie the dough around the egg mixture to shape a

purse and pinch the seams along with the dough.

3. Put dough purses in air fryer baskets in a single layer, cover with cooking spray. Cook for 5 to 6 minutes at 350 ° F until golden brown, checking after 5 minutes.

24. Air Fryer Breakfast Biscuit Bombs

Ingredients

- ❖ Vegetable oil 1 tablespoon
- ❖ Bulk breakfast sausage 1 / 4 lb
- ❖ Eggs 2
- ❖ Salt 1 / 8 teaspoon
- ❖ Pepper 1 / 8 teaspoon
- ❖ Biscuits bomb
- ❖ Pillsbury 1 can
- ❖ Cheddar cheese 2 oz
- ❖ Egg wash and water 1 tablespoon

Steps

1. Break the cooking parchment paper into two 8-inch rounds. Set one round at the bottom of the basket of the air fryer.

2. Heat oil over medium to high heat in a 10-inch nonstick skillet. Cook the sausage in oil for 2 to 5 minutes, frequently stirring to crumble, till it is no longer pink; transfer to a medium bowl with a slotted spoon. Decrease the heat to medium. To skillet drippings, add pounded eggs, salt, and pepper; cook until eggs are thickened, but still moist, stirring regularly. Stir the eggs in the cup onto the sausage. Cool for five minutes.

3. Meanwhile, divide the dough into five biscuits; divide each biscuit into two layers. Push into a 4-inch round each. Spoon 1 into the middle of each circular heaping tablespoonful of the egg mixture. Cover it with one of the cheese bits. Fold the sides carefully up and over the filling, press to seal. Beat most of the egg and water in a shallow cup. Rub the biscuits with egg wash on both ends.

4. Put 5 of the biscuit bombs on the parchment in the air fryer bowl, seam side down. With cooking water, water all sides of the second round of parchment. Cover the second parchment round biscuit bombs in the bowl, then cover it with the leftover 5 biscuit bombs.

5. Set to 325 degrees F; cook for 8 minutes. Remove the circular

parchment; use tongs to carefully transform the biscuits and position them in a single layer in the basket. Heat again 4 to 6 minutes longer or (at least 165 ° F) before cooked through.

25. Air Fryer Stuffed Breakfast Bombs with Eggs & Bacon

Ingredients

- ❖ Bacon ½ cup
- ❖ Eggs 1 cup
- ❖ Cheddar cheese ½ cup
- ❖ Salt and pepper
- ❖ Freeze biscuits 1 package

Steps

1. Merge the fried eggs, baked bacon, and melted Cheddar cheese in a little bowl.

2. Add a few teaspoons of combination to the biscuit and put it in the middle of it.

3. Just use and cover another biscuit or surround the biscuit on itself and cover the corners by pushing tightly. Put on the air fryer bowl.

4. Adjust the temperature to an air fryer level of 320 degrees F for 5 minutes.

5. Table, eat and enjoy.

26. Air Fryer Breakfast Burritos

Ingredients

- ❖ Ground sausage ½ lb.
- ❖ Bacon bits 1/3 cup
- ❖ Bell pepper ½
- ❖ Shredded cheese ½ cup
- ❖ Spraying oil
- ❖ Flour tortillas 6 medium
- ❖ Eggs 6

Steps

1. In a large bowl, mix the fried sausage, scrambled eggs, cheese, bell pepper, bacon bits. Stir to blend.

2. Spoon about half a cup of the combination into the flour tortilla core.

3. Fold the ends, and then move.

4. With the remaining ingredients, repeat.

5. Put filled burritos in the basket of the air fryer & liberally spray with oil.

6. Cook for 5 minutes at 330 degrees.

27. Air Fryer Breakfast Frittata

Ingredients

- ❖ Cheddar cheese ½ cup

- Breakfast sausage ¼ pound
- Eggs 4 large
- Red Bell pepper 2 tablespoon
- Green onion 1
- Cayenne pepper 1 pinch
- Cooking spray

Steps

1. Mix all the ingredients in a bowl.
2. Heat the air fryer at 360 degrees.
3. Put the mixture in already ready cake pan.
4. Cook till frittata is adjusted for 19-20 mins.

28. Air Fryer Crispy Bacon

Ingredients

- Thick one bacon ¾ lb.

Steps

1. Put bacon within the air fryer in the form of a thin layer.
2. Heat the air fryer to 400 degrees and cook for 8-10 mins till become crispy in taste.

29. Air Fryer Raspberry Muffins

Ingredients

- Baking powder 1 teaspoon
- Flour 1 cup
- Orange zest ½ teaspoon
- Sugar 1/3 cup
- Milk 1/3 cup
- Egg 1

- Vegetable oil 2.5 tablespoons
- Salt 1/8 teaspoon
- Vanilla essence ½ teaspoon
- Raw vanilla sugar ½ tablespoon
- Raspberries ½ cup

Steps

1. Put a muffin paper inside the muffin tray.
2. Blend baking powder, salt, and flour in a bowl.
3. In another bowl, blend sugar, egg, vanilla, and milk properly until mix.
4. Add the wet ingredients into dry ones and softly cover them in raspberries.
5. Split the muffin batter having surface covering of vanilla sugar into muffin cups.
6. Put them in an air fryer and bake them for 15 mins till muffins come out. Keep them aside to cool down properly.

30. Air Fryer Tofu

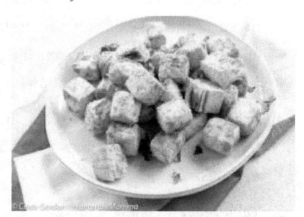

Ingredients

- ❖ Soy sauce 2 tablespoons
- ❖ Black firm tofu 453 g
- ❖ Olive oil 1 tablespoon
- ❖ Sesame oil 1 tablespoon
- ❖ Garlic 1 clove

Steps

1. Push the tofu for at least 14 mins, using either a hard pan or placing it on top, enabling the moisture to drain away. When done, bite-sized chunks of tofu are cut and moved to a dish.

2. In a tiny cup, combine all the leftover ingredients. Drizzle and throw over the tofu to coat. Let the tofu marinate for 15 more minutes.

3. Heat the air-fryer to 190-degree C. In a single layer, apply tofu blocks to the Air Fryer bowl. Cook for 15 minutes, frequently shaking the pan to facilitate frying. Before transferring a rack to them, let the muffins cool a bit in the baking pan to cool completely.

31. Air Fryer Brussel Sprouts

Ingredients

- ❖ Brussel sprouts 1 pound
- ❖ Olive oil 1 tablespoon
- ❖ Shallot 1 medium
- ❖ Salt ½ teaspoon
- ❖ Unsalted butter 2 tablespoons
- ❖ Red wine vinegar 1 teaspoon

Steps

1. Heat an air fryer at 375ºF. Meanwhile, cut 1 pound of sprouts from Brussels and halve any sprouts longer than an inch across. Apply 1 tablespoon of olive oil and 1/2 teaspoon of kosher salt to a medium bowl and blend.

2. To the air fryer, add the Brussels sprouts and shake them into one single plate. Air fry, stopping to move the bowl around midway through, for a total of 15 minutes. Begin preparing the shallot butter, meanwhile.

3. Chop 1 medium shallot finely. In a medium microwave-safe dish, put 2 tablespoons of unsalted butter and heat it in the microwave. Add the shallots and 1 tsp vinegar of red wine and mix to incorporate.

4. When the Brussels sprouts are set, move the shallot butter into the bowl or saucepan and toss to mix. Immediately serve.

Air Fryer Main Dishes

1. Parmesan Breaded Air Fryer Chicken Tenders

Ingredients

- ❖ Chicken tenders 8
- ❖ Egg 1
- ❖ Water 2 tablespoon
- ❖ Canola cooking spray

For Dredge coating

- ❖ Panko breadcrumbs 1 cup
- ❖ Salt ½ tsp
- ❖ Black pepper ¼ tsp
- ❖ Garlic powder 1 tsp
- ❖ Onion powder ½
- ❖ Parmesan ¼ cup

Steps

1. In a shallow bowl or baking pan wide enough to accommodate the chicken bits, mix the dredge-coating ingredients.

2. Put the egg and water in a second shallow bowl or baking pan and whisk to mix.

3. Dip the chicken tenders in the egg wash and then into the combination of the panko dredge.

4. In the fry basket, bring the breaded tenders in it.

5. Over the panko, spray a light coat of canola oil.

6. Fix the temperature and fry for 12 minutes at 400 degrees. Half through the cooking time, check the chicken and switch the chicken off to brown the other side.

2. Air Fryer Garlic Mushrooms Steaks

Ingredients

- ❖ Mushrooms, washed and dried, 8 oz.
- ❖ Olive oil 2 tablespoons
- ❖ Garlic powder ½ teaspoon
- ❖ Soy sauce 1 teaspoon
- ❖ Salt and pepper according to taste
- ❖ Sliced parsley 1 tablespoon

Steps

1. Slice out the mushrooms in half and add to a bowl and mix with garlic powder, oil, pepper, salt, and soy sauce.

2. Heat the air fryer at 380-degree F for 12 mins and move it midway thoroughly.

3. Sprinkle lemon and cover it with sliced parsley.

3. Air Fryer Falafels

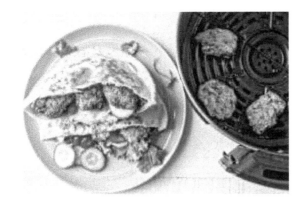

Ingredients

- ❖ Chickpeas 2 cans
- ❖ Fresh parsley ¼ cup
- ❖ Cilantro ¼ cup
- ❖ Garlic 2 cloves
- ❖ Shallot 1 large
- ❖ Flour 3 tablespoons
- ❖ Ground cumin 2 teaspoons
- ❖ Paprika 1 teaspoon
- ❖ Lemon juice ½
- ❖ Salt 1 teaspoon
- ❖ Olive oil spray

Steps

1. Add the shallot, chickpeas, parsley, garlic, cilantro, sesame seeds, rice, paprika, salt, lemon, and cumin to a food processor bowl.

2. Form the falafel mixture, around 1-inch in diameter, into tablespoon-sized discs. Repeat this before enough of the falafel combination is used. Get 25 to 30 discs of falafel.

3. Spray the basket with non-adhesive olive oil for your air fryer. Add as many falafel discs to the basket as you can without hitting them and gently brush them with olive oil. Air fried the falafel for 8 minutes at 350 ° F. Flip and fried the second side for an extra 6 minutes.

4. Repeat before you have all the falafel fried.

5. Serve falafel in a warm pita. Serve with some toppings you want and tahini yogurt sauce.

4. Air Fryer Pita Bread Pizza

Ingredients

- ❖ Pita bread 1
- ❖ Olive oil 1 tsp
- ❖ Tomato sauce 1 ½ tsp
- ❖ Shredded mozzarella cheese ¼ cup

Steps

1. Sprinkle the air fryer bowl within from cooking oil spray.

2. Place the pita in the air fryer bowl.

3. Rub the pita with olive oil.

4. Spread out the tomato sauce on the pita.

5. Spray the pita with shredded cheese.

6. Heat the pita pizza in the air fryer at 400-degree F for 5 mins.

5. Air Fryer Chicken Quesadilla

Ingredients

- ❖ Soft taco shells
- ❖ Chicken fajita strips
- ❖ Green pepper sliced ½ cup
- ❖ Shredded Mexican cheese
- ❖ Sliced onion ½ cup

Steps

1. For around 3 minutes, heat the Air Fryer to 370 degrees.

2. Lightly coat the plate with vegetable oil, and in the bowl, position 1 soft taco shell.

3. Put on the shell with shredded cheese.

4. Layout the strips of fajita chicken until they are in a continuous layer.

5. On top of your chicken, place your onions and green peppers on top.

6. Apply more cheese that is shredded.

7. Put on the top of another soft taco shell and gently spray with vegetable oil.

8. Set a four-minute timer.

9. Flip the broad spatula over cautiously.

10. Lightly spray with vegetable oil and set the rack on top of the shell to support it in line.

11. Set a four-minute timer.

12. Leave in for a few more minutes if it's not crispy enough for you.

13. Remove and break into 4 or 6 slices, respectively.

14. If needed, serve with salsa and sour cream.

6. Crispy Golden Air Fryer Fish

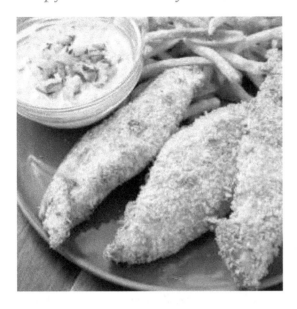

Ingredients

- ❖ Salt and black pepper
- ❖ Flour ½ cup
- ❖ Catfish 4 strips around 1 lb.
- ❖ Egg 1 large
- ❖ Old Bay seasoning 1 tsp.
- ❖ Panko breadcrumbs 2 cup
- ❖ Lemon wedges and Tartar sauce

Steps

1. Heat an air fryer at 400-degree F.

2. Mix the first 5 ingredients and add them to a Ziploc bag.

3. Wash the catfish, pat it off, and add the Ziploc bag to the fillets.

4. Enclose the bag, and then shake until it is thoroughly coated with the fillets.

5. Insert the coated fillets into the basket of the air fryer.

6. Spray the low-calorie spray on the fish fillets, cover the air fryer and cook for 9-10 mins.

7. Switch over the fillets of air fryer fish and continue to cook 3-4 mins, or until finished.

8. Serve the fillets of air fryer fish with a small salad.

7. Air Fryer Chicken Fried Rice

Ingredients

- ❖ Cold cooked white rice 3 cups
- ❖ Frozen peas and carrots 1 cup
- ❖ Soy sauce 6 tablespoons
- ❖ Vegetable oil 1 tablespoon
- ❖ Packed cup chicken 1
- ❖ Onion ½ cup

Steps

1. Put in the mixing bowl with the cold cooked white rice.

2. Add the soy sauce and vegetable oil, then mix well.

3. Add the onion and the diced ham, the frozen peas & carrots and blend completely.

4. In the nonstick plate, dump the rice mixture into it.

5. Place the Air Fryer in the bowl.

6. With a cooking period of 20 minutes, set the Air Fryer to 360-degree F.

7. Take off the pan from the Air Fryer as soon as the timer goes off.

8. Serve with your meat of preference, or just take a bowl and enjoy it.

8. Air Fryer Steak Bites and Mushrooms

Ingredients

- ❖ Sirloin fillet 1 pound
- ❖ Olive oil 1 tablespoon
- ❖ Montreal seasoning 1 tablespoon
- ❖ Mushrooms 8 ounces
- ❖ Blue cheese sauce

Steps

1. Heat the empty air fryer at 390 ° F for 3 minutes with the crisper plate.

2. Toss the beef cubes with the olive oil and Montreal seasoning when the air fryer is heating up.

3. Chop halves or thirds of the mushrooms.

4. In the hot oven air fryer, pour the beef cubes and mushrooms and gently shake to combine.

5. Set the temperature of the air fryer to 390 ° F and set the timer for 7 minutes.

6. Pause and shake the basket after 3 minutes. Do this again at intervals of 2 minutes until the beef cubes achieve the desired doneness. Dependent on the thickness of the cubes, the period can differ by machine. Lift a large piece out and test it to see the progress with a meat thermometer. Once it is removed from the air fryer, note that the meat will continue to cook. The meat is medium and has a warm pink center at 145 ° F.

7. Allow the meat a few minutes before serving to rest and then enjoy it.

9. Juicy Air Fryer Pork Chops with Rub

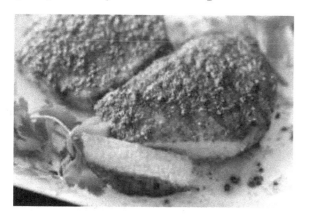

Ingredients

- ❖ Boneless pork chops 2-4

- ❖ Pork rub 2 tablespoon

- ❖ Olive oil 1 tablespoon

Steps

1. Rub both sides of the pork chops with olive oil.

2. Spread seasoning on all sides of the pork chops with pork rub. To get the seasoning to adhere, it works best to push the rub softly into the pork chops.

3. To help make clean-up easier, spray the aluminum air fryer basket with cooking spray.

4. Insert 2-4 boneless pork chops into the basket of the air fryer.

5. Set the temperature setting to 400-degree F with a total cooking time of 12 minutes.

6. Cook the pork chops for 7 minutes on one side of the air fryer.

7. Flip them over and cook for another 5 minutes, or until the internal temperature hits 145-degree F.

8. If you are frying 4 pork chops in an air fryer, make sure to turn and ROTATE the pan to maintain an even cooking period. In other words, the pork chops that were in the front for the first 7 minutes, turn them and position them in the back of the pan for when they are finished frying.

9. Before serving, rest for 5 + minutes. It is important.

10. Air Fryer Steak with Garlic Mushrooms

Ingredients

- ❖ Avocado oil 1 tablespoon

- ❖ Ribeye steak 16 oz.

- ❖ Mushrooms 2 cup

- ❖ Salt ½ teaspoon

- ❖ Black pepper ½ teaspoon

- ❖ Unsalted butter 2 tablespoon

- ❖ Minced garlic 2 tablespoon

- ❖ Red pepper flakes ¼ teaspoon

Steps

1. For 4 minutes, heat the Air Fryer at 400 ° F.

2. Dry the steaks and split them into 1/2-inch pieces. Pass the pieces of steak to a wide bowl.

3. Cut out the fresh mushrooms in half and move them into the large bowl with the cubed steak.

4. Add the garlic, salt, melted butter, pepper and red pepper flakes, and toss to cover the steak bites and mushrooms equally to the wide bowl.

5. In an even, non-overlapping layer, pass the mixture to an air fryer basket.

6. Air fried for 7-15 minutes, tossing the steak and mushrooms twice during this period. Test the steak after 7 minutes to see whether it's according to taste. If it's too pink, proceed to cook as required.

7. Garnish with parsley and serve with the finest taste and feel right away.

8. Turn them over and continue to cook for 5 more minutes or until 145-degree F is hit in the inner temperature.

9. Make sure to turn and ROTATE the pan and maintain an equal cooking period while you're frying 4 pork chops in an air fryer.

10. Before serving, leave to rest for 5 + minutes. Quite necessary.

11. Low Carb Coconut Shrimp

Ingredients

- ❖ Large shrimp, peeled off, 1 lb.
- ❖ Coconut flour ¼ cup
- ❖ Eggs 2
- ❖ Unsweetened flaked coconut 1 cup

Steps

1. Add coconut flour in a tiny bowl. In a 2nd cup, put eggs and mix well. In a 3rd tub, incorporate flaked coconut.

2. In the coconut flour, dip the shrimp. Then dip the eggs, making sure the excess egg is removed. Finally, add the shrimp to the coconut bowl and push to coat the whole coconut shrimp.

3. Put covered shrimp in the air fryer bowl. Continue to add shrimp until the basket has a full layer of shrimp.

4. Cook in an air fryer for 6-8 minutes at 400 degrees. To flip the shrimp, stop cooking midway through. When the shrimp is yellow, and the coconut is golden brown, they are finished.

12. Tandoori Fish Tikka

Ingredients

For Tikka

- ❖ Fish (Salmon) 1 lb.
- ❖ Nell pepper 1
- ❖ Onion 1 medium

Tandoori Marinade

- ❖ Light olive oil 2 tablespoon
- ❖ Plain yogurt 4 tablespoons
- ❖ Ginger 2 teaspoon
- ❖ Garlic 2 teaspoon
- ❖ Lime juice 1 tablespoon
- ❖ Salt 1 teaspoon
- ❖ Turmeric ½ teaspoon
- ❖ Coriander 2 teaspoon
- ❖ Cumin powder 1 teaspoon
- ❖ Garam masala 1.5 teaspoon
- ❖ Kashmiri red chili powder 1 teaspoon
- ❖ Kasoori methi 2 teaspoon

Steps

1. Mix the yogurt, oil, ginger-garlic paste, and lemon juice all the spices together in a mixing bowl.

2. In the marinade, incorporate fish bits, capsicum and onion and toss well before it gets covered.

3. Use an air fryer for cooking Tikka

4. For quick clean-up, cover the drip pan with aluminum foil. Place the basket of fried food in the drip pan.

5. In a single layer, place the tuna, peppers, and onions in the basket. Otherwise, they will not crisp up while cooking.

6. Reinsert the basket. Use the 360°F temperature set-button. Depending on the thickness of the fish, set the timer for 8-10 mins.

13. Bharwa Bhindi (Stuffed Okra)

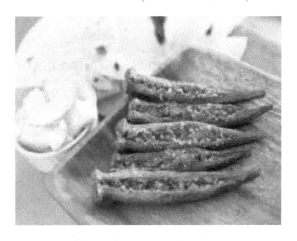

Ingredients

- ❖ Okra (bhindi) 10.5 oz.

❖ Oil for frying 2 tablespoons

❖ Lime ½

Spice stuffing

❖ Coriander powder 2 tablespoon

❖ Ground cumin 2 teaspoon

❖ Dry mango powder 1 teaspoon

❖ Kashmiri red chili powder 1 teaspoon

❖ Garam masala 1 teaspoon

❖ Ground turmeric ¼ teaspoon

❖ Salt 1 teaspoon

❖ Oil 2 teaspoon

Steps

1. Use water to wash the bhindi and let it air dry.

2. Trim the ends and slit each bhindi lengthwise.

3. Mix all the stuffed spices in a bowl.

4. Take one bhindi at a time and use the spice blend to stuff it. With all the slit bhindi, repeat. When filling the bhindi, be generous; it's all right with some masala falls out.

1. In the air-fryer basket, put the stuffed okra in a single sheet. Cook for 12 mins at 360-degree F. To flip the okra, cut the basket after about 8 minutes.

2. It can be served by Bharwa bhindi. With a generous squeeze of lime juice on top, we enjoy it. Represent with warm roti or paratha.

14. Greek-Style Chicken Wings

Ingredients

❖ Extra virgin olive oil ½ cup

❖ Fresh lemon juice ¼ cup

❖ Minced garlic 2 cloves

❖ Dried oregano 2 teaspoon

❖ Dried thyme 1 teaspoon

❖ Salt 1 teaspoon

❖ Ground pepper ½ teaspoon

❖ Red pepper flakes ½ teaspoon

❖ Crushed red pepper flakes ¼ teaspoon

❖ Chicken wings drumettes 2 lb.

❖ Tzatziki sauce

Steps

1. Mix all the ingredients, except the Tzatziki sauce and chicken. Put the marinade in a large bag that can be resealed and add the chicken.

2. Refrigerate overnight for 4 hours, turning over occasionally.

3. Heat the air fryer to 370 ° F.

4. Add half of the chicken and simmer for 20 minutes, flipping the chicken midway through.

5. After 20 minutes, offer the air fryer bowl a shake to throw the chicken a bit. Cook 1-2 minutes more or till juices run clear and meat is no longer pink.

6. Repeat for the chicken that remains. Represent with Tzatziki sauce.

15. Air Fryer Garlic Ranch Wings

Ingredients

❖ Ranch seasoning mix 3 tablespoons

❖ Butter melted ¼ cup

❖ Fresh garlic minced 6 cloves

❖ Chicken wings 2 pounds

Steps

1. Melt the butter and mix with Ranch dry seasoning mix as well as minced garlic.

2. Put wings into a bowl and marinade it.

3. Put the bag into the freezer for the whole night.

4. Put wings in the air fryer and heat up to 360 degrees for 15-20 mins, while shaking two times.

5. Increase the temperature to 390 degrees and heat more for 5 mins.

16. Air Fryer Crispy Buffalo Chicken Hot Wings

Ingredients

❖ Chicken wings drumettes 16

❖ Low sodium soy sauce 2 teaspoons

❖ Montreal Grill Mate chicken seasoning

❖ Garlic powder 1 teaspoon

❖ Pepper according to taste

❖ Cooking spray

❖ Frank's Red-hot buffalo wing sauce ¼ cup

Steps

1. Drizzle over the chicken with the soy sauce.

2. To eat, prepare the chicken with the garlic powder, chicken seasoning, and pepper.

3. Put the chicken in a fryer in the air. Stacking the chicken on top of each other is fine.

4. Over the top of the meat, spray cooking oil.

5. Simmer the chicken at 400 degrees for five minutes. To ensure all the parts are thoroughly prepared, cut the pan, and shake the meat.

6. Throw the chicken back into an air fryer. Give an extra five minutes for the chicken to cook.

7. Take the chicken out of an air fryer.

8. Glaze the buffalo wing sauce with each slice of meat.

9. Throw the chicken back into an air fryer. Cook for 7-12 minutes till the chicken reaches the crisp you want and is not pink on the inside anymore.

17. Air Fryer Marinated Steak

Ingredients

- ❖ Butcher Box New York Strip Steaks 2

- ❖ Soy sauce 1 tablespoon

- ❖ Liquid smoke 1 teaspoon

- ❖ McCormick's Grill Mates seasoning 1 tablespoon

- ❖ Unsweetened cocoa powder ½ tablespoon

- ❖ Salt and pepper to taste

- ❖ Melted butter as an option

Steps

1. Drizzle the liquid smoke and soy sauce with the Butcher Box Steak.

2. With the seasonings, season the steak.

3. Refrigerate, ideally overnight, for a minimum of a couple of hours.

4. In an air fryer, put the steak. Cook two steaks at a time. An accessory grill tray, sheet shelf, or the regular air fryer basket may be used.

5. Cook it at 370 degrees for 5 minutes. Open the air fryer after 5 minutes and check your steak. Based on the target thickness, cooking time can differ. Cook to 125 ° F for rare, 135 ° F for medium-rare, 145 ° F for medium, 155 ° F for medium-well, and 160 ° F for well cooked. Using a meat thermometer.

6. For an extra 2 minutes of medium-done beef, I grilled the beef.

7. Remove the steak and drizzle with the melted butter from the air-fryer.

18. Air Fryer Bacon and egg Bite Cups

Ingredients

- ❖ Eggs 6 large

- Milk 2 tablespoons
- Salt and pepper to taste
- Sliced green peppers ¼ cup
- Red peppers sliced ¼ cup
- Sliced onions ¼
- Fresh spinach sliced ¼ cup
- Shredded cheese ½ cup
- Mozzarella cheese ¼ cup
- Cooked and crumbled bacon 3 slices

Steps

1. Add eggs in a bowl along with salt, pepper, and cream. Whisk together.

2. Spray green and red peppers, onions, cheeses, spinach, and bacon. Whisk them.

3. Put silicone molds in the air fryer before this mixture preparation.

4. Add the egg mixture into every silicon molds. Sprinkle all the remaining veggies.

5. Heat the air fryer for 12-15 minutes at 300 degrees till the toothpick comes out clearly from the egg mixture.

19. Air Fryer Tender Juicy Smoked BBQ Ribs

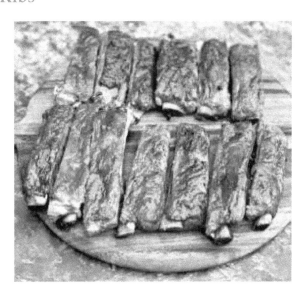

Ingredients

- Ribs rack 1
- Liquid smoke 1 tablespoon
- Pork rub 2-3 tablespoons
- Salt and pepper according to taste
- BBQ sauce ½ cup

Steps

1. There is a thin film that can be difficult to strip. Remove the skin from the back of the ribs. It can peel straight off occasionally. You should split it, too, and then take it off. Break the ribs in half so that the ribs will fit into the air fryer.

2. Drizzle along all sides of the ribs with the liquid smoke, and with

the pork paste, salt and pepper, season all ends.

3. Wrap the ribs and enable the ribs to rest for 30 minutes at room temperature.

4. Use an air fryer to add the ribs. Stacking the ribs is okay.

5. Simmer at 360 degrees for 15 minutes.

6. Open a fryer in the air. The ribs flip. For an extra 15 minutes, cook.

7. Remove from the air fryer from the ribs. Drizzle BBQ sauce on the ribs.

20. Air Fryer Bacon and Cream Cheese Stuffed Jalapeno Poppers

Ingredients

- ❖ Fresh jalapenos 10
- ❖ Cream cheese 6 oz.
- ❖ Shredded cheddar cheese ¼ cup
- ❖ Bacon 2 slices
- ❖ Cooking oil spray

Steps

1. To produce 2 halves per jalapeno, break the jalapenos in two, vertically.

2. Put it in a bowl with the cream cheese. 15 seconds in the oven to soften.

3. Remove the jalapeno and seeds from the inside.

4. In a cup, mix the crumbled bacon, cream cheese, and grilled cheese. Mix thoroughly.

5. With the cream cheese mixture, stuff each of the jalapenos.

6. Through the Air Fryer, fill the poppers. With cooking oil, brush the poppers.

7. Air Fryer Close Up. Cook the poppers for 5 minutes at 370 degrees.

8. Remove and cool from the Air Fryer before serving.

21. Air Fryer Italian Herb Pork loin

Ingredients

- ❖ Boneless pork loin (not tenderloin), 3-4 pound
- ❖ Italian Vinaigrette Marinade 1/4 cup
- ❖ Garlic 4 cloves, minced
- ❖ Rosemary (crushed) 1 teaspoon
- ❖ Thyme 1 teaspoon
- ❖ Italian Seasoning 1/2 teaspoon

❖ Salt and pepper to taste

Steps

1. Drizzle both sides of the pork loin with the Italian marinade. The leftover seasoning is sprinkled on both ends.

2. It is recommended, though optional, to marinate the pork loin for 2 hours. Marinate the covered pork loin in a bowl or the refrigerator in a sealable bag.

3. Place the pork loin on parchment paper in the air fryer basket.

4. Fry the pork loin at 360 degrees for 25 minutes.

5. Open and rotate the pork loin with the air fryer. Cook for a further 12-15 minutes or until the pork loin's internal temperature hits at least 145 degrees. Use a thermometer for meat.

6. Use the air fryer to cut the pork loin. Until slicing, enable the meat to rest for at least 9-10 minutes. If wanted, you may glaze them with extra vinaigrette.

22. Air Fryer Grilled Chicken Kebabs

Ingredients

❖ Skinless chicken breasts, cut into 1-inch cubes, 16 oz

❖ Soy sauce 2 tablespoons

❖ McCormick's Grill Mates Chicken Seasoning 1 tablespoon

❖ McCormick's Grill Mates BBQ Seasoning 1 teaspoon

❖ Salt and pepper to taste

❖ Green pepper sliced ½

❖ Red pepper sliced ½

❖ Yellow pepper sliced ½

❖ Zucchini sliced ½

❖ Red onion sliced ¼

❖ 4-5 grape tomatoes

❖ Cooking oil spray optional

Steps

1. Marinating the chicken is desired but not needed. Put the chicken in a sealable plastic bag or wide bowl with chicken seasoning, soy sauce, BBQ seasoning, salt, and pepper to taste if you intend to marinate the

chicken. Shake the bag to ensure that it is evenly covered and seasoned with the chicken.

2. Remove and thread the chicken onto a skewer.

3. Layer the zucchini, tomatoes, and onions with the chicken. Cover each skewer with a grape tomato.

4. With cooking oil, spray the chicken and vegetables.

5. Line up the air fryer with parchment paper liners for simple clean up.

6. Put the skewers on a grill rack in the air fryer bowl. Cook at 350 degrees for 10 minutes.

7. Open and rotate the skewers with the air fryer. Cook for a further 7-10 minutes before the chicken hits an internal temperature of 165 degrees. Evaluate the interior of one of the chicken parts by using a meat thermometer.

23. Air Fryer Shrimp and Vegetables

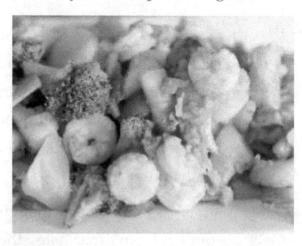

Ingredients

❖ Small shrimp

❖ Frozen mixed vegetables 1 bag

❖ Gluten-free Cajun seasoning 1 tablespoon

❖ Olive oil spray

❖ Cooked rice

Steps

1. Add vegetables and the shrimp to the air fryer.

2. Cover it with Cajun seasoning and sprinkle it with oil spray.

3. Heat it at 355 degrees for 10 mins.

4. Now open and mix the vegetables and shrimp.

5. Continue to cook for extra 10 mins. Serve on cooked rice.

24. Air Fryer Bratwurst and Vegetables

Ingredients

❖ Bratwurst 1 package

❖ Red bell pepper 1

❖ Green bell pepper 1

❖ Red onion ¼ cup

❖ Gluten-free Cajun seasoning ½ tablespoon

Steps

1. Line up the air fryer with foil and add vegetables.

2. Break down the bratwurst into ½ inch size and put on top of the vegetables.

3. Spray the Cajun seasoning smoothly on it.

4. Air fryer at 390 degrees for 5-10 mins. Now open and mix it well.

5. Remove an air fryer after another extra 10 mins and serve.

25. Air Fryer Turkey Legs

Ingredients

❖ Turkey drumsticks 1 package

❖ Olive oil cooking spray

❖ BBQ sauce

Steps

1. Put the turkey legs in the bowl of an air fryer and sprinkle it with olive oil cooking spray.

2. Heat it to 390 degrees for 5-10 mins. Turn on and cook for more than 10 mins till 165-degree temperature.

3. Add sauce and roll it in foil. Let it cool and serve.

26. Air Fryer Roasted Edamame

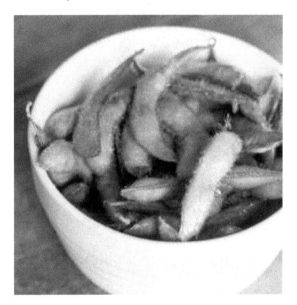

Ingredients

❖ Edamame 2 cups

❖ Olive oil spray

❖ Garlic salt

Steps

1. Put edamame in the air fryer bowl, and it can be fresh or frozen.

2. Cover it with olive spray and pinch of garlic salt.

3. Heat the air fryer at 390 degrees for 10 mins.

4. Mix midway through the cooking time and roasted it more for extra 5 mins. Serve it.

27. Air Fryer Bulgogi Burgers

Ingredients

For the Bulgogi Burgers

- ❖ Lean ground beef 1 pound
- ❖ Gochujang 2 tablespoon
- ❖ Dark soy sauce 1 tablespoon
- ❖ Minced garlic 2 teaspoon
- ❖ Minced ginger 2 teaspoon
- ❖ Sugar 2 teaspoon
- ❖ Sesame oil 1 tablespoon
- ❖ Chopped green Scallions ¼ cup
- ❖ Salt ½ teaspoon

For the Gochujang Mayonnaise

- ❖ Mayonnaise ¼ cup
- ❖ Gochujang 1 tablespoon
- ❖ Sesame oil 1 tablespoon
- ❖ Sesame seeds 1 tablespoon
- ❖ Chopped green Scallions ¼ cup
- ❖ Hamburger buns 4

Steps

1. Mix the ground beef, soy sauce, gochujang, garlic, sugar, ginger, sesame oil, minced onions and salt in a big bowl and let the mixture sit in the refrigerator for 30 minutes up to 24 hours.

2. With a small depression in the center, divide the beef into four portions and create circular patties to keep the burgers from puffing out during cooking into a dome-shape.

3. For 10 minutes, set the air fryer to 360-degree F and put the patties in the air fryer bowl in one single sheet.

4. Make the Gochujang Mayonnaise: Mix the gochujang, mayonnaise, sesame oil, scallions, and sesame seeds while the patties are cooking.

5. Ensure that the beef has achieved an internal temperature of 160F using a meat thermometer and remove it onto a serving tray.

6. Serve the patties and the gochujang mayonnaise with hamburger buns.

28. Air Fryer Carne Asada

Ingredients

- ❖ Limes juiced 2 mediums

- ❖ Orange peeled 1 medium
- ❖ Cilantro 1 cup
- ❖ Jalapeno pepper 1
- ❖ Vegetable oil 2 tablespoons
- ❖ White vinegar 2 tablespoons
- ❖ Ancho chile powder 2 teaspoons
- ❖ Sugar 2 teaspoon
- ❖ Salt 1 teaspoon
- ❖ Cumin seeds 1 teaspoon
- ❖ Skirt steak 1.5 pound
- ❖ Coriander powder 1 teaspoon

Steps

1. In a blender, put all the ingredients except the skirt steak and combine until a smooth sauce is obtained.

2. Split the skirt steak into four sections and put it in a plastic zip-top container.

3. Add the marinade on the steak and keep the beef marinated for 30 minutes.

4. Place the steaks in the air fryer basket and adjust the air fryer to 400-degree F.

5. Cook for 8 minutes, or until your steak's internal temperature has hit 145-degree F. It is necessary not to overcook skirt steak to toughen the beef.

6. For 10 minutes, let the steak rest. Don't hurry at this stage.

7. Slice (this aspect is important) the steak against the grain and serve.

29. Keto Steak Nuggets

Ingredients

- ❖ Beefsteak 1 pound
- ❖ Egg1 large
- ❖ Palm oil for frying
- ❖ Parmesan cheese ½ cup
- ❖ Pork panko ½ cup
- ❖ Homemade seasoned salt ½ teaspoon
- ❖ Mayonnaise ¼ cup
- ❖ Sour cream ¼ cup
- ❖ Chipotles paste 1 teaspoon
- ❖ Dip mix ½ teaspoon
- ❖ Lime juiced ¼ medium

Steps

1. For the Chipotle Ranch Dip: Add all the ingredients together and mix properly. A medium-spice version produces 1 teaspoon of chipotle paste. Before serving,

refrigerate for at least 30 minutes and hold for up to 1 week.

2. Combine Panko pork, parmesan cheese and seasoned salt-use my homemade stuff again, not the store-bought.

3. Beat the egg 1. Place 1 bowl of beaten egg and another breading mix in another.

4. Dip the steak chunks into the egg, then bread it. Place it on a sheet pan or plate lined with wax paper.

5. FREEZE breaded bites of raw steak 30 minutes before frying.

6. Heat your lard to approximately 325 degrees F. Fry steak nuggets (from frozen or chilled) once browned, around 2-3 minutes, working in batches as needed.

7. Switch to a lined plate with paper towels, season with a salt spray, and serve with Chipotle Ranch.

30. Korean Short BBQ Ribs

Ingredients

❖ Short ribs

❖ Korean BBQ sauce

❖ Pineapple 2 tablespoon

Steps

1. Mix all the ingredients and leave for 24 hours.

2. Put the rack in the air fryer bowl. Heat the air fryer at 360-degree F for 12 minutes. Switch the other side. Serve it.

31. Air Fryer Korean Hot Dogs

Ingredients

❖ Hot dogs 6
❖ Mozzarella cheese and sausages
❖ Wooden chopsticks 3 pairs
❖ Panko breadcrumbs 1 cup
❖ Oil spray, sugar, and mustard sauce

Steps

1. Without cutting open, cut a slice down each hot dog; cut the slice with a half cheese handle.

2. Heat the air fryer at 350 °. Mix the butter, rice, vinegar, jalapenos, chili powder, and half a cup of broken tortilla chips in a wide bowl to form a smooth mixture. On a lightly floured board, position the dough; divide into sixths. Roll the dough into 15-inch large pieces; tie the cheese-stuffed hot dog along one strip. Repeat with the dough and the hot dogs that remain. Spray the cooking spray on the dogs and

move softly onto the leftover smashed chips. Spray the air fryer container with cooking spray and, without contact, put the dogs in the bowl, leaving space for expansion.

3. Cook in batches for 8-10 minutes until the dough is finely browned, and the cheese begins to melt. Represent with extra chips, sour cream and guacamole if needed.

Chapter 3: Lunch

1. Air Fryer Sweet Chili Chicken Wings

Ingredients

- ❖ Chicken Wings 12
- ❖ Baking Powder ½ Tbsp
- ❖ Black Pepper 1 Tsp
- ❖ Sea Salt ½ Tsp
- ❖ Garlic Powder 1 Tsp
- ❖ Onion Powder ¼ Tsp
- ❖ Paprika ¼ Tsp

Steps

1. Dry the chicken wings with a paper towel. With baking powder and seasoning, add the chicken wings to a zip-lock container. Cover the bag (make sure all the air is out) and chuck it around until it covers the wings.

2. Spray with cooking spray on the metal rack and place the chicken wings into a single layer. Close the Ninja Foody lid and press AIR CRISP, then set the TEMP to 400 ° F, set the Period to 20 minutes, and then press START. The sweet chili sauce is made when frying the chicken wings.

3. Open the cover for 10 minutes and toss/flip the chicken wings with tongs to keep them from sticking. Cover the lid and allow the remaining 10 minutes to cook for them.

4. However, monitor the internal temperature to guarantee that they are cooked after the time has passed. Before tossing in the sweet chili sauce, encouraged to rest for 5 minutes.

Warm Sauce with Chili

1. In a shallow saucepan, mix all ingredients and cook over medium heat on the burner. Carry the sauce to a boil and then reduce heat until the sauce has decreased and thickened gradually to a simmer, stirring. Hold the sauce warm before you're done with the chicken wings.

2. In the gravy, toss or drop the fried chicken wings. I want to make sure that they are coated thoroughly.

3. Put a single layer of the sauced chicken wings on a greased baking sheet with a wire rack cover. Broil the chicken wings for 2-4 minutes at HIGH on the top rack. Stay

tight to the oven and periodically. Check the wings till they burn easily. Remove them from the oven till the sauce is crispy, and the wings have some flavor. Serve immediately.

2. Air Fryer Fish

Ingredients

- ❖ Fish fillets 8
- ❖ Olive oil 1 tablespoon
- ❖ Garlic powder ¼ tsp
- ❖ Dry breadcrumbs 1 cup
- ❖ Black pepper ¼ tsp
- ❖ Paprika ½ teaspoon
- ❖ Chili powder ¼ tsp
- ❖ Salt ½ teaspoon
- ❖ Onion powder ¼ teaspoon

Steps

1. Blend the breadcrumbs with chili powder, paprika, black pepper, onion powder, garlic powder, and salt in a shallow bath.
2. Coat-fillet of fish with breadcrumbs and move to the bowl of the air fryer.
3. Cook in an air fryer for 12-15 minutes at 390 ° f (200 ° c). Open the air fryer for the first 8-10

minutes and then turn the fish fillets on the opposite side and cook.

3. Air Fryer Wonton Mozzarella Sticks

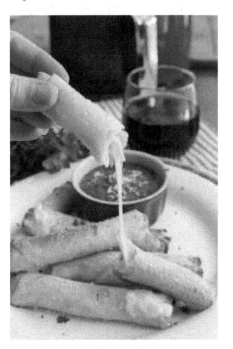

Ingredients

- ❖ Mozzarella cheese sticks 6
- ❖ Egg roll 6
- ❖ Olive oil spray
- ❖ Salt

Steps

1. Put a slice of string cheese on the egg roll wrapper's bottom corner. Roll up halfway and fold the sides over the cheese carefully into the middle. Soak finger in water and examine the wrapper's edges. Roll over the mozzarella stick with the

remaining wrapper. Repeat for the leftover cheese and wrappers.

2. In the air fryer, put 6 of the mozzarellas sticks and spray with an olive oil spray. Using kosher salt to sprinkle.

3. Fry for 3 minutes at 350 degrees, flip, sprinkle the other side with a spray of olive oil and sprinkle with salt, and proceed to fry for another 3 minutes. If needed, provide with a marinara sauce for soaking.

4. Air Fryer Steak

Ingredients

- ❖ Loin steaks 2 strip
- ❖ Salt 2 tsp
- ❖ Black pepper 2 tsp
- ❖ Butter 2 tsp

Steps

1. Spray with pepper and salt on the steaks, put on a plate and refrigerate, uncovered, for 2-3 days. Flip it with a paper towel every 11-12 hours or so, blotting the fluids.

2. For advanced tenderness and enriched taste, this stage is suggested, but one may miss it if pressed for time.

3. 45-60 minutes before serving, take the steaks from the fridge and allow them to stay at room temperature.

4. Rub the steaks on both sides with melted butter and put on the rack of the air fryer. For medium thickness, steam at 410F for 14 minutes, without raising the temperature.

5. If air-fried steaks are thicker or thinner than 1,25 "thick, the times may need to be modified.

6. This cooking time is an estimate, so use an instant reading thermometer in the Notes segment in conjunction with the bowl.

7. Remove the steaks from the air fryer, cover them in foil or wax paper, and let them sit for 10 minutes, then eat.

5. Air Fryer Caramelized Bananas

Ingredients

- ❖ Bananas 2
- ❖ Lemon 1/4
- ❖ Coconut sugar 1 tbsp

Steps

1. Wash bananas, then cut them straight down the center, lengthwise

2. Try squeezing the lemon juice over each banana's top.

3. When combined with coconut sugar using cinnamon, rub the bananas' surface until covered with coconut sugar.

4. At 400F, put in the parchment-lined air fryer for 7-9 minutes.

5. Eat as is or top up with favorite toppings until removed from the air fryer and enjoy.

6. Air Fryer Sesame Chicken

Ingredients

* ❖ Boneless Chicken Thighs 6

* ❖ Cornstarch 1/2 Cup

* ❖ Olive Oil Spray

Steps

1. Break the chicken into cubed pieces, then add the cornstarch into a dish.

2. Put it in the air fryer and cook it according to the chicken air fryer manual. So, when chicken is in the air fryer, put a good even layer of olive oil spray; it works well to mix things up midway through cooking time and add an extra coat of spray.

3. While the chicken is frying, start preparing the sauce in a tiny saucepan.

4. On a medium-high fire, add sugar, orange juice, ginger, hoisin sauce, garlic, and soy sauce to the saucepan. When well mixed, whisk this away.

5. Stir in the water and cornstarch till the sugar has fully melted, and a low boil is achieved.

6. Mix the sesame seeds in it and take the sauce from the heat. Put aside to thicken for 5 minutes.

7. Take from the air fryer and put in a bowl until the chicken is cooked, and then cover with the sauce.

8. Topped over rice and beans and eat.

7. Air Fryer Donuts

Ingredients

* ❖ Milk 1 cup

* ❖ Instant yeast 2 ½ tsp.

* ❖ Sugar ¼ cup

* ❖ Salt ½ tsp

* ❖ Egg 1

* ❖ Butter ¼ cup

* ❖ Flour 3 cups

❖ Oil spray

Steps

1. Gently whisk together milk, 1 tsp of sugar, and yeast in the bowl of a stand mixer equipped with a dough handle. Let it stay for 10 minutes until it is foamy

2. To the milk mixture, add the cinnamon, egg, and sugar, melted butter and 2 cups of flour. Mix until mixed at a low level, then add the remaining cup of flour slowly with the mixer going, until the dough no longer sticks to the pipe. Increase the pace to medium-low and knead until the dough is elastic and smooth for 5 minutes.

3. Place the dough and cover it with plastic wrap in a greased bowl. In a warm spot, let it grow before it doubles.

4. Place the dough on a floured board, punch it down and stretch it out softly to a thickness of around 1/2 inch. 1- To extract the middle, cut out 11-13 donuts.

5. Switch to thinly floured parchment paper donuts and donut holes and cover loosely with oiled plastic wrap. Let the donuts grow for about 30 minutes before the amount has doubled. Preheat the 350F Air Fryer.

6. Spray the Air Fryer bowl with oil spray and gently move the donuts in a single layer to the Air Fryer jar. Using oil spray to spray donuts and cook at 350F until golden brown, around 4 minutes. Repeat for donuts and gaps left.

7. Melt butter over medium heat in a shallow saucepan while the donuts are in the Air Fryer. Stir in the sugar and vanilla extract powder until smooth. Remove from the heat and mix one tablespoon at a time in hot water until the icing is a little thin, still not watery.

8. Using forks to dip hot donuts and donut holes into the glaze to submerge them. To encourage the excess glaze to drip off, position it on a wire rack placed over a rimmed baking sheet. Let it hang for about 10 minutes before the glaze hardens.

8. Bang Bang Chicken

Ingredients

❖ Mayonnaise 1/2 cup

- ❖ <u>Honey </u>2 tablespoons
- ❖ Sriracha sauce 1/2 tablespoon
- ❖ Buttermilk 1 cup
- ❖ Flour ¾
- ❖ Cornstarch ½ cup
- ❖ Egg 1
- ❖ Oil

Steps

1. Add all ingredients in a mixing bowl to create bang bang chicken sauce. Whisk before it's all mixed.

2. In the air fryer, first create buttermilk batter by mixing flour, egg, corn starch, pepper, salt, sriracha sauce, and buttermilk to produce bang bang meat. And whisk until mixed.

3. Before inserting the poultry, grease your Air Fryer with some oil of your choosing. Next, work in plenty, drop bits of chicken in buttermilk batter and then apply breadcrumbs to the Air Fryer. Air Fried for 8-10 minutes at 375F or until chicken is boiling thru. When on the other hand, rotate the chicken bits.

4. Drizzle over the chicken with the sauce and serve with leafy greens or Eggs and Green Onion Fried Rice Recipe.

9. Crispy Air Fryer Eggplant Parmesan

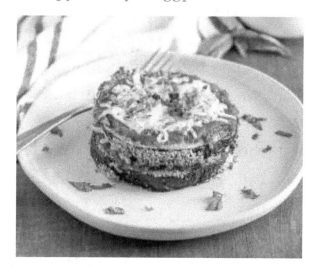

Ingredients

- ❖ Eggplant 1 large
- ❖ Wheat breadcrumbs ½ cup
- ❖ Parmesan cheese 3 tbsp
- ❖ Salt
- ❖ Italian seasoning 1 tsp
- ❖ Flour 3 tbsp
- ❖ Water 1 tbsp
- ❖ Olive oil spray
- ❖ Marinara sauce 1 cup
- ❖ Mozzarella cheese ¼ cup
- ❖ Fresh parsley

Steps

1. Break the eggplant into slices of approximately 1/2. "Add some salt on both ends of the slices and hold for at least 10-15 minutes.

2. Meanwhile, combine the egg with water and flour in a small bowl to make the batter.

3. Put cheese, breadcrumbs, Italian seasoning, and salt in a medium shallow bowl. Mix thoroughly.

4. Now equally add the batter to every eggplant slice. To cover it equally to both sides, add the battered halves in the breadcrumb mix.

5. On a clean, dry flat plate, put breaded eggplant slices and spray oil on them.

6. Heat the Air Fryer to 360F. Then place the slices of eggplant on the wire mesh and fry for around 8 minutes.

7. With around 1 tsp of marinara sauce and fresh mozzarella cheese thinly scattered on it, cover the air fried slices with around 1 tablespoon. Fry the eggplant for another 2 min or till the cheese melts.

8. On the side of your favorite pasta, serve soft.

10. Air Fryer Shrimp Fajitas

Ingredients

- ❖ Medium Shrimp 1 Pound
- ❖ Red Bell Pepper 1
- ❖ Green Bell Pepper 1
- ❖ Sweet Onion 1/2 Cup
- ❖ Gluten-Free Fajita 2 Tbsp
- ❖ Olive Oil Spray
- ❖ White Corn Tortillas or Flour Tortillas

Steps

1. Spray with olive oil or cover with foil on the air fryer bowl.

2. To get the ice off, pass cold water over it if the shrimp is stuck with ice on it.

3. Add to the bowl the tomatoes, seafood, seasoning, and cabbage.

4. Attach a layer with a mist with olive oil.

5. Mix everything.

6. Cook for 12 minutes at 390 degrees using the Ninja Foody Air Fryer.

7. Place the cap open and sprinkle it again and blend it up.

8. Cook for 10 more minutes.

9. On soft tortillas, eat.

11. Honey Glazed Air Fryer Salmon

Ingredients

- ❖ Salmon Fillets 4
- ❖ Salt
- ❖ Black Pepper

- ❖ Soy Sauce 2 teaspoons
- ❖ Honey 1 tablespoon
- ❖ Sesame Seeds 1 teaspoon

Steps

1. Heat the air fryer (it takes 1-2 mins).
2. Additionally: Season with pepper and salt on each salmon fillet. Rub the fish with soy sauce.
3. Put the fillets in the air fryer's bowl and cook for 8 minutes or till ready at 375 ° F (190 ° C).
4. Glaze every fillet with honey around a minute or two until the time is up and spray with sesame seeds. Bring them back in to have the cooking finished.
5. With a side of your choosing, serve.

12. Crispy Air Fryer Roasted Brussels Sprouts With Balsamic

Ingredients

- ❖ Brussels sprouts 1 pound
- ❖ Olive oil 2 Tablespoons
- ❖ Balsamic vinegar 1 Tablespoon
- ❖ Salt and Black pepper

Steps

1. Place the cut sprouts in a bowl. Sprinkle the vinegar and oil generously over the sprouts in Brussels. Don't pour vinegar and oil in one place, or just brush one of the sprouts in Brussels.
2. Sprinkle generously with pepper and salt around the Brussels sprouts. Mix to combine all and long enough so that the marinade soaks up all the Brussels sprouts.
3. Add the Brussels to the bowl of the air fryer. For around 15-20 minutes, fry the air at 359 ° F. Shake and softly stir halfway through to cook for about 7-8 minutes. At the halfway point, make sure the shaking. Shake and flip a third time if necessary, to ensure sure it cooks equally.
4. For the rest of the period, aim to air-fried Brussels completely. To make sure nothing burns, you should search earlier if necessary.
5. If needed, add extra salt, and pepper to the Brussels sprouts and enjoy.

13. Air Fryer Chicken Nuggets

Ingredients

- ❖ Cooking spray
- ❖ Chicken breasts 2

❖ Olive oil 1/3 cup

❖ Panko 1.5 cup

❖ Parmesan ¼ cup

❖ Sweet paprika 2 tsp

Steps

1. Break the chicken breasts into cubes from 1 "to 1.5" and put them aside and with one dish holding olive oil, while the other carrying panko, parmesan, and paprika, set up the station.

2. Lightly spritz the interior of your air fryer with some grease.

3. Dip the cube of chicken in the olive oil, then placed it on the top of the suit. Make sure you have a well-covered nugget and put it in the air fryer. Repeat until it's complete on your air fryer.

4. Adjust air fryer to 400F and cook for 8 minutes with homemade chicken nuggets.

5. Serve with the side of your choosing.

14. Air Fryer Baked Apples

Ingredients

❖ Apples 2

❖ Butter 1 tsp

❖ Cinnamon ½ tsp

Steps

1. Break the chicken breasts into cubes from 1 "to 1.5" and put them aside.

2. With one dish holding olive oil, the other carrying parmesan, paprika blend, and panko, set up the station.

3. Lightly spritz the interior of your air fryer with some grease.

4. Dip the cube of chicken in the olive oil, then placed it on the top of the suit. Make sure you have a well-covered nugget and put it in the air fryer. Repeat until it's complete on your air fryer.

5. Adjust air fryer to 400F and cook for 8 minutes with homemade chicken nuggets.

6. Serve with the side of your choosing.

15. Air Fryer Fish Tacos

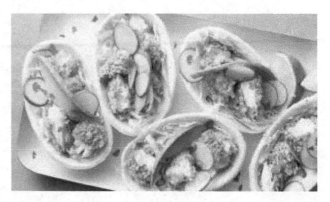

Ingredients

❖ Firm white fish fillets 24 oz

- ❖ Grill seasoning 1 tbsp
- ❖ Avocado 1 large
- ❖ Oranges 2 medium
- ❖ Red onion 1/4 cup
- ❖ Fresh cilantro 2 tbsp
- ❖ Salt 1 tsp
- ❖ Mayonnaise 1/4 cup
- ❖ Chipotle sauce 1/4 cup
- ❖ Lime juice 1 tbsp
- ❖ Corn tortillas

Steps

1. Mix the orange, avocado, cilantro, cabbage, and half a teaspoon of salt.

2. Stir the chipotle sauce, mayonnaise, lime juice and half a teaspoon of salt together.

3. Spray the fish generously, mostly with grill seasoning.

4. To stop sticking, quickly spray the air-fryer basket with vegetable oil.

5. Organize the fish in the bowl in a single sheet. Cook for 8-12 minutes at 400 degrees f, or until the fish's internal temperature exceeds 145 degrees f. Flipping the fish during frying is not required.

6. To make tacos, eat the fish with warmed avocado citrus salsa, corn tortillas, and chipotle mayonnaise.

16. Air Fryer Dumplings

Ingredients

- ❖ Chicken dumplings 8 ounces
- ❖ Soy sauce 1/4 cup
- ❖ Water 1/4 cup
- ❖ Maple syrup 1/8 cup
- ❖ Garlic powder 1/2 teaspoon
- ❖ Rice vinegar 1/2 teaspoon
- ❖ Small pinch of red pepper flakes

Steps

1. Preheat the air fryer for about 4 minutes to 370 degrees.

2. Put the frozen dumplings in one layer within the air fryer and spray them with gasoline.

3. Fry for 5 minutes, rotate the bowl and then apply a little more oil to the mist.

4. For another 4-6 minutes, cook the dumplings.

5. Meanwhile, make the dipping sauce by adding together the ingredients.

6. Take the fried dumplings from the bowl and let stay before enjoying for another 2 minutes.

17. Air Fryer Pork Chops

Ingredients

- ❖ Boneless 4 pork chops
- ❖ Grill seasoning 1 tbsp
- ❖ Maple syrup 1/4 cup
- ❖ Dijon mustard 2 tbsp
- ❖ Lemon juice 2 tsp
- ❖ Salt 1/2 tsp
- ❖ Vegetable oil

Steps

1. Rub air-fryer basket lightly with vegetable oil.

2. Clean pork chops with towels and generously brush with the barbecue seasoning on both sides.

3. Place the pork chops in one layer in the basket of the air fryer. You can need to bake the pork chops in two batches, depending on your air fryer's capacity.

4. Cook the pork chops for 12-15 minutes at 375 degrees F (more time is required if your pork chops are thick). Halfway into cooking time, turn over the pork chops.

5. Test the pork chops' internal temperature-when they are 145 degrees F, and they are finished frying.

6. In an air fryer, mix the vinegar, lemon juice, maple syrup, and salt while the pork chops are frying.

7. After extracting them from the air fryer, dump the sauce over the pork chops instantly.

8. Until eating, cause the pork chops to rest for 2 minutes.

18. Air Fryer Chicken Chimichangas

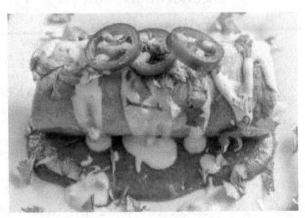

Ingredients

- ❖ Rotisserie chicken white meat 1
- ❖ Cooked rice 1 1/2 cups
- ❖ Salsa 1 cup
- ❖ Salt 1/2 tsp
- ❖ Soft taco size flour tortillas about 8 inches across
- ❖ Vegetable oil 2 tbsp

Steps

1. Rub the bottom of the basket with vegetable oil for the air fryer. The air fryer should be preheated to 360 degrees.
2. Mix the rice, chicken, salt, and salsa in a big bowl until well mixed.
3. In the middle of each tortilla, position about 1/2 cup of the chicken filling. With the ends bent in to lock in the lining, firmly wrap them back.
4. Place the chimichangas in the oiled bowl, two at a time and seam side down. With vegetable oil, gently clean the tops of the chimichangas.
5. Air-fry the chimichangas at 360 degrees for around 4 minutes. To flip the chimichangas, open an air fryer and use metal tongs. Once the chimichangas are crispy and browned, proceed to air fry for another 4 minutes.
6. The filling will be stored for up to two days in the refrigerator in an air-tight container so that the chimichangas can be prepared as desired.
7. Placed sour cream, white cheese sauce, onion, spinach, and guacamole on top of the chimichangas.

19. Simple Chicken Burrito Bowls

Ingredients

- ❖ Rotisserie chicken 1
- ❖ Black beans 1 15 oz
- ❖ Corn 1 15 oz
- ❖ Taco Skillet Sauce 1 8 oz packet
- ❖ Vegetable oil 1 tbsp
- ❖ White rice 1 cup
- ❖ Salt 1 tsp
- ❖ Water 1 3/4 cup
- ❖ Taco sauce 2 tbsp
- ❖ Iceberg lettuce 1 cup
- ❖ Avocado 1
- ❖ Lime wedges 4
- ❖ Medium cheddar cheese 6 oz
- ❖ Sour cream ½ cup

❖ Jalapenos 4 oz

Steps

1. Add the corn, chicken, taco skillet sauce, and black beans to a wide saucepan. Mix, cover, and heat until simmering, over medium-low heat.

2. Meanwhile, over medium-high pressure, heat the oil in a different saucepan. Add the rice and cook for a minute, sometimes stirring, before the rice begins to toast. Add the sauce to the water, salt and taco and bring it to a boil. Cover and boil the rice for 15-20 minutes or until the water is absorbed. Lower the pressure.

3. Add a large scoop of rice to the cups, then cover with the mixture of meat, beans, then maize. Add lime wedge, diced avocado, shredded lettuce, shredded cheese, sliced jalapeños, and sour cream to the option. Immediately serve.

20. Chicken Soft Tacos

Ingredients

❖ Unsalted butter 3 tbsp

❖ Garlic 4 cloves

❖ Chipotle chiles 2 tsp

❖ Orange 1/2 cup

❖ Worcestershire sauce 1/2 cup

❖ Cilantro 3/4 cup

❖ Boneless, skinless chicken breasts 4

❖ Yellow mustard 1 tsp

❖ Salt and pepper

❖ Flour tortillas 12 4-inch

Steps

1. In a broad skillet over the medium-high fire, melt the butter.

2. Add the garlic and chipotle and roast for around 1 minute before it is fragrant.

3. Stir in Worcestershire, orange juice, and 1/2 cup of cilantro and bring to a simmer.

4. Add the chicken and boil, covered, over medium-low heat for 10 to 15 minutes, until the meat is 160 degrees, flipping the chicken midway through cooking. Move to the foil-plate and tent.

5. Increase the heat to medium-high and simmer for around 5 minutes, until the liquid is reduced to 1/4 cup.

6. Whisk in the mustard, off the heat.

7. Shred the chicken into bite-sized bits using 2 forks, then return to the skillet.

8. In a pot, apply the remaining cilantro and mix until well mixed. With salt and pepper, season.

9. Serve with shredded cabbage, tortillas, sauce, cheese, sour cream, and wedges of lime.

21. Ground Pork Tacos - Al Pastor Style

Ingredients

- ❖ Pork 1 1/3 lbs.
- ❖ Orange 1/3 cup
- ❖ Canned chipotle sauce 3 tbsp
- ❖ Smoked paprika 1 tsp
- ❖ Cumin 1 tsp
- ❖ Salt 1 tsp
- ❖ Garlic powder 1/2 tsp
- ❖ Cayenne pepper 1/4 tsp
- ❖ Pineapple 1 1/2 cups
- ❖ Red onion finely diced 1/3 cup
- ❖ Cilantro 1/3 cup
- ❖ Juice of one-half lime
- ❖ Salt 1/2 tsp
- ❖ Pepper Jack cheese 6 oz
- ❖ Corn tortillas

Steps

1. Place the red onion, pineapple, lime juice, cilantro, and

1/2 tsp together in a bowl and set aside.

2. Add the chopped pork and cook till it is no longer pink in a non-stick skillet on medium heat, cutting ties the meat with a spatula.

3. Stir the chipotle sauce, orange juice, smoked paprika, garlic powder, cumin, and the remaining tsp and cayenne pepper into the fried pork. Stir well and allow for about 5 minutes to simmer.

4. Serve with tortillas, organic pineapple salsa and sliced Pepper Jack cheese on the pork taco meat.

22. Air-Fryer Southern-Style Chicken

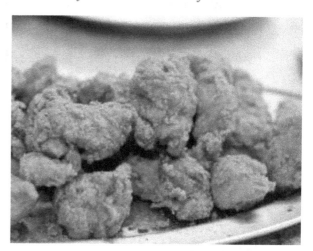

Ingredients

- ❖ Crushed Ritz crackers 2 cups
- ❖ Fresh parsley 1 tablespoon
- ❖ Garlic salt 1 teaspoon

- Paprika 1 teaspoon
- Pepper 1/2 teaspoon
- Cumin 1/4 teaspoon
- Rubbed sage 1/4 teaspoon
- Egg 1 large
- 1 broiler/fryer chicken
- Cooking spray

Steps

1. Heat an air fryer at 375 °. Blend the first seven ingredients in a small dish. Put the egg in a different shallow bowl. Dip the chicken in the shell, then pat in the cracker combination to help adhere to the coating. Place the chicken in batches in a thin layer on the oiled tray in the air-fryer bowl and sprinkle with the cooking mist.

2. Cook for 10 minutes. With cooking oil, transform the spritz and chicken; cook until the chicken is lightly browned, and the juices are transparent, 15-20 mins longer.

23. Air-Fryer Fish and Fries

Ingredients

- Potatoes 1 pound
- Olive oil 2 tablespoons
- Pepper 1/4 teaspoon
- Salt 1/4 teaspoon

FISH:

- Flour 1/3 cup
- Pepper 1/4 teaspoon
- Egg 1 large
- Water 2 tablespoons
- Cornflakes 2/3 cup
- Parmesan cheese 1 tablespoon
- Cayenne pepper 1/8 teaspoon
- Salt 1/4 teaspoon
- Haddock 1 pound

Steps

1. Heat air fryer at 400 °. Lengthwise, peel and cut the potatoes into 1/2-in.-thick slices; cut the slices into 1/2-in.-thick sticks.

2. Toss the potatoes with oil, pepper, and salt in a wide bowl. Place potatoes in batches in a single layer on the air-fryer basket tray; cook until only soft, 5-10 minutes to redistribute tossed potatoes; cook until slightly golden brown and crisp, 5-10 minutes longer.

3. Meanwhile, combine the flour and pepper in a small dish. Mix the egg with water in another small dish.

Toss the cornflakes with the cheese and cayenne in a third bowl. Sprinkle salt on the fish; dip in the flour mixture to cover all sides; shake off the residue. Dip in the mixture of shells, then pat in the cornflake mixture to bind to the coating.

4. Take the fries out of the bowl and stay warm. In an air-fryer bowl, put the fish in a single layer on the plate. Cook until fish is gently browned and, 9 minutes, turning midway through cooking, only begins to flake easily with a fork. Do not overcook it anymore. To heat up, return the fries to the basket. Immediately serve. Serve with tartar sauce if needed.

24. Air-Fryer Ground Beef Wellington

Ingredients

- ❖ Butter 1 tablespoon
- ❖ Mushrooms 1/2 cup
- ❖ Flour 2 teaspoons
- ❖ Pepper 1/4 teaspoon
- ❖ Half-and-half cream 1/2 cup
- ❖ Egg yolk 1 large
- ❖ Onion 2 tablespoons
- ❖ Salt 1/4 teaspoon

- ❖ Beef 1/2 pound
- ❖ Freeze Crescent rolls 1 tube (4 ounces)
- ❖ Egg 1 large
- ❖ Parsley flakes 1 teaspoon

Steps

1. Heat the air fryer at 300 °. Heat the butter over medium-high heat in a saucepan. Insert mushrooms; boil and mix for 5-6 minutes, until soft. Add flour and 1/8 of a teaspoon of pepper when combined. Add cream steadily. Cook and whisk until thickened, about 2 minutes.

2. Combine the egg yolk, carrot, 2 teaspoons of salt, mushroom sauce, and 1/8 teaspoon of pepper in a cup. Crumble over the mixture of beef and blend properly. Unroll and divide the crescent dough into 2 rectangles; force the perforations to close. Place each rectangle with the meatloaf. Bring together the sides and press to cover. Clean the broken egg if needed.

3. Put Wellingtons in a thin layer in an air-fryer basket on a greased plate. Cook until a thermometer placed into the meatloaf measures

160 °, 18-22 minutes, until golden brown.

4. Meanwhile, over low heat, steam the remaining sauce; mix in the parsley. With Wellingtons, serve the sauce.

25. Air-Fryer Ravioli

Ingredients

- ❖ Breadcrumbs 1 cup
- ❖ Parmesan cheese 1/4 cup
- ❖ Dried basil 2 teaspoons
- ❖ Flour 1/2 cup
- ❖ Eggs 2 large
- ❖ 1 package frozen beef ravioli
- ❖ Cooking spray
- ❖ 1 cup marinara sauce, warmed

Steps

1. Heat the air fryer at 350 °. Mix the breadcrumbs, the cheese, and the basil in a small dish. In different shallow cups, position the flour and eggs. To cover all ends, dip the ravioli in flour; shake off the waste. Dip in the shells, then pat in the crumb mixture to help bind to the coating.

2. Arrange the ravioli in batches on a greased tray in the air-fryer basket in a single layer; spritz with olive oil. Cook for 3-4 minutes before it's golden brown. Flip; spritz with spray for cooking. Fry till lightly browned, for 3-4 more minutes. Sprinkle instantly with basil and extra Parmesan cheese if needed. With marinara sauce, eat warm.

26. Popcorn Shrimp Tacos with Cabbage Slaw

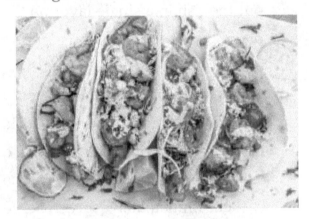

Ingredients

- ❖ Coleslaw 2 cups
- ❖ Cilantro 1/4 cup
- ❖ Lime juice 2 tablespoons
- ❖ Honey 2 tablespoons
- ❖ Salt 1/4 teaspoon
- ❖ Eggs 2 large
- ❖ 2% Milk 2 tablespoon
- ❖ Flour 1/2 cup
- ❖ Panko breadcrumbs 1-1/2 cups
- ❖ ground cumin 1 tablespoon

- ❖ Garlic powder 1 tablespoon
- ❖ Non cooked shrimp 1 pound
- ❖ Cooking spray
- ❖ Corn tortillas 8
- ❖ Avocado 1 medium

Steps

1. Combine the cilantro, coleslaw blend, sugar, lime juice, salt, and jalapeno, if needed, in a small bowl; toss to cover.

2. Heat an air fryer at 375 °. Whisk the eggs and milk together in a small dish. Place flour in a different shallow bowl. Cumin, Panko, and garlic powder are combined in a final small cup. To cover all ends, dip the shrimp in flour; shake off the waste. Dip in the egg mixture, then pat onto the panko mixture to help bind to the coating.

3. Organize shrimp in a thin layer in an oiled air-fryer bowl in batches, dust with cooking spray. For 2-3 minutes, cook till lightly browned. Turn; spritz with spray for cooking. Cook until the shrimp turns pink and lightly browned, 3 minutes longer.

4. Serve shrimp in coleslaw blend and avocado in tortillas.

27. Bacon-Wrapped Avocado Wedges

Ingredients

- ❖ Avocados 2 medium
- ❖ Bacon strips 12
- ❖ Mayonnaise 1/2 cup
- ❖ Sriracha chili sauce 2 to 3 tablespoons
- ❖ Lime juice 1 to 2 tablespoons

Steps

1. Heat the air fryer at 400 degrees. Break each avocado in half; peel and extract the pit. Break the halves into thirds each. Wrap over each avocado wedge with 1 bacon slice. If required, operate in batches, put slices in a thin layer in the fryer basket and cook 10-15 minutes until the bacon is fried through.

2. Meanwhile, whisk together the sriracha sauce, mayonnaise, lime juice and zest in a shallow dish. Serve with sauce on the wedges.

28. Air-Fryer Steak Fajitas

Ingredients

- ❖ Tomatoes 2 large

- Red onion 1/2 cup

- Lime juice 1/4 cup

- Pepper 1 jalapeno

- Cilantro 3 tablespoons

- Cumin 2 teaspoons

- Salt 3/4 teaspoon

- 1 beef flank steak

- Onion 1 large

- 6 whole-wheat tortillas (8 inches), warmed

Steps

1. Place five ingredients in a little bowl for salsa first; mix in 1 tsp cumin and 1/4 tsp salt. Let it stand until you serve.

2. Heat an air fryer at 400 °. Sprinkle the residual cumin and salt with the steak. Place the air-fryer basket on a greased plate. Cook until the meat hits the appropriate thickness (a thermometer can read 135 ° for medium-rare; medium, 140 °; moderate-well, 145 °), 6-8 minutes on each hand. Remove from the basket and quit for 5 minutes to stand.

3. Meanwhile, put the onion in the air-fryer basket on the counter. Cook till crisp-tender, stirring

once, 2-3 minutes. Thinly slice the steak around the grain; eat with salsa and onion in tortillas. Serve with lime and avocado slices if needed.

29. Air-Fryer Sweet and Sour Pork

Ingredients

- Pineapple 1/2 cup

- Cider vinegar 1/2 cup

- Sugar 1/4 cup

- Dark brown sugar 1/4 cup

- Ketchup 1/4 cup

- Reduced-sodium soy sauce 1 tablespoon

- Dijon mustard 1-1/2 teaspoons

- Garlic powder 1/2 teaspoon

- 1 pork tenderloin

- Salt 1/8 teaspoon

- Pepper 1/8 teaspoon

- Cooking spray

Steps

1. Integrate the first eight ingredients in a shallow saucepan. Get it to a boil; lower the flame. Simmer, exposed, for 6-8 minutes till thickened, stirring periodically.

2. Heat the air fryer at 350 °. Sprinkle salt and pepper on the bacon. Place the pork in the air-fryer bowl on a greased tray; spritz with the cooking mist. Cook for 7-8 minutes before the pork starts to brown around the edges. Place 2 teaspoons of sauce over the pork. Heat till at least 145 ° is read by a thermometer placed into the bacon, 11-13 minutes longer. Let the pork stand before slicing for 5 minutes. Serve with the sauce that exists. Cover with chopped green onions if needed.

30. Air-Fryer Taco Twists

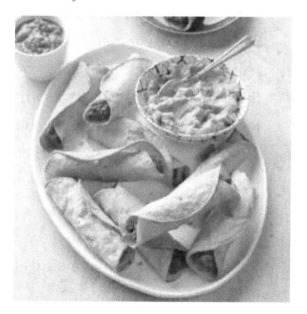

Ingredients

* Beef 1/3 pound

* Onion 1 large

* Cheddar cheese 2/3 cup

* Salsa 1/3 cup

* Canned chopped green chiles 3 tablespoons

* Garlic powder 1/4 teaspoon

* Hot pepper sauce 1/4 teaspoon

* Salt 1/8 teaspoon

* Cumin 1/8 teaspoon

* Freeze Crescent rolls 1 tube

Steps

1. Heat the air fryer at 300 °. Cook the beef and onion on medium heat in a large skillet until the meat is no longer pink, rinse. Integrate salsa, garlic powder, cheese, salt, and cumin with sweet pepper sauce.

2. Unroll and divide the crescent roll dough into 4 rectangles; push the sealing perforations. Put in the middle of each rectangle with 1/2 cup of meat mixture. Twist and put 4 corners to the center: pinch to cover. Place in a thin layer on the greased tray in the air-fryer bowl in batches. Cook for 18-22 minutes before it is golden brown. Serve with condiments of your choosing, if needed.

31. Air-Fryer Potato Chips

Ingredients

- ❖ Potatoes 2 large
- ❖ Olive oil spray
- ❖ Sea salt ½ teaspoon

Steps

1. Preheat the air fryer at 360 °. Cut the potatoes into thinly sliced using a mandolin or vegetable peeler. Switch to a wide bowl; to fill, add sufficiently ice water. Take a 15-minute soak, rinse. Soak for 15 more minutes.

2. Drain potatoes, put, and pat dry on towels. Sprinkle with cooking spray on the potatoes; sprinkle with salt. Put potato slices in batches in a thin layer on the oiled air-fryer basket plate. Cook for 15-17 minutes until it is crisp and lightly browned, stirring and rotating every 6 minutes. Sprinkle with parsley if needed.

32. Air-Fryer Greek Breadsticks

Ingredients

- ❖ Marinated quartered artichoke hearts 1/4 cup
- ❖ Pitted Greek olives 2 tablespoons
- ❖ Frozen puff pastry 1 package
- ❖ Spreadable spinach and artichoke cream cheese 1 carton
- ❖ Parmesan cheese 2 tablespoons
- ❖ Egg 1 large
- ❖ Water 1 tablespoon
- ❖ Sesame seeds 2 teaspoons

Steps

1. Heat an air fryer at 325 °. In a food processor, put the artichokes and olives; cover and pulse till finely chopped. On a lightly floured board, unfold 1 pastry sheet; scatter half the cream cheese on half of the pastry. Comb with a variation of half the artichoke. Sprinkle the Parmesan cheese with half of it. Fold the simple half over the filling; pressure to close softly.

2. Repeat with the remaining cookie, cream cheese, Parmesan cheese and artichoke mixture. Whisk the water and egg; clean the tips. Sprinkle the seeds with sesame. Split into 16 3/4-in.-wide strips for each rectangle.

3. Adjust bread pieces in a single sheet in batches on a greased tray in the air-fryer basket. Cook for 12-15 minutes until it is golden brown.

33. Air-Fryer Crumb-Topped Sole

Ingredients

- ❖ Mayonnaise 3 tablespoons
- ❖ Parmesan cheese 3 tablespoons
- ❖ Mustard seed 2 teaspoons
- ❖ Pepper 1/4 teaspoon
- ❖ Sole fillets 4
- ❖ Soft breadcrumbs 1 cup
- ❖ Onion 1
- ❖ Mustard 1/2 teaspoon
- ❖ Butter 2 teaspoons
- ❖ Cooking spray

Steps

1. Heat an air fryer at 375 °. Combine mayonnaise, bacon, mustard seed, pepper, 2 tablespoons: place over the fillets' tops.
2. In the air-fryer bowl, put the fish in a single layer on the greased plate. Cook for 3-5 minutes before the fish quickly flakes with a fork.
3. Meanwhile, mix breadcrumbs, carrot, ground mustard and 1 remaining tablespoon of cheese in a small bowl: whisk in butter. Cook until golden brown, for 2-3 more minutes. Sprinkle with additional green onions if needed.

34. Air-Fried Radishes

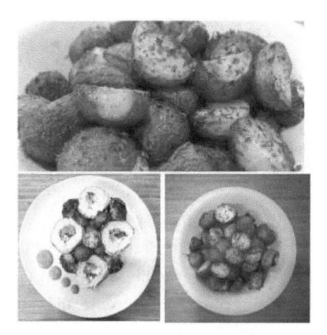

Ingredients

- ❖ Radishes 2-1/4 pounds
- ❖ Olive oil 3 tablespoons
- ❖ Oregano 1 tablespoon
- ❖ Salt 1/4 teaspoon
- ❖ Pepper 1/8 teaspoon

Steps

1. Heat the air fryer at 375 degrees. Mix all the ingredients.
2. Place radishes on an oiled tray in the air fryer bowl. Fry till crispy, 15 minutes, blend frequently.

35. Air-Fryer Ham and Egg Pockets

Ingredients

- Egg 1 large
- 2% Milk 2 teaspoons
- Butter 2 teaspoons
- Sliced deli ham 1 ounce
- Cheddar cheese 2 tablespoons
- Freeze Crescent rolls 1 tube

Steps

1. Heat the air fryer at 300 °. Combine the egg and milk in a shallow dish. Heat the butter in a small skillet until sweet. Add the egg combination; cook and stir until the eggs are formed, over medium heat. Distance yourself from the steam. Fold in the cheese and ham.

2. Divide the crescent dough into two rectangles. Fold the dough over the filling, close with a squeeze. In the air-fryer basket, put it in a single layer on a greased plate. Cook for 8-10 minutes until it is lightly browned.

36. Air-Fryer Eggplant Fries

Ingredients

- Eggs 2 large
- Parmesan cheese 1/2 cup
- Toasted wheat germ 1/2 cup

- Italian seasoning 1 teaspoon
- Garlic salt 3/4 teaspoon
- Eggplant 1 medium
- Cooking spray
- Meatless pasta sauce 1 cup

Steps

1. Heat an air fryer at 375 °. Whisk the eggs together in a small dish. Mix the cheese, seasonings, and wheat germ in another small dish.

2. Trim the eggplant ends; split the eggplant into 1/2-in.-thick pieces lengthwise. Split elongated into 1/2-in pieces. Dip the eggplant in the eggs, then cover with the mixture of cheese.

3. Adjust eggplant in batches on a greased tray in the air-fryer bowl in a single layer; spritz with olive oil. Cook for 4-5 minutes until it is golden brown. Turn; spritz with spray for cooking. Cook for 4-5 minutes until it is golden brown. Serve with pasta sauce directly.

37. Air-Fryer Turkey Croquettes

Ingredients

- Mashed potatoes 2 cups
- Parmesan cheese 1/2 cup

- Swiss cheese 1/2 cup

- Shallot 1

- Rosemary 2 teaspoons

- Sage 1 teaspoon

- Salt 1/2 teaspoon

- Pepper 1/4 teaspoon

- Cooked turkey 3 cups

- Egg 1 large

- Water 2 tablespoons

- Panko breadcrumbs 1-1/4 cups

- Butter-flavored cooking spray

Steps

1. Heat the air fryer at 350 °. Mix the cheese, sage, pepper, salt, mashed potatoes, shallot, and rosemary in a big bowl, whisk in the turkey.

2. Whisk the egg and water in a small dish. In another shallow cup, position the breadcrumbs. Dip the croquettes in the egg mixture, then pat them onto the breadcrumbs to make the coating hold.

3. Place croquettes in batches on a greased tray in the air-fryer bowl in a single layer; spritz with olive oil. Cook for 4-5 minutes until it is golden brown. Turn; spritz with spray for cooking.

Cook for 4-5 minutes, until golden brown. Serve with sour cream if needed.

38. Garlic-Herb Fried Patty Pan Squash

Ingredients

- Small pattypan squash 5 cups

- Olive oil 1 tablespoon

- Garlic cloves 2

- Salt 1/2 teaspoon

- Oregano 1/4 teaspoon

- Dried thyme 1/4 teaspoon

- Pepper 1/4 teaspoon

- Parsley 1 tablespoon

Steps

1. Heat the air fryer at 375 degrees and put the squash in a bowl. Blend salt, oil, garlic, pepper, oregano, and thyme. Toss to coat.

2. Put the squash on an oiled tray in the air fryer bowl. Fry till tender, 15 mins, stirring frequently. Spray with parsley.

39. Air-Fryer Quinoa Arancini

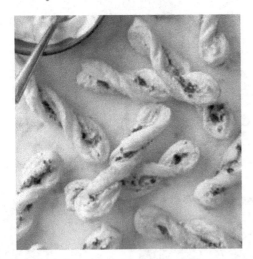

Ingredients

- ❖ Cooked quinoa 1-3/4 cups

- ❖ Eggs 2 large

- ❖ seasoned breadcrumbs 1 cup

- ❖ Parmesan cheese 1/4 cup

- ❖ Olive oil 1 tablespoon

- ❖ Basil 2 tablespoons

- ❖ Garlic powder 1/2 teaspoon

- ❖ Salt 1/2 teaspoon

- ❖ Pepper 1/8 teaspoon

- ❖ Mozzarella cheese 6 cubes

- ❖ Cooking spray

Steps

1. Heat an air fryer at 375 °. Prepare quinoa. Incorporate 1 white, 1/2 cup of cheese, breadcrumbs, basil oil and seasonings.

2. Split into 6 parts. To cover entirely, shape each part around a cheese ball, creating a ball.

3. In separate shallow cups, position the leftover egg and 1/2 cup of breadcrumbs. Dip the quinoa balls into the egg, then apply the breadcrumbs to the roll. Put in the air-fryer bowl on a greased tray; spritz with the cooking mist. Cook for 6-8 minutes until it is golden brown. Represent with pasta sauce if needed.

40. Air-Fryer General Tso's Cauliflower

Ingredients

- ❖ Flour 1/2 cup

- ❖ Cornstarch 1/2 cup

- ❖ Salt 1 teaspoon

- ❖ Baking powder 1 teaspoon

- ❖ Club soda 3/4 cup

- ❖ Head cauliflower 1 medium

Steps

1. Heat an air fryer at 400 °. Toss the rice, cornstarch, baking powder, and salt together. Just when mixed, stir in club soda (batter would be thin). Toss the florets in the batter, transfer on a baking sheet to a wire rack. Let the 5

minutes stand. Place cauliflower in batches on a greased tray in the air-fryer basket. Heat till soft and lightly browned, 10-12 minutes.

2. Meanwhile, whisk the sauce ingredients together, whisk until smooth in the cornstarch.

3. Steam canola oil on medium-high heat in a big saucepan. Add the chiles; cook and mix for 1-2 minutes, until fragrant. Add the ginger, white onions, garlic, and orange zest; simmer for around 1 minute, until fragrant. Stir in the mixture of orange juice; return to the saucepan. Put to a boil; fry and mix for 2-4 minutes before it thickens.

4. To the sauce, add cauliflower, toss to cover. Represent with rice; scatter with green onions, thinly cut.

41. Air-Fryer Pork Chops

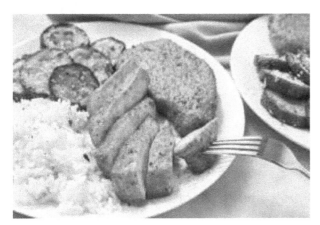

Ingredients

- ❖ Boneless pork loin chops 4
- ❖ Almond flour 1/3 cup
- ❖ Parmesan cheese 1/4 cup
- ❖ Garlic powder 1 teaspoon
- ❖ Creole seasoning 1 teaspoon
- ❖ Paprika 1 teaspoon
- ❖ Cooking spray

Steps

1. Heating air fryer to 375 degrees; frying spray spritz fryer basket. Toss the garlic powder, almond flour, creole seasoning, cheese, and paprika in a small dish. Cover pork chops with a combination of flour; shake off the surplus. Working as needed in batches, place chops in the air-fryer bowl in a single layer; spritz with cooking spray.

2. Heat till lightly browned, 12-15 minutes or until a 145 degrees thermometer registers, changing with additional cooking spray midway through cooking and spritzing. Remove it and remain wet. Repeat with the chops that remain.

42. Air-Fryer Nacho Hot Dogs

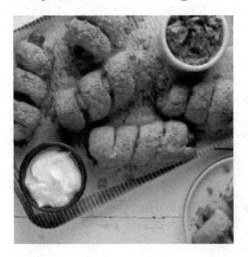

Ingredients

- ❖ Hot dogs 6
- ❖ Cheddar cheese sticks 3
- ❖ Flour 1-1/4 cups
- ❖ Greek yogurt 1 cup
- ❖ Salsa 1/4 cup
- ❖ Chili powder 1/4 teaspoon
- ❖ Chopped seeded jalapeno pepper 3 tablespoons
- ❖ Nacho-flavored tortilla chips 1 cup

Steps

1. Without cutting open, cut a slice down each hot dog; cut the slice with a half cheese handle.
2. Heat the air fryer at 350 °. Mix the butter, rice, vinegar, jalapenos, chili powder, and half a cup of broken tortilla chips in a wide bowl to form a smooth mixture.

On a lightly floured board, position the dough; divide into sixths. Roll the dough into 15-inch large pieces; tie the cheese-stuffed hot dog along one strip. Repeat with the dough and the hot dogs that remain. Spray the cooking spray on the dogs and move softly onto the leftover smashed chips. Spray the air fryer container with cooking spray and, without contact, put the dogs in the bowl, leaving space for expansion.

3. Cook in batches for 8-10 minutes until the dough is finely browned, and the cheese begins to melt. Represent with extra chips, sour cream and guacamole if needed.

43. Air-Fryer Raspberry Balsamic Smoked Pork Chops

Ingredients

- ❖ Eggs 2 large
- ❖ 2% milk 1/4 cup
- ❖ Panko breadcrumbs 1 cup
- ❖ Pecans 1 cup
- ❖ Smoked bone-in pork chops 4
- ❖ Flour 1/4 cup
- ❖ Cooking spray
- ❖ Balsamic vinegar 1/3 cup

- ❖ Brown sugar 2 tablespoons
- ❖ Seedless raspberry jam 2 tablespoons
- ❖ Frozen orange juice 1 tablespoon

Steps

1. Heat an air fryer at 400 °. Whisk the eggs and milk together in a small dish. Toss the breadcrumbs with the pecans in another small dish.
2. Cover the chops of pork with flour; shake off the fat. Dip in the mixture of shells, then pat onto the crumb mixture to help stick. In batches, on an oiled tray in an air-fryer rack, put chops in a single layer; spritz with cooking spray.
3. Heat till light brown and a thermometer placed into the pork reads 145 °, 12-15 minutes, turning with extra cooking spray midway across cooking and spritzing. Meanwhile, put in a small saucepan the remaining ingredients; bring to a boil. Cook and mix until it thickens slightly, 6-8 minutes. With chops, eat.

44. Air-Fryer Chickpea Fritters with Sweet-Spicy Sauce

Ingredients

- ❖ Yogurt 1 cup
- ❖ Sugar 2 tablespoons
- ❖ Honey 1 tablespoon
- ❖ Salt 1/2 teaspoon
- ❖ Pepper 1/2 teaspoon
- ❖ Red pepper flakes 1/2 teaspoon
- ❖ Garbanzo beans 15 ounces
- ❖ Cumin 1 teaspoon
- ❖ Salt 1/2 teaspoon
- ❖ Garlic powder 1/2 teaspoon
- ❖ Ginger 1/2 teaspoon
- ❖ Egg 1 large
- ❖ Baking soda 1/2 teaspoon
- ❖ Cilantro 1/2 cup
- ❖ Onions 2

Steps

1. Heat an air-fryer at 400 °. Integrate the ingredients in a small bowl; refrigerate before they are eaten.
2. Put in a food processor with seasonings and chickpeas; pulse unless finely ground. Also include baking soda and egg, pulse until combined. Then shift to a bowl,

whisk in the green onions and cilantro.

3. Drop rounded teaspoons of bean combination on the greased tray in the air-fryer basket in batches. For 5-6 minutes, fry till golden brown. Serve with the gravy.

45. Air-Fryer Crispy Sriracha Spring Rolls

Ingredients

- Coleslaw 3 cups
- Onions 3
- Soy sauce 1 tablespoon
- Sesame oil 1 teaspoon
- Boneless skinless chicken breasts 1 pound
- Salt 1 teaspoon
- Cream cheese 2 packages
- Sriracha chili sauce 2 tablespoons
- Spring roll wrappers 24
- Cooking spray

Steps

1. Heat the air fryer at 360 °. Toss with the mixture of coleslaw, green onions, soy sauce and sesame oil; leave stand while the chicken is frying. In an air-fryer bowl, put the chicken in a single layer on an oiled plate. Cook until a chicken-inserted thermometer reads 165 °, 18-20 minutes. Chicken removal; cold slightly. Chop the chicken finely; toss with seasoned salt.

2. Increase the temperature of the air-fryer to 400 °. Combine the cream cheese and the Sriracha chili sauce in a large bowl, whisk in the chicken and coleslaw mixture. Place about 2 teaspoons of filling just below the middle of the wrapper with 1 side of a spring roll wrapper facing you. Fold the bottom corner over the filling; wet the remaining edges with water. Overfilling, fold side corners towards the center; tightly roll up, pressing the tip to seal.

3. Arrange spring rolls in batches on a greased tray in the air-fryer bowl in a single layer; spritz with cooking spray. For 5-6 minutes, cook until lightly browned. Turn; spritz with spray for cooking. Cook until crisp and golden brown, 5-6 minutes longer. Serve with sweet chili sauce if needed.

4. Freeze 1 inch of uncooked spring rolls. Separating layers with waxed paper and in freezer cases.

To use, cook frozen spring rolls as instructed, as required, increasing the time.

46. Air-Fryer Pork Schnitzel

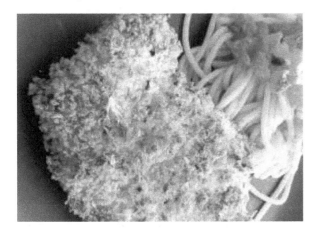

Ingredients

* Flour 1/4 cup

* Salt 1 teaspoon

* Pepper 1/4 teaspoon

* Egg 1 large

* 2% milk 2 tablespoons

* Dry breadcrumbs 3/4 cup

* Paprika 1 teaspoon

* Pork sirloin cutlets 4

* Cooking spray

Steps

1. Heat an air fryer at 375 °. Mix the flour and the seasoned salt and pepper in a small dish. Whisk the egg and milk in a second shallow bowl until well mixed. Mix the breadcrumbs and paprika in a third bowl.

2. Pound pork cutlets with a 1/4-in beef mallet. Dip the cutlets to cover all sides in the flour mixture; shake off the excess. Dip in the mixture of shells, then pat in the crumb mixture to help adhere to the coating.

3. Put the pork in a single layer in an air-fryer bowl on an oiled tray; spritz with olive oil. Cook for 4-5 minutes until it is lightly browned. Turn; spritz with spray for cooking. Heat till lightly browned, for 4-5 more minutes. Set aside in a serving dish; hold hot.

4. Meanwhile, mix the flour and broth in a shallow saucepan until creamy. Put to a boil, continuously stirring; simmer and mix for 2 minutes or thickened. Reduce the heat to low amounts. Stir in the dill and sour cream; heat up (do not boil). With bacon, eat.

47. Air-Fryer Green Tomato Stacks

Ingredients

* Mayonnaise 1/4 cup

* Lime zest 1/4 teaspoon

* lime juice 2 tablespoons

- ❖ Thyme 1 teaspoon

- ❖ Pepper 1/2 teaspoon

- ❖ Flour 1/4 cup

- ❖ Egg whites 2 large

- ❖ Cornmeal 3/4 cup

- ❖ Salt 1/4 teaspoon

- ❖ Green tomatoes 2 medium

- ❖ Red tomatoes 2 medium

- ❖ Cooking spray

- ❖ 8 slices Canadian bacon

Steps

1. Heat an air fryer at 375 °. Mix the lime zest, thyme, mayonnaise, juice, and 1/4 of a teaspoon of pepper; cool until ready to eat. Place the flour in a shallow bowl, place in a different shallow bowl the egg whites. Mix the cornmeal, salt and the remaining 1/4 of a teaspoon of pepper in a third dish.

2. Break into 4 slices of each tomato crosswise. Coat each slice thinly with flour; shake off the waste. Dip in the egg whites, then the combination of cornmeal.

3. Place tomatoes in batches in an air-fryer basket on a greased tray; spritz with olive oil. Cook for 4-6 minutes before it's lightly browned. Turn; spritz with spray for cooking. Cook until golden brown, for 4-6 more minutes.

4. Stack 1 slice of green tomato, bacon, and red tomato for each meal. Represent with the gravy.

48. Air-Fryer Pretzel-Crusted Catfish

Ingredients

- ❖ Catfish fillets 6 oz

- ❖ Salt 1/2 teaspoon

- ❖ Pepper 1/2 teaspoon

- ❖ Eggs 2 large

- ❖ Dijon mustard 1/3 cup

- ❖ 2% milk 2 tablespoons

- ❖ Flour 1/2 cup

- ❖ Honey mustard small pretzels 4 cups

- ❖ Cooking spray

Steps

1. Heat an air fryer at 325 °. Sprinkle salt and pepper with the catfish. In a small dish, whisk in the mustard, eggs, and milk. Put in different shallow bowls of flour and pretzels. Cover the flour fillets, then drop in the mixture of the eggs and coat with the pretzels.

2. Put fillets in a thin layer on the greased tray in the air-fryer basket in batches, spray with olive oil. Cook for 10-12 minutes before the fish quickly flakes with a fork. Represent with lemon slices if needed.

49. Air-Fryer French Toast Cups with Raspberries

Ingredients

- ❖ Italian bread 2 slices
- ❖ Raspberries 1/2 cup
- ❖ Cream cheese 2 ounces
- • Eggs 2 large
- • Milk 1/2 cup
- • Maple syrup 1 tablespoon

Steps

1. Divide half the bread cubes into 2 8-oz greased cubes. Cups of custard. Using raspberries and cream cheese to scatter. Cover with leftover pasta. Whisk the sugar, eggs, and syrup in a small bowl, sprinkle over the toast. For at least 1 hour, cover and refrigerate.

2. Heat an air fryer at 325 °. Put custard cups in an air-fryer basket on a plate. Cook for 12-15 minutes, until golden brown and puffy.

3. Meanwhile, mix cornstarch and water in a shallow saucepan until smooth. Add 1-1/2 cups of raspberries, lemon juice, lemon zest and syrup. Get it to a boil; lower the flame. Cook and mix for around 2 minutes, until thickened. Strain and extract the seeds; lightly cool off.

4. Stir the remaining 1/2 cup of berries into the syrup gently. Sprinkle the French toast cups with cinnamon if desired; serve with syrup.

50. Air Fryer Ham and Cheese Turnovers

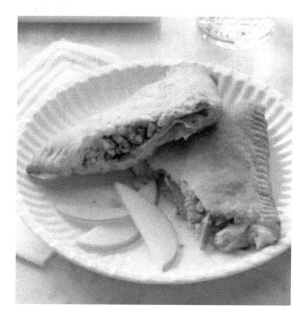

Ingredients

- ❖ Freeze pizza crust 1 tube

- ❖ Black forest deli ham 1/4 pound
- ❖ Pear 1 medium
- ❖ Walnuts 1/4 cup
- ❖ Blue cheese 2 tablespoons

Steps

1. Heat an air fryer at 400 °. Unroll the pizza base into a 12-in section on a thinly floured board. Round into 4 triangles. Layer pork, half pear strips, walnuts, and blue cheese on half of every square diagonally within 1/2. From the margins. Fold 1 corner to the opposite side, creating a triangle over the filling; force the edges to close with a fork.

2. Adjust turnovers in batches on an oiled tray in the air-fryer bowl in a single layer; spritz with a cooking mist. Heat till lightly browned, on either hand, for 4-6 minutes. Garnish with the remaining slices of pear.

51. Air-Fryer Shrimp Po'Boys

Ingredients

- ❖ Mayonnaise 1/2 cup
- ❖ Creole mustard 1 tablespoon
- ❖ Cornichons 1 tablespoon

- ❖ Shallot 1 tablespoon
- ❖ Lemon juice 1-1/2 teaspoons
- ❖ Cayenne pepper 1/8 teaspoon

Steps

1. Add the ingredients in a shallow dish. Refrigerate until consumed, sealed.

2. Heat an air fryer at 375 °. Combine the rice, garlic powder, sea salt, pepper, and cayenne in a small dish. Whisk the egg, milk, and spicy pepper sauce together in a small shallow dish. In a third shallow bowl, put the coconut in it. To cover all ends, dip the shrimp in flour; shake off the waste. Dip in the egg mixture, then pat in the coconut to help hold to it.

3. Arrange shrimps in batches on a greased tray in the air-fryer bowl in a single layer; spritz with olive oil. Cook for 3-4 minutes on either side until the coconut is gently browned and the shrimp turns yellow.

4. Spread cut side of remoulade for buns. Place the seafood, lettuce, and tomato on top.

52. Air-Fryer Papas Rellenas

Ingredients

- ❖ Potatoes 2-1/2 pounds
- ❖ Lean ground beef 1 pound
- ❖ Green pepper 1 small
- ❖ Onion 1 small
- ❖ Tomato sauce 1/2 cup
- ❖ Green olives with pimientos 1/2 cup
- ❖ Raisins 1/2 cup
- ❖ Salt 1-1/4 teaspoons
- ❖ Pepper 1-1/4 teaspoons
- ❖ Paprika 1/2 teaspoon
- ❖ Garlic powder 1 teaspoon
- ❖ Eggs 2 large
- ❖ seasoned breadcrumbs 1 cup
- ❖ Cooking spray

Steps

1. Place the potatoes and cover them with water in a large saucepan. Just get it to a simmer. Reduce heat; cover and simmer for 15-20 minutes, till tender. In the meantime, add green pepper, cook beef, and onion on medium heat in a broad skillet until the meat is no longer pink, rinse. Add olives, tomato sauce, raisins, 1/4 of a teaspoon of cinnamon, 1/4 of a teaspoon of pepper and paprika; combine well.

2. Drain the potatoes; mash with garlic powder and 1 teaspoon of salt and pepper left. Put a tbsp of filling in the middle and form 2 tablespoons of potatoes into a patty. Form the potatoes around the filling, making a ball. Only repeat.

3. Put in different shallow bowls of eggs and breadcrumbs. Dip the potato balls into the eggs, then apply the breadcrumbs to the roll. Preheat the fryer to 400 degrees. Place in batches in an air-fryer bowl on an oiled tray in a thin layer; sprinkle with cooking spray. Cook until the brown is translucent, 14-16 minutes.

53. Air-Fryer Herb and Cheese-Stuffed Burgers

Ingredients

- ❖ Green onions 2
- ❖ Parsley 2 tablespoons
- ❖ Dijon mustard 4 teaspoons
- ❖ Breadcrumbs 3 tablespoons
- ❖ Ketchup 2 tablespoons

- ❖ Salt 1/2 teaspoon

- ❖ Rosemary 1/2 teaspoon

- ❖ Sage leaves 1/4 teaspoon

- ❖ Lean ground beef 1 pound

- ❖ Cheddar cheese 2 ounces

- ❖ Hamburger buns 4

Steps

1. Heat an air fryer at 375 °. Combine the parsley, green onions, and 2 teaspoons of mustard in a shallow dish. Combine the ketchup, breadcrumbs, seasonings and the remaining 2 teaspoons of mustard in another cup. To the bread crumb mixture, add beef, blend gently yet thoroughly.

2. Shape 8 thin patties into the mixture. Place the sliced cheese in the middle of four patties; spoon the green onion mixture over the cheese. Top with the remaining patties, tightly pushing the edges close, making sure to completely cover.

3. Place burgers in batches in a thin layer on the tray in the air-fryer bowl. Eight minutes of cooking. Flip: cook for 9 minutes further before the thermometer inserted into the burger measures 160 °.

Serve burgers, with toppings if needed, on buns.

54. Air-Fryer Nashville Hot Chicken

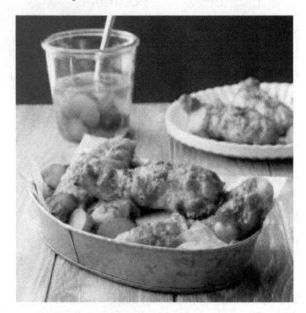

Ingredients

- ❖ Pickle juice 2 tablespoons

- ❖ Hot pepper sauce 2 tablespoons

- ❖ Salt 1 teaspoon

- ❖ Chicken tenderloins 2 pounds

- ❖ Flour 1 cup

- ❖ Pepper 1/2 teaspoon

- ❖ Egg 1 large

- ❖ Buttermilk 1/2 cup

- ❖ Cooking spray

- ❖ Olive oil 1/2 cup

- ❖ Cayenne pepper 2 tablespoons

- ❖ Dark brown sugar 2 tablespoons

- ❖ Paprika 1 teaspoon

❖ Chili powder 1 teaspoon

❖ Garlic powder 1/2 teaspoon

❖ Pickle slices

Steps

1. Combine 1 tablespoon pickle juice, 1 tablespoon hot sauce and 1/2 teaspoon salt in a cup or shallow bath. Connect the bird, then switch the coat over. Freeze, sealed, for 1 hour. Drain, tossing out some marinade.

2. Heat an air fryer at 375 °. Mix the starch, the remaining 1/2 teaspoon salt, and the pepper in a small dish. Whisk together the bacon, buttermilk, 1 tablespoon of pickle juice and 1 tablespoon of hot sauce in another small cup. To cover all ends, dip the chicken in flour; shake off the waste. Dip in the egg mixture, then the flour mixture again.

3. Organize the chicken in batches on a well-greased tray in the air-fryer bowl in a single layer; spritz with cooking spray. Cook for 5-6 minutes until it is golden brown. Turn; spritz with spray for cooking. Cook until golden brown, for 5-6 more minutes.

4. Mix milk, cayenne pepper, brown sugar, seasonings, spillover warm chicken and cover with the flip. With pickles, eat.

55. Air-Fryer Salmon with Maple-Dijon Glaze

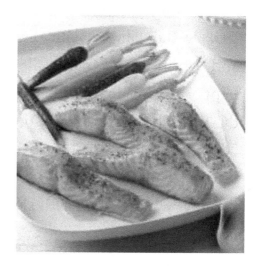

Ingredients

❖ Butter 3 tablespoons

❖ Maple syrup 3 tablespoons

❖ Dijon mustard 1 tablespoon

❖ Lemon 1 medium

❖ Garlic clove 1

❖ Olive oil 1 tablespoon

❖ Salt 1/4 teaspoon

❖ Pepper 1/4 teaspoon

❖ Salmon fillets 4 ounces

Steps

1. Heat an air fryer at 400 degrees.

2. Meanwhile, melt butter over medium to high heat in a deep saucepan. Add the mustard, lemon juice, maple syrup, and minced garlic. Lower the flame and boil for 2-3 minutes before the mixture thickens significantly.

3. Drizzle the salmon with olive oil and sprinkle it with salt and pepper. In an air fryer bowl, put the fish in a single sheet. Cook for 5-7 minutes until the fish is gently browned and only starts to flake quickly with a fork. Drizzle just before eating with sauce.

56. Air Fryer Tortellini with Prosciutto

Ingredients

- ❖ Olive oil 1 tablespoon
- ❖ Onion 3 tablespoons
- ❖ Garlic cloves 4
- ❖ Tomato puree 15 ounces
- ❖ Basil 1 tablespoon
- ❖ Salt 1/4 teaspoon
- ❖ Pepper 1/4 teaspoon

Steps

1. Heat oil on medium-high heat in a shallow saucepan. Add the garlic and onion; cook and mix for 3-4 minutes, until soft. Add the basil, tomato puree, salt and pepper and stir. Get it to a boil; lower the flame. Simmer, 10 minutes, open. Only stay wet.

2. Meanwhile, preheat the 350 ° air fryer. Whisk the eggs and milk together in a shallow cup. Combine the parsley, garlic powder, breadcrumbs, cheese, and salt in another dish.

3. Dip the tortellini into the egg mixture and then cover in the bread crumb combination. Organize tortellini in batches in a single layer in an air-fryer basket on a greased tray, dust with olive oil. Cook for 4-5 minutes until it is golden brown. Turn; spritz with spray for cooking. Heat till lightly browned, for 4-5 more minutes. Serve with sauce; apply extra minced fresh basil to scatter.

57. Air-Fryer Cumin Carrots

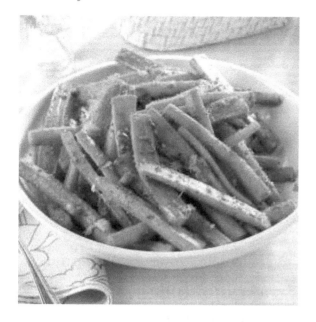

Ingredients

- ❖ Coriander seeds 2 teaspoons

- ❖ Cumin seeds 2 teaspoons

- ❖ Carrots 1 pound

- ❖ Coconut oil 1 tablespoon

- ❖ Garlic cloves 2

- ❖ Salt 1/4 teaspoon

- ❖ Pepper 1/8 teaspoon

Steps

1. Heat an air fryer at 325 °. Toast the coriander and cumin seeds in a small dry skillet over medium heat for 50-60 seconds or till aromatic, stirring regularly. Grind in a spice grinder until finely ground, or with a mortar and pestle.

2. Place the carrots in a wide bowl. Mix melted garlic, coconut oil, salt, cloves, and pepper; swirl to cover. Place the air-fryer bowl on an oiled plate.

3. Cooked, stirring regularly, till crispy and golden brown, 12-15 minutes. Sprinkle with cilantro if necessary.

58. Air-Fryer Mini Chimichangas

Ingredients

- ❖ Beef 1 pound

- ❖ Onion 1 medium

- ❖ Taco seasoning 1 envelope

- ❖ Water 3/4 cup

- ❖ Monterey Jack cheese 3 cups

- ❖ Sour cream 1 cup

- ❖ Green chiles 4 ounces

- ❖ Roll wrappers 14 egg

- ❖ Egg white 1 large

- ❖ Cooking spray

- ❖ Salsa

Steps

1. Cook the beef and onion on medium heat in a large skillet until the meat is no longer pink, wash. Stir in water and taco seasoning.

Just get it to a simmer. Reduce heat; boil, open, for 5 minutes, sometimes stirring. Remove from heat; mildly cold.

2. Heat an air fryer at 375 °. Combine the sour cream, cheese, and chiles in a wide cup. Stir in the blend of meat. With 1 point facing you, put an egg roll wrapper on the work surface. Place 1/3 of the filled cup in the center. Fold one-third of the bottom of the wrapper over the filling; fold sideways.

3. Top point brush with egg white; wrap up to secure. Repeat for the filling and leftover wrappers.

4. Place chimichangas in batches on a greased tray in the air-fryer bowl in a thin layer; spritz with olive oil. Heat till lightly browned, on either hand, for 3-4 minutes. With salsa and extra sour cream, serve immediately.

59. Air-Fryer Fiesta Chicken Fingers

Ingredients

- ❖ Boneless skinless chicken breasts 3/4 pound
- ❖ Buttermilk 1/2 cup
- ❖ Pepper 1/4 teaspoon
- ❖ Flour 1 cup

- ❖ Corn chips 3 cups
- ❖ Taco seasoning 1 envelope
- ❖ Salsa

Steps

1. Heat an air fryer at 400 °. Pound the chicken breasts with a 1/2-in meat mallet. Slice into 1-in. Strips big.

2. Whisk together the buttermilk and pepper in a small dish. Place flour in a different shallow bowl. In the third bowl, combine the corn chips with the taco seasoning. To cover all ends, dip the chicken in flour; shake off the waste. Dip in the buttermilk combination, then pat in the corn chip mixture to help adhere to the coating.

3. Arrange the chicken in batches on an oiled tray in the air-fryer bowl in a single layer; spritz with olive oil. Cook for 7-8 minutes on either side until the covering is lightly browned and the chicken is no longer pink. Repeat for the chicken that remains. Serve with dip or salsa from the ranch.

60. Air-Fryer Everything Bagel Chicken Strips

Ingredients

- Bagel 1 day-old

- Panko breadcrumbs 1/2 cup

- Parmesan cheese 1/2 cup

- Red pepper flakes 1/4 teaspoon

- Butter 1/4 cup

- Chicken tenderloins 1 pound

- Salt 1/2 teaspoon

Steps

1. Heat an air fryer at 400 °. In a food processor, pulse the broken bagel until coarse crumbs develop. In a shallow bowl, put 1/2 cup bagel crumbs; toss with panko, pepper flakes, and cheese.

2. Microwave butter once molten in a microwave-safe small dish. Sprinkle salt on the chicken. To aid bind, dip in hot butter, then cover with crumb mixture, patting. Place the chicken in a thin layer on an oiled tray in the air-fryer bowl in batches.

3. Cook for 7 minutes; switch the chicken around. Continue to cook for 7-8 minutes until the covering is lightly browned and the chicken is no longer yellow.

61. Quentin's Air-Fryer Peach-Bourbon Wings

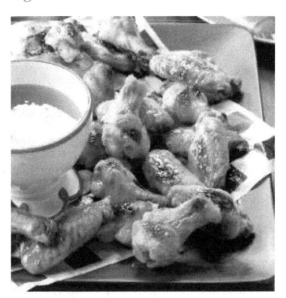

Ingredients

- ❖ Peach preserves 1/2 cup

- ❖ Brown sugar 1 tablespoon

- ❖ Garlic cloves 1

- ❖ Salt 1/4 teaspoon

- ❖ White vinegar 2 tablespoons

- ❖ Bourbon 2 tablespoons

- ❖ Cornstarch 1 teaspoon

- ❖ Water 1-1/2 teaspoons

- ❖ Chicken wings 2 pounds

Steps

1. Heat an air fryer at 400 °. In a food processor, put the preserves, brown garlic, sugar, and salt, until blended. Move it to a tiny casserole. Remove bourbon and

vinegar; heat it. Reduce heat; boil, uncovered, for 4-6 minutes, until lightly thickened.

2. Mix the cornstarch and water in a small bowl until smooth, whisk in the mixture of preserves. Return to a boil, continuously stirring; cook and stir for 1-2 minutes or until thickened. For serving, save 1/4 cup sauce.

3. Breakthrough the 2 joints on each chicken wing with a sharp knife; cut the wings' tips. Place wing parts in a single layer on an oiled tray in the air-fryer bowl in batches. Cook for 6 minutes, switch and spray with a blend of preserves. Cooked 6-8 minutes longer, before browned and juices run free. Serve the wings with the reserved sauce immediately.

62. Turkey Breast Tenderloins in the Air Fryer

Ingredients

- ❖ Dill weed 1 teaspoon
- ❖ Dried thyme 1 teaspoon
- ❖ Oregano dried 1 teaspoon
- ❖ Salt ¾ teaspoon
- ❖ Onion sliced 1 teaspoon
- ❖ Butter ¼ cup
- ❖ Pepper ¼ teaspoon

- ❖ Carrots 3 cups
- ❖ Celery ribs 4
- ❖ Olive oil 1 tablespoon
- ❖ Onions 2 medium
- ❖ Water ¼ cup
- ❖ Cornstarch 2 teaspoons
- ❖ Turkey Breast Tenderloins 8

Steps

1. Heat the stove to 425 °. Blend the first six ingredients in a shallow bowl. Combine the butter with 2 teaspoons of the seasoning combination; toss with the vegetables. Move to a plate for roasting. Bake for 15 minutes, uncovered.

2. Rub oil over turkey, meanwhile, dust with the remaining mixture of seasoning. Shift the vegetables to the sides of the pan; in the center, put the turkey. Cook, uncovered, 20-25 minutes or till 165 ° is read by a thermometer inserted into turkey and vegetables are soft.

3. Save half the turkey with Linguine for Buffalo Turkey or save for another use. Remove the leftover turkey and vegetables and hold warm on a serving platter.

4. Onto a shallow saucepan, add the cooking juices. Combine the

cornstarch and water until it is smooth, swirl in the pan gradually. Cook and stir until thickened, about 2 minutes. Serve with carrots and turkey.

63. Air Fryer Rotisserie Roasted Whole Chicken

Ingredients

- ❖ Whole chicken 5 pounds
- ❖ Lemon ½
- ❖ Onion whole ¼
- ❖ Thyme 4 springs
- ❖ Rosemary 4 springs
- ❖ Olive oil spray
- ❖ Thyme ground 1 teaspoon
- ❖ Onion powder 1 teaspoon
- ❖ Garlic powder 1 teaspoon
- ❖ Salt and pepper to taste

Steps

1. Cut the excess fat, usually the neck and tail section, from around the chicken.
2. Pat the chicken dry.
3. Drizzle with seasonings and olive oil.
4. Air Fried and to rest before slicing, remove the chicken from the air fryer.

Chapter 4: Appetizers

1. Coconut Shrimp with Spicy Marmalade Sauce

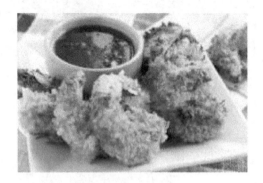

Ingredients

- ❖ Shrimp (1 pound)
- ❖ Flour (1/2 cup)
- ❖ Cayenne pepper (1/2 tsp.)
- ❖ Salt (1/4 tsp.)
- ❖ Pepper (1/4 tsp.)
- ❖ Panko bread (1/2 cup)
- ❖ Coconut milk (8 ounces)
- ❖ 1 egg
- ❖ Sweetened shredded coconut (1/2 cup)

Ingredients for the Sauce

- ❖ Marmalade of orange (1/2 cup)
- ❖ Honey (1 tbsp.)
- ❖ Mustard (1 tsp.)
- ❖ Sweet sauce (1/4 tsp.)

Steps

1. Let all the shrimps wash and put aside.

2. The rice, pepper, salt, panko breadcrumbs and cayenne are mixed.

3. Whisk the coconut milk and the egg in a shallow bowl. With the shredded coconut, fill a third shallow bowl.

4. In the flour mixture, soak the shrimp and the coconut milk one and then cover in the coconut.

5. Place the shrimp in the air-fryer basket and heat up to 400 °. Bake for 12 - 15 minutes until the shrimp is crispy and golden. Work in different batches.

6. When frying the shrimp, whisk the sugar, marmalade, hot sauce and mustard together.

7. Serve the shrimp directly with the sauce.

2. Air Fried Shishito Peppers

Ingredients

- ❖ Shishito peppers (6 oz. package)
- ❖ Salt and pepper
- ❖ Avocado oil (1/2 tbsp.)
- ❖ Asiago Cheese (1/3 cup)
- ❖ Lemons

Steps

1. Wash the peppers and pat them dry with a paper towel. Place the avocado salt, oil and pepper in a bowl and mix. Put the air fryer and cook for ten minutes at 349. Watch attentively. They need to come out looking lacerated, but not burned.

2. Put Shishito peppers on the dish to eat. Sprinkle with a slight quantity of lime juice and finish with rubbed asiago cheese.

3. Air Fryer Beet Root Chips

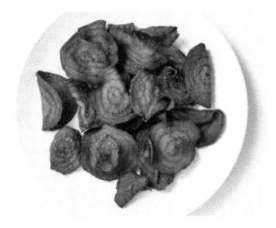

Ingredients

- ❖ Beetroot (1 medium-sized)
- ❖ Olive oil (1 tsp.)
- ❖ Salt
- ❖ Pepper

Steps

1. Clean the beetroot, peel, and set aside the skin. Cut into finely using a mandolin slicer. If you're not using a slicer, instead, cut into evenly thin with your knife.

2. Place the slices of beetroot on the paper and put another piece of paper on top. For ten min, hold it aside. This method helps the thin beetroot to retain some excess moisture.

3. Mix the beetroot sliced in oil and sprinkle with the salt on the beet and place it in the air fryer's basket.

4. To change the time and temperature to 165 ° c and fifteen minutes, switch the + /- buttons in the air fryer. After every 5 minutes, rotate and switch the beet chips around until they dry out equally. Set the timer for 10 minutes and raise the temperature to 182C. The Beet Chips are going to curl overall. Allow five min of cooling for the chips, and they will crisp well.

5. If you want, season with sea salt, freshly ground pepper.

4. Air Fryer Weight Watchers Pork Taquitos

Ingredients

- ❖ Shredded pork (3 cups)
- ❖ Shredded mozzarella (2 1/2 cups)
- ❖ Tortillas (10 little)
- ❖ Lime juiced with sugar (1 tbsp.)
- ❖ Cooking mist

Steps

1. Heat the air fryer to 385 degrees.
2. Spray the lime juice over the pork and swirl gently.
3. Oven 5 tortillas at a time and melt it for ten seconds, with a wet paper towel over it.
4. Apply   Pork and 1/4 cup tortilla cheese.
5. Roll the tortillas firmly and softly.
6. Line up all tortillas on a plate covered with greased foil.
7. Spray the tortillas with a coat of cooking oil spray.
8. Air Fried until the tortillas are a dark golden color for 7-8 minutes, turning halfway through.
9. But they can also be cooked in the oven at 450 ° for 7-10 minutes if you're not using an air fryer.

5. Air Fryer Pickles

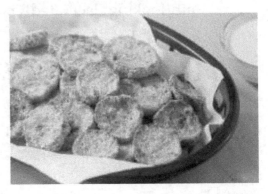

Ingredients

- ❖ Dill pickle (32 pieces)
- ❖ Flour (1/2 cup)
- ❖ Salt (1/2 tsp.)
- ❖ Lightly beaten eggs (3)
- ❖ Juice for dill pickle (2 tsp.)
- ❖ Garlic (1/2 tsp.)
- ❖ Panko breadcrumbs (2 cups)
- ❖ Dill snipped (2 tsp.)
- ❖ Cooking mist
- ❖ Ranch   sauce   with sandwiches

Steps

1. Heat the air fryer at 400 °. Let the pickles stay on a paper towel for around 15

minutes, till the liquid is almost drained.

2. Meanwhile, mix the flour and salt in a small dish. Whisk the eggs, cayenne, pickle juice, and garlic powder together in another small dish. In a third small dish, combine the panko and dill.

3. Dip the pickles to cover all sides in the flour mixture; shake off the excess. Dip in the mixture of shells, then pat in the crumb mixture to help adhere to the coating. Put pickles in one layer on an oiled tray in the air-fryer basket in batches. Cook until brown and crispy golden, 7-10 mins. Pickles to turn; spritz with cooking oil. Cook for 7-10 mins, until crispy and light brown. Immediately serve. Serve with BBQ sauce if needed.

6. Air Fryer Crispy Sriracha Spring Rolls

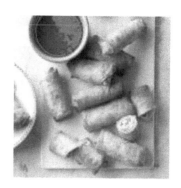

Ingredients

- ❖ Coleslaw mix (3 cups)
- ❖ Chopped onions (3 big)
- ❖ Soy sauce (1 tbsp.)
- ❖ Sesame oil (1 tsp.)
- ❖ Boneless chicken breasts without skin (1 pound)
- ❖ Salt (1 tsp.)
- ❖ 2 boxes of cream cheese (8 ounces each)
- ❖ Sriracha chili sauce (2 tbsp.)
- ❖ 24 roll wrappers for spring
- ❖ Cooking mist
- ❖ Sweet sauce of chili and additional green onions

Steps

1. Heat the air fryer at 360 °. Toss with the mixture of green onion, coleslaw, sesame oil and soy sauce; leave stand while the chicken is frying. In an air-fryer basket, put the chicken

in a single layer on a greased plate. Cook until a chicken-inserted thermometer reads 160 ° at about 20 minutes. Chop the chicken finely; toss with salt.

2. Increase the temperature of the air-fryer to 402 °. Mix the cream cheese and the Sriracha chili sauce in a large bowl; mix in the chicken and coleslaw mixture. Place about 2 tsp. Of stuffing just below the middle of the wrapper with 1 corner of a spring roll wrapper. (Until fit for usage, cover the remaining wrappers with a moist paper towel.) Fold the bottom corner over the filling; wet the remaining edges with water. Overfilling, fold side corners into the middle; firmly roll back, forcing tip to seal.

3. Arrange spring rolls in batches on an oiled tray in the air-fryer basket in a single layer; spritz with cooking oil spray. For 4-5 minutes, cook until lightly browned. Turn; spritz with spray for cooking. Cook until crisp and golden brown, 5-6 minutes longer. Serve with sweet chili sauce if needed.

4. Choice: Freeze 1 inch of uncooked spring rolls. Separating layers with waxed paper and in freezer containers.

7. Air Fryer Fiesta Chicken Fingers

Ingredients

- ❖ Boneless chicken breasts without skin (3/4 pound)
- ❖ Buttermilk (1/2 cup)
- ❖ Pepper (1/4 tsp.)
- ❖ Flour (1 cup)
- ❖ Chips of maize, smashed (3 cups)
- ❖ Taco seasoning envelope (1)
- ❖ Sour cream ranch or tomato dip

Steps

1. Heat the air fryer at 402°. Strike the chicken breasts with a 1/2-in meat mallet. Slice it into 1-in. Long Strips

2. Whisk together the buttermilk and pepper in a small dish. Place flour in a different shallow bowl. In the third bowl, combine the corn chips with the taco sauce. To cover all ends, dip the chicken in flour; shake off the excess. Dip in the buttermilk mixture, then pat in the corn chip mixture to help adhere to the coating.

3. Arrange the chicken in batches on an oiled tray in the air-fryer basket in a single layer, spray with vegetable oil. Cook for 7-8 minutes on either side until the covering is lightly browned and the chicken is no longer pink. Repeat for the chicken that remains. Serve with dip or salsa from the ranch.

8. Air Fryer Cheeseburger Onion Rings

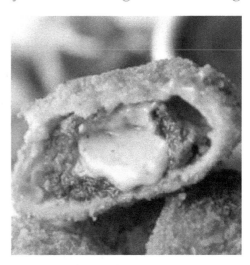

Ingredients

- Lean ground beef (1 pound)
- ketchup (1/3 cup)
- Mustard (2 tsp.)
- Salt (1/2 tsp.)
- 1 large onion
- Cheddar cheese (4 ounces)
- Flour (3/4 cup)
- Garlic powder (2 tbsp.)
- Lightly beaten eggs (2 big)
- Panko crumbs for bread (1-1 ½)
- Cooking mist
- Hot ketchup

Steps

1. Preheat the air fryer at 335 °. Combine the ketchup, meat, salt, and mustard in a wide bowl, mixing gently but thoroughly. Cut a 1/2-in onion. Slices; Split into

circles. Cover half of the beef mixture with 8 slices (save the leftover onion rings for another use). Cover each with a slice of cheese and a variation of the leftover meat.

2. Mix the flour and garlic powder in a small dish. In different shallow bowls, place the eggs and breadcrumbs. Dip filled onion rings in flour; shake off the waste. Dip in the egg, then pat in the breadcrumbs to make the coating stick.

3. Place onion rings in batches on an oiled tray in the air-fryer basket in a single layer; sprinkle with cooking oil spray. Cook until lightly browned, and a beef thermometer measures 163 °, 12-15 minutes. Serve with spicy ketchup if needed.

9. Air Fryer Garlic Rosemary Brussels Sprouts

Ingredients

- ❖ Olive oil (3 tbsp.)
- ❖ Diced garlic (3 cloves)
- ❖ Salt (1/2 tsp.)
- ❖ Pepper (1/4 tsp.)

- ❖ Trimmed and halved Brussels sprouts (1 pound)
- ❖ Crumbs of panko bread (1/2 pound)
- ❖ New rosemary minced (1 tsp.)

Steps

1. Heat the air fryer at 352 °. Put the first 4 ingredients in a tiny microwave-safe dish first: microwave for 30 seconds or more.

2. Toss Brussels sprouts with an oil combination of 2 teaspoons. In the air-fryer basket, put the Brussels sprouts on the tray; cook for 5-6 minutes. Stir-up sprouts. Cook until the sprouts are finely browned and almost tender, about Eight minutes longer, stirring during the cooking process.

3. Toss the rosemary and remaining oil mixture with breadcrumbs, scatter with sprouts. Continue cooking for 4-5 minutes, until the crumbs are golden brown, and the sprouts are soft. Immediately serve.

10. Air Fryer Ravioli

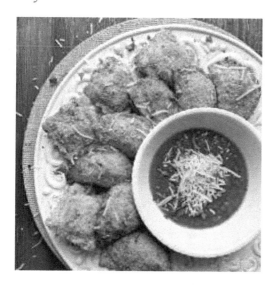

Ingredients

- ❖ Breadcrumbs (1 cup)
- ❖ Parmesan sliced cheese (1/4 cup)
- ❖ Dried basil (2 tsp.)
- ❖ Flour (1/2 cup)
- ❖ Lightly beaten eggs (2 big)
- ❖ 1 bag Frozen beef ravioli (9 ounces)
- ❖ Cooking mist
- ❖ New basil minced
- ❖ 1 cup of sauce of marinara

Steps

1. Heat the air fryer at 350 °. Mix the parmesan cheese, breadcrumbs, and the basil in a small dish. In different shallow cups, position the flour and eggs. To cover all ends, dip the ravioli in flour; shake off the excess. Dip in the shells, then pat in the crumb mixture to help bind to the coating.

2. Arrange the ravioli in batches on an oiled tray in the air-fryer basket in a single layer, sprinkle with cooking oil spray. Cook for 4-5 minutes before it's golden brown. Turn; spritz with spray for cooking. Cook until lightly browned, for 4-5 more minutes. Sprinkle instantly with basil and extra Parmesan cheese if needed.

11. Air Fryer Taquitos

Ingredients

- ❖ Eggs (2 big)
- ❖ Crumbs of dry bread (1/2 cup)
- ❖ Seasoning taco (3 tsp.)
- ❖ Lean ground beef (1 pound)
- ❖ 6 tortillas of corn (6 inches)
- ❖ Cooking mist
- ❖ Guacamole and salsa

Steps

1. Heat the air fryer at 352 °. Combine the breadcrumbs, eggs, and taco seasoning in a

wide dish. Add beef, blend deeply, but lightly.

2. Spoon down the middle of each tortilla with 1/4 cup of beef mixture. With toothpicks, coil up tightly and stable. Arrange taquitos in batches on an oiled tray in the air-fryer basket in a single layer, spray with cooking oil spray. Cook for six minutes; switch and bake until meat is cooked, and taquitos are 7-8 minutes longer, lightly browned, and crispy. Before serving, remove the toothpicks.

12. Air Fryer General Tso's Cauliflower

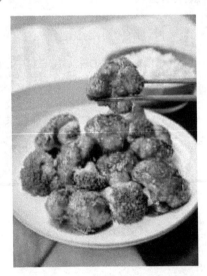

Ingredients

- ❖ Flour (1/2 cup)
- ❖ Cornstarch (1/2 cup)
- ❖ Salt (1 tsp.)

- ❖ Powder for baking (1 tsp.)
- ❖ Soda club (3/4 tsp.)
- ❖ 1 cauliflower with a medium head

Ingredients for sauce

- ❖ Fruit juice (1/4 cup)
- ❖ Sugar (3 tsp.)
- ❖ Soy sauce (3 tbsp.)
- ❖ Vegetable broth (3 tsp.)
- ❖ Vinegar for rice (2 tbsp.)
- ❖ Sesame oil (2 tbsp.)
- ❖ Cornstarch (2 tsp.)
- ❖ Canola oil (2 tsp.)
- ❖ Minced pasilla or other spicy chiles (2-6)
- ❖ 3 green onions
- ❖ Garlic (3 cloves)
- ❖ Freshly grated ginger root (1 tsp.)
- ❖ Orange zest grated (1/2 tsp.)
- ❖ Hot cooked rice (4 cups)

Steps

1. Heat the air fryer at 402 °. Toss the rice, salt, baking powder and cornstarch together. Just when mixed, stir in club soda (batter would be thin). Toss the florets in the batter, transfer over a baking sheet to a wire rack. Let the

ingredients to stand for 5 minutes. Place cauliflower in batches on an oiled tray in the air-fryer basket. Cook until soft and lightly browned, 8-12 minutes.

2. Meanwhile, whisk the first 6 ingredients of the sauce together: whisk in cornstarch until smooth.

3. Heat canola oil over medium-high heat in a big saucepan. Apply the chilies; cook and mix for 1-2 minutes, until tangy. Add the white onions, ginger, garlic, and orange zest; cook for about 2 minutes until tangy. Stir in the mixture of orange juice; add to the saucepan. Put to a boil; cook and mix for 2-4 minutes before it thickens.

4. For the sauce, add cauliflower and serve it rice and green onions.

13. Air Fryer Nashville Hot Chicken

Ingredients

- ❖ Dill pickle juice (2 tsp.)
- ❖ Spicy pepper sauce (2 tsp.)
- ❖ Salt (1 tsp.)

- ❖ Tenderloin chicken (2 pounds)
- ❖ Flour (1 cup)
- ❖ Mustard (1/2 tsp.)
- ❖ Egg
- ❖ Buttermilk (1/2 cup)
- ❖ Cooking mist
- ❖ Olive oil (1/2 cup)
- ❖ Cayenne pepper (2 tsp.)
- ❖ Dark brown sugar (2 cups)
- ❖ Paprika (1 tsp.)
- ❖ Chili powder (1 tsp.)
- ❖ Garlic (1/2 tsp.)
- ❖ Pieces of dill pickle

Steps

1. Mix 1 tbsp. Pickle juice, 1 tbsp. Hot sauce and 1/2 tsp. Salt in a cup or shallow dish. Add chicken and refrigerate for a minimum of 1 hour. Discharge, tossing out some marinade.

2. Heat a 375 ° air fryer. Mix the flour, the remaining 1/2 tsp salt, and the pepper in a small dish. Whisk together the egg, buttermilk, 1 tbsp of pickle juice and 1 tbsp of hot sauce in another small cup. To cover all ends, dip the chicken in flour; shake off the waste. Dip in the egg

mixture, then the flour mixture again.

3. Arrange the chicken in batches on a well-oiled tray in the air-fryer bowl in a single layer, spray with vegetable oil. Heat for 6-7 minutes until it is nicely browned. Turn, spray with spray for cooking. Cook until lightly browned, for 6-7 more minutes.

4. Mix milk, brown sugar, cayenne, pepper, and spices together, splash over warm chicken.

14. Air Fryer Pumpkin Fries

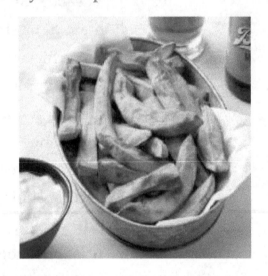

Ingredients

❖ Plain Greek yogurt (1/2 cup)

❖ Maple syrup (2 cups)

❖ Minced chipotle peppers (3 tsp.)

❖ Sodium (1/8 tsp.)

❖ 1 pumpkin

❖ Garlic (1/4 tsp.)

❖ Ground cumin (1/4 tsp.)

❖ Chili powder (1/4 tsp.)

❖ Pepper (1/4 tsp.)

Steps

1. Mix the maple syrup, chipotle peppers, yogurt, and 1/6 tsp salt in a shallow cup. Refrigerate till the serving.

2. Heat a 402 ° air fryer. Peel off the pumpkin and break lengthwise in half. Discard the seeds for toasting. Slice into 1/4-in long strips. Transfer to a spacious bowl. Sprinkle with 1/4 tsp. of remaining salt, cumin, garlic powder, pepper, and chili powder.

3. Arrange pumpkin in batches on an oiled tray in an air-fryer basket. Cook for 8 mins until just soft. Cook until crisp and light brown.

15. Sweet and Spicy Air Fryer Meatballs

Ingredients

- ❖ Oats for quick cooking (2/3 cup)
- ❖ Ritz crackers (1/2 cup)
- ❖ Beaten eggs (2)
- ❖ Milk (5 ounces)
- ❖ Minced onion (1 tbsp.)
- ❖ Salt (1 tsp.)
- ❖ Garlic (1 tsp.)
- ❖ Cumin ground (1 tsp.)
- ❖ Honey (1 tsp.)
- ❖ Mustard (1/2 tsp.)
- ❖ Beef (2 pounds)

Ingredients for sauce

- ❖ Brown sugar (1/3 cup)
- ❖ Honey (1/3 cup)
- ❖ Orange marmalade (1/3 cup)
- ❖ Cornstarch (2tsp.)
- ❖ Soy sauce (2 tsp.)
- ❖ Louisiana-style hot sauce (1 -2 tsp.)
- ❖ Worcestershire sauce (1 tbsp.)

Steps

1. Heat the air fryer at 380 °. Mix the first ten ingredients in a wide bowl. Add beef, blend deeply, but lightly. Mold to 1-1/4-in balls.
2. In a single layer, arrange the meatballs on an oiled

tray in an air-fryer basket. Cook for 14-15 minutes, until browned and fully baked. Meanwhile, combine the sauce components in a small saucepan. Cook and stir until it thickens, over medium heat.

16. Air Fryer Ham and Cheese Turnovers

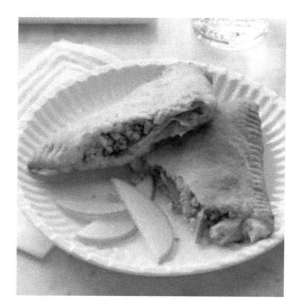

Ingredients

- ❖ Refrigerated pizza crust (13.8 ounces)
- ❖ Black forest deli ham (1/4 pound)
- ❖ 1 medium pear
- ❖ Sliced, toasted walnuts (1/4 cup)
- ❖ Blue cheese crumbled (2 tsp.)

Steps

1. Heat the air fryer at 400 °. Roll up the pizza crust into a 14-in section on a thinly floured board. Slice into 4 triangles. Layer ham, walnuts, half pear strips, and blue cheese over half of each square diagonally to within 1/4 in. from the margins. Fold 1 corner to the opposite corner, creating a triangle over the filling; force the edges to close with a fork.

2. Arrange turnovers in batches on an oiled tray in the air-fryer basket in a single layer, spray with a cooking mist. Cook until lightly browned for 5-6 minutes. Garnish with the remaining pieces of pear.

17. Air Fryer Pepper Poppers

Ingredients

- ❖ 1 bag of cream cheese (8 ounces)
- ❖ Cheddar cheese (3/4 cup)
- ❖ Monterey jack cheese sliced (3/4 cup)
- ❖ 6 fried and crumbled bacon strips

- ❖ Salt (1/4 tsp.)
- ❖ Garlic (1/4 tsp.)
- ❖ Chili powder (1/4 tsp.)
- ❖ Paprika (1/4 tsp.)
- ❖ Fresh jalapenos (1 pound)
- ❖ Breadcrumbs (1/2 cup)
- ❖ Optional: sour cream, French onion dip and seasoning for ranch salad

Steps

1. Heat the air fryer at 325 °. Mix the bacon, cheeses and spices in a wide bowl, blend well. For each half of the pepper, fill to about 1 tbsp and merge into breadcrumbs.

2. If necessary, operate in batches and put poppers in a single layer in the basket. For a spicy taste, cook for 14 minutes, medium for 22 minutes and moderate for 26 minutes. Serve it with sour cream or sauce if needed.

18. Air Fryer Wasabi Crab Cakes

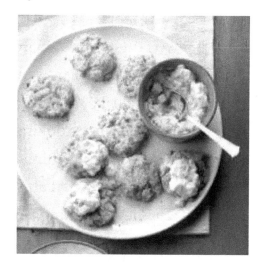

Ingredients

- ❖ Red pepper (1 medium)
- ❖ 1 celery rib
- ❖ 3 green onions
- ❖ 2 big egg whites
- ❖ Mayonnaise (3 tsp.)
- ❖ Wasabi (1/4 tsp.)
- ❖ Salt (1/4 tsp.)
- ❖ Breadcrumbs (1/3 cup)
- ❖ Lump crabmeat (1-1 ½ cup)
- ❖ Cooking mist

Ingredients for sauce

- ❖ 1 celery diced
- ❖ Mayonnaise (1/3 cup)
- ❖ 1 green onion
- ❖ Pickle (1 tbsp.)
- ❖ Wasabi (1/2 tsp.)
- ❖ Salt (1/4 tsp.)

Steps

1. Heat the air fryer at 370°. Mix 7 ingredients first: substitute 1/4 of a cup of breadcrumbs. Fold in the crab softly.

2. In a small dish, put the remaining breadcrumbs. Drop crumbs into piling teaspoons of crab mixture. Form and cover softly into 3/4-in.-thick patties. Place crab cakes in batches in a single layer on an oiled tray in an air-fryer tray. Spritz crab cakes with spray for frying. Heat until lightly browned, 12 minutes, gently turning with extra cooking oil spray halfway through cooking and spraying.

3. Meanwhile, in the food processor, put sauce ingredients; pulse 3-4 times to blend or perfect consistency. Serve the crab cakes with the dipping sauce promptly.

19. Air Fryer Caribbean Wontons

Ingredients

- ❖ Cream cheese (4 ounces)
- ❖ Shredded coconut (1/4 cup)
- ❖ Banana mashed (1/4 cup)
- ❖ Diced walnuts (2 tsp.)

- ❖ Crushed canned pineapple (2 tbsp.)
- ❖ Marshmallow cream (1 cup)
- ❖ 24 wonton wrappers
- ❖ Cooking mist

Ingredients for sauce

- ❖ Strawberries (1 pound)
- ❖ Sugar (1/4 cup)
- ❖ Cornstarch (1 tsp.)
- ❖ Sugar and ground cinnamon of confectioners

Steps

1. Heat the air fryer at 350 °. Stir the cream cheese in a small bowl until smooth. Stir in the pineapple, banana, coconut, and walnuts.
2. Place a wonton wrapper with 1 point in your direction. Keep the remaining wrappers covered until ready for use with a damp paper towel. In the middle of the wrapper, position 2 tsp. Of filling. Moisten the sides with water; fold the opposite corners over the filling and push to seal together. Repeat for the filling and leftover wrappers.
3. Arrange wontons in batches on a greased tray in the air-fryer basket in a single layer, spray with cooking spray. Cook for 8-12 minutes, until lightly browned and crisp.
4. In the meantime, in a food processor, put strawberries, cover, and process until pureed. Combine the sugar and cornstarch in a shallow saucepan. Stir in the strawberry purée. Bring to a boil; cook and stir for 3 minutes until it thickens. Remove the mixture if desired, sauce reserve, discard seeds. Sprinkle wontons with sugar and cinnamon from confectioners.

20. Air fryer Beefy Swiss Bundles

Ingredients

- ❖ Beef (1 pound)
- ❖ Mushrooms (1 – 1 ½)
- ❖ Sliced onion (1- 1 ½ tsp.)
- ❖ Garlic (1- 1 ½ tsp.)
- ❖ Sauce from Worcestershire (2 cups)

- ❖ Dry rosemary (3/4 tsp.)
- ❖ Paprika (3/4 tsp.)
- ❖ Salt (1/2 tsp.)
- ❖ Pepper (1/4 tsp.)
- ❖ 1 frozen puff pastry
- ❖ Mashed potatoes (2/3 cup)
- ❖ 1 cup Swiss cheese shredded
- ❖ 1 large egg
- ❖ Water (2 tbsp.)

Steps

1. Preheat the air fryer at 380 °. Cook the beef, mushrooms, and onion over medium heat in a broad skillet until the meat is no longer pink and the vegetables are soft, 10-12 minutes. Stir in garlic; simmer for 1 minute longer. Mix in the sauce and spices from Worcestershire.

2. Roll puff pastry into a 16x13-in on a thinly floured table, for a square. Split into four 7-1/2x6-1/2-in, with rectangles. Over each rectangle, put around 2 tsp of potatoes; spread to within 1 inch from the margins. Cover each with 3/4 cup beef mixture; scatter with 1/4 cup cheese.

3. Whip the egg and water; brush some over the edges of the pastry. Place opposite pastry corners over each bundle; pinch the seams to seal. Rub for the leftover combination of shells. Place the pastries in batches in a single layer on the tray in the air-fryer basket; cook for 10-12 minutes until golden brown.

4. Store options: unbaked pastries until stable on a parchment-lined baking sheet. Shift to a watertight bag; return to the freezer. Cook frozen pastries until light brown and cook, increasing time to 20-25 minutes.

21. Air Fryer Tortellini with Prosciutto

Ingredients

- ❖ Olive oil (1 tbsp.)
- ❖ Finely chopped onion (3 tbsp.)
- ❖ Garlic (4 cloves)
- ❖ 1 can of puree tomato (15 ounces)
- ❖ Fresh basil minced (1 tbsp.)
- ❖ Salt (1/4 tsp.)

❖ Pepper (1/4 tsp.)

Ingredients for tortellini

- ❖ 2 large eggs
- ❖ Milk (2 tbsp.)
- ❖ Breadcrumbs (2/3 cup)
- ❖ Garlic (1 tsp.)
- ❖ Pecorino Romano grated cheese (2 tsp.)
- ❖ Minced fresh parsley (1 tbsp.)
- ❖ Salt (1/2 tsp.)
- ❖ 1 package tortellini prosciutto ricotta
- ❖ Cooking mist

Steps

1. Heat oil over medium-high heat in a small saucepan. Add the onion and garlic; cook and stir for 4-5 minutes, until soft. Add the tomato puree, salt, basil and pepper and mix. Boil and heat to about ten minutes.

2. Besides that, preheat the air fryer to 350 °. Whisk the eggs and milk together in a shallow cup. Mix the garlic powder, breadcrumbs, cheese, parsley, and salt in another dish.

3. Dip the tortellini into the egg mixture and then coat in the bread crumb blend. Arrange tortellini in batches in a single layer in an air-fryer basket on a greased tray, sprinkle with cooking spray. Cook for 5-6 minutes until it is golden brown. Turn, sprinkle with spray for cooking. Cook until lightly browned, 5-6 minutes.

22. Air Fryer Crispy Curry Drumsticks

Ingredients

- ❖ Drumsticks of chicken (1 pound)
- ❖ Salt (3/4 tsp.)
- ❖ Olive oil (2 tbsp.)
- ❖ Curry powder (2 tsp.)
- ❖ Onion salt (1/2 tsp.)
- ❖ Garlic (1/2 tsp.)
- ❖ Minced coriander

Steps

1. Place the chicken and water in a large bowl to cover it. Add 1/2 tsp salt and allow to stand at room temperature for 20 minutes.

2. Preheat a 380° air fryer. Combine curry powder, oil, garlic powder, onion salt and remaining 1/4 tsp salt in another bowl; add chicken and coat with the toss. Place the chicken in batches in a single layer on the tray in the air-fryer tray. Cook until a chicken-inserted thermometer reads 175-180°, 17-18 minutes, rotating halfway through. Sprinkle with cilantro if desired.

23. Air Fryer Rosemary Sausage Meatballs

Ingredients

- ❖ Olive oil (2 tbsp.)
- ❖ Garlic (4 cloves)
- ❖ Powdered curry (1 tsp.)
- ❖ 1 large egg
- ❖ 1 jar diced peppers (4 ounces)
- ❖ Breadcrumbs (1/4 cup)
- ❖ Fresh parsley minced (1/4 cup)
- ❖ New rosemary minced (1 tbsp.)
- ❖ Pork sausage (2 kilos)

Steps

1. Heat the air fryer at 450°. Heat the oil over a moderate flame in a small baking dish, stir-frying curry powder and garlic until tender, 2-3 minutes.

2. Combine the egg, breadcrumbs, pepper, rosemary, parsley, and garlic mixture in a dish. Mix sausage; mix thoroughly but lightly.

3. Form 1-1/3 in. to shape. Make the small balls. In the air-fryer basket, put in a single layer on the tray; cook till golden brown and cooked through, 8-10 minutes. Serve with pretzels if desired.

24. Air Fryer Egg Rolls

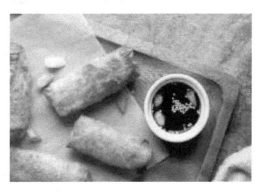

Ingredients

- ❖ Boiling water (2 cups)
- ❖ Sprouts for beans (3 cups)
- ❖ Chicken (1 pound)

- ❖ 6 sliced green onions
- ❖ Gingerroot minced (1 tbsp.)
- ❖ Garlic (3 cloves)
- ❖ 1 container of Chinese-style sauce
- ❖ Soy sauce (1 tbsp.)
- ❖ Soya sauce (1 tsp.)
- ❖ 1 bag of coleslaw mix (14 ounces)
- ❖ 1 bag of frozen chopped spinach (10 ounces)
- ❖ 18 wrappers or egg roll

Steps

1. Pour warm water in a small bowl over the bean sprouts; let sit for 5 minutes. Besides that, cook chicken over a moderate flame in an oven until no longer pink, breaking into crumbles for 6-10 minutes. Add the garlic, green onions, and ginger. For 2 minutes, cook and then rinse. Stir in 1/2 cup fish sauce and soy sauce in Chinese style: switch to a wide bowl. Clean the pan.

2. Cook and stir the mixture of spinach, coleslaw, and drained bean sprouts in the same pan until crisp-tender, 5-6 minutes.

3. Preheat an air fryer to 400 degrees. Place the 1/4 cup filling just below the wrapper's middle with one corner of an egg roll wrapper. (Until fit for usage, cover the remaining wrappers with a wet paper towel.) Fold the lower corner over the filling; moisten the excess wrapping sides with water. Fold side corners over the filling into the middle. Roll the egg securely and push on the tip to close.

4. Arrange egg rolls in batches in a single layer in the greased air-fryer basket; coat them with cooking spray. For 12-14 minutes, cook until lightly browned. Turn, sprinkle with spray for additional cooking. Golden brown, 5-6 minutes longer to roast. Serve with the remaining sauce.

25. Air Fryer Turkey Croquettes

Ingredients

- ❖ Mashed potatoes (2 cups)

- ❖ Parmesan grated cheese (1/2 cup)
- ❖ Swiss cheese shredded (1/2 cup)
- ❖ 1 shallot, thinly sliced
- ❖ Fresh rosemary minced (2 tsp
- ❖ Fresh minced sage (1 tsp)
- ❖ Salt (1/2 tsp.)
- ❖ Pepper (1/4 tsp.)
- ❖ Cooked turkey (3 cups)
- ❖ 1 big egg
- ❖ Water (2 tsp.)
- ❖ Breadcrumbs (1/4 cup)
- ❖ Frying mist with butter fragrance

Steps

1. Preheat the air fryer at 355 °. Mix the cheese, mashed potatoes, rosemary, shallot, pepper, salt, and sage in a big bowl; mix in the turkey. Form 1-in.-thick patties.
2. Whisk the egg and water in a small dish. In another deep cup, position the breadcrumbs. Dip the croquettes in the egg mixture, then pat them onto the breadcrumbs to make the coating stick.
3. Place croquettes in batches on a greased tray in the air-fryer basket in a single layer; spray with cooking oil. Cook for 5-6 minutes until it is lightly browned. Turn, sprinkle with spray for cooking. Cook for 5-6 minutes, until golden brown. Serve with sour cream if needed.

26. Air Fryer Cauliflower Tots

Ingredients

- ❖ 1 nonstick spray for cooking
- ❖ 1 box of cauliflower tots (16 ounces)

Steps

1. Pre - heat to 450 degrees F for the air fryer. Spray with non - stick cooking spray on the air fryer basket.
2. Place as many tots of cauliflower in the basket as you can, make sure they do not touch.
3. Cook for 8 minutes in the preheated air fryer. Take the basket out, switch the tots over, and simmer for around 3 more minutes until golden brown and cooked.

27. Air Fryer Spicy Dill Pickle Fries

Ingredients

- ❖ Spicy dill pickle jar (16 ounces)
- ❖ Flour (1 cup)
- ❖ Paprika (1/2 tsp.)
- ❖ Milk (1/4 cup)
- ❖ 1 egg
- ❖ Breadcrumbs (1 cup)
- ❖ Cooking mist

Steps

1. Wash and pat the pickles off.
2. Mix flour and paprika in a bowl. Mix milk and beaten egg in another bowl. Put the panko in a third bowl.
3. Heat an air-fryer to 410 degrees f
4. Mix a pickle first in the flour mix, then in egg mix, and then in breadcrumbs until fully covered and put on a tray. Repeat for the pickles that remain. Lightly spray the coated pickles with cooking spray.
5. In the air fryer basket, put pickles in a single layer; if appropriate, cook in batches to prevent overcrowding the fryer. Set a 16-minute timer; switch the pickles halfway through the cooking period.

28. Stuffed Mushroom with Sour Cream

Ingredients

- ❖ 24 medium mushrooms
- ❖ 1/2 Bell pepper green, diced
- ❖ 1/2 Onion, sliced
- ❖ 1 thin, diced carrot
- ❖ Two bacon strips, sliced
- ❖ 1 cup of Cheddar cheese shredded
- ❖ 1/2 cup of sour cream
- ❖ 1 1/2 teaspoons sliced, or to taste, Cheddar cheese

Steps

1. Over moderate flame places the orange bell pepper, mushroom, stems, cabbage, bacon, and carrot in a skillet. Cook and stir until tender, 5min. Stir in 1 cup of sour cream and cheddar cheese; cook for about two min until the stuffing is well mixed and the cheese melts.
2. Preheat the fryer to 180 degrees C.
3. On the baking tray, place the mushroom caps. To each mushroom cap, in a grated

fashion, add stuffing. Sprinkle on top of 1 1/2 tsp of Cheddar cheese.

4. Put the mushroom tray in the air fryer's basket. Cook before cheese melts, around eight minutes.

29. Honey Sriracha Air Fryer Wings

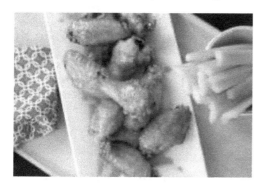

Ingredients

❖ Chicken wing drumettes (12 each)

❖ Salt (1/2 tsp.)

❖ Powdered garlic (1/2 tbsp.)

❖ Butter (1 tbsp.)

❖ Honey (1/4 cup)

❖ Vinegar (2 tsp.)

❖ Sriracha sauce (1 tbsp.)

Steps

1. Pre - heat to 365 degrees F with an air fryer.

2. Put the chicken wings, season with garlic powder, and salt and toss to cover in a cup.

3. Place the wings in the basket of an air fryer. Set the 27-minute timer and cook the wings and shake the basket every 8-9 minutes. Switch the air fryer off when the timer stops, and let the wings stand for 5 more minutes in the basket.

4. Meanwhile, over medium heat, melt the butter in a shallow saucepan. Whisk in the butter with the sugar, vinegar, rice, and sriracha sauce and bring to a simmer. Switch off the heat.

5. In a bowl, toss the fried wings and sauce together.

30. Air Fryer Buffalo Ranch Chickpeas

Ingredients

❖ Chickpeas (15 ounces)

❖ Buffalo wing sauce (2 tbsp.)

❖ Ranch dressing (1 tbsp.)

Steps

1. Heat up to 325 degrees F with an air fryer.

2. Use paper towels to cover a baking sheet. Spread on the paper towels with chickpeas. Over the

chickpeas, place a sheet of paper towels and push softly to extract excess moisture.

3. Put the chickpeas in a saucepan. To mix, apply wing sauce and toss. Mix and apply a dressing of the salad

4. Place the chickpeas in an even layer in the basket of an air fryer.

5. For 8 min. cook it. For an extra five min, shake and cook. Shake for another five minutes and cook. For the final two min, shake and cook. Enable five min to cool and serve.

31. Air Fryer Sweet Potato Tots

Ingredients

- ❖ 2 sweet potatoes
- ❖ Seasoning Cajun (1/2 tsp.)
- ❖ Cooking mist with olive oil
- ❖ Sea salt to favor

Steps

1. Boil a pot of water and add some potatoes. Cook till a fork will pierce the potatoes, but they are still solid around 20 min. Let it soak and cool.

2. A box grater is used to grind potatoes into a dish. Mix in the Cajun spice carefully. Transform the mixture into cylinders that are tot shaped.

3. Spray olive oil at the basket of air fryers. Place the tots in a single row in the basket without reaching the container's edges or each other. Spray the tots with a spray of olive oil and sprinkle them with sea salt.

4. Heat the 400 degrees F air fryer and cook the tots for 8 min. Switch, spray with a little spray of olive oil and spray salt. Cook for an extra 8 min.

32. Air Fryer Korean Chicken Wings

Ingredients

- ❖ Hot honey (1/4 cup)
- ❖ Gochujang (3 tsp.)
- ❖ Brown sugar (1 tbsp.)
- ❖ Soy sauce (1 tbsp.)
- ❖ Lemon juice (1 tsp.)
- ❖ Garlic minced (2 tsp.)
- ❖ Fresh ginger (1 tsp.)

- ❖ Salt (1/2 tsp.)
- ❖ Black pepper (1/4 tsp.)
- ❖ Finely chopped green onions (1/4 tsp.)
- ❖ Ingredients for wings
- ❖ Chicken wings (2 kg)
- ❖ Salt (1 tsp.)
- ❖ Garlic (1 tsp.)
- ❖ Onion powder (1 tsp.)
- ❖ Black pepper (1 tsp.)
- ❖ Cornstarch (1/2 cup)

Ingredients for garnishes

- ❖ Sliced green onions (2 scoops)
- ❖ Sesame seed (1 tsp.)

Steps

1. In a saucepan, blend the gochujang, hot honey, soy sauce, brown sugar, lemon juice, ginger, garlic, salt, and black pepper. Over moderate pressure, raise the sauce to a boil, reduce heat and simmer for 6 minutes. Garnish with green onions and stir.

2. Heat up to 450 degrees F for the air fryer.

3. In a wide cup, put the wings and mix in the salt, onion powder, garlic powder, and black pepper. Apply cornstarch and throw the wings until they're fully covered. Shake each wing and put in the air fryer's basket to ensure that they do not touch; if appropriate, cook in batches.

4. Fry for 15 minutes in a preheated air fryer, shake the basket and fry for an extra 12 minutes. Flip the wings over and fry for 7 - 10 more minutes until the chicken is cooked.

5. Soak each wing in the sauces and marinade with the sesame seeds and the sliced green onions. Serve on the hand with the leftover sauce.

33. Air Fried Mozzarella Sticks

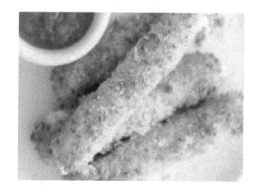

Ingredients

Ingredients for batter

- ❖ Water (1/2 cup)

- ❖ Flour (1/4 cup)
- ❖ Cornstarch (5 tsp.)
- ❖ Cornmeal (1 tbsp.)
- ❖ Garlic (1 tsp.)
- ❖ Salt (1/2 tsp.)

Ingredients for coatings

- ❖ Breadcrumbs (1 cup)
- ❖ Salt (1/2 tsp.)
- ❖ Black pepper (1/2 tsp.)
- ❖ Flakes of parsley (1/2 tsp.)
- ❖ Powdered garlic (1/2 tsp.)
- ❖ Onion (1/4 tsp.)
- ❖ Oregano dried (1/4 tsp.)
- ❖ Dry basil (1/4 tsp.)
- ❖ Mozzarella cheese (5 ounces)
- ❖ Flour (1 tbsp.)
- ❖ Cooking mist

Steps

1. In a large, shallow cup, put cornstarch, water, flour, garlic powder, cornmeal, and salt; blend the pancake batter's consistency into a batter. If necessary, change the ingredients to get the correct quality.

2. In another large, shallow cup, whisk together the salt, panko, pepper, parsley, garlic powder, oregano, onion powder and basil.

3. Cover each stick of mozzarella thinly with flour. In the batter, dip each stick and throw it in the panko mixture. On a baking sheet, put the sticks in a single layer. Freeze for one hour, at least.

4. Warm an air-fryer to 450 degrees F as instructed by the maker. Place a series of sticks of mozzarella in the basket of the fryer. Spray with a layer of light spray for frying. Cook for six minutes on sticks. Open the fryer and use a spatula to flip the sticks. Continue to cook for9-10 minutes, until lightly browned.

34. Air Fryer Pakoras

Ingredients

- ❖ Sliced cauliflower (2 cups)
- ❖ Potatoes diced (1 cup)
- ❖ Chickpea flour (1 1/4 cups)
- ❖ Water (3/4 cup)
- ❖ Red onion, chopped (1/2 tbsp.)
- ❖ Salt (1 tbsp.)

- ❖ Garlic (1 clove)
- ❖ Powdered curry (1 tsp.)
- ❖ Cilantro (1 tsp.)
- ❖ Cayenne pepper (1/2 tsp.)
- ❖ Cumin (1/2 tsp.)
- ❖ Cooking spray

Steps

1. In a large bowl, mix the potatoes, curry powder, cauliflower, water, red onion, cilantro, cayenne, chickpea flour, salt, garlic, and cumin. Put aside for 10 mins to relax.

2. Heat the air-fryer to 180 degrees C.

3. Spray the air-fryer basket with the cooking spray. Fill the basket with 2 tsp of the cauliflower mixture and flatten it. Repeat this without touching the pakoras.

4. Flip and cook 8 minutes. Transfer it to a plate lined with paper towels. Repeat for the batter that remains.

35. Air Fryer Bacon Wrapped Scallops with Sriracha Mayo

Ingredients

- ❖ Mayonnaise (1/2 cup)

- ❖ Sriracha sauce (2 tbsp.)
- ❖ Bay scallops (1 pound)
- ❖ Salt (1 pinch)
- ❖ Black pepper (1 pinch)
- ❖ 12 bacon strips
- ❖ Cooking mist with olive oil

Steps

1. In a shallow bowl, mix the Sriracha sauce and mayonnaise. Sriracha mayo can be refrigerated before ready to eat.

2. Heat up to 395 degrees F for the air fryer.

3. Spread the scallops on a tray and use a paper towel to rinse them. With pepper and salt, season. Using a 1/4 piece of bacon to seal each scallop.

4. Spray a basket of air fryers with vegetable oil. Put scallops that are bacon wrapped in a single layer in the basket; break if necessary, into two rounds.

5. In an air fryer, cook for seven minutes. Test for doneness; it should be translucent for scallops and crisp for bacon. If required, cook 1 - 2 mins longer,

testing every min. Carefully pick the scallops with tongs and extract the bacon's excess grease. Serve with mayo from Sriracha.

36. Air Fryer Balsamic Glazed Chicken Wings

Ingredients

Ingredients for coatings

- ❖ Cooking mist
- ❖ Baking powder (3 tbsp.)
- ❖ Salt (2 tbsp.)
- ❖ Freshly ground black pepper (1 tbsp.)
- ❖ Paprika (1 tsp.)
- ❖ Chicken legs (2 pounds)

Ingredients for glaze

- ❖ Water (1/3 cup)
- ❖ Balsamic vinegar (1/3 cup)
- ❖ Soy sauce (2 tsp.)
- ❖ Honey (2 tsp.)
- ❖ Chili sauce (2 tsp.)
- ❖ Garlic, minced (2 cloves)
- ❖ Water (1 tsp.)
- ❖ Cornstarch (1 tsp.)

Ingredients for Garnish

- ❖ 1 onion
- ❖ Sesame seeds (1/4 tsp.)

Steps

1. Heat up to 385 degrees F with an air fryer. Cover the basket of the fryer with cooking oil.

2. In a shallow cup, mix the pepper, baking powder, cinnamon, and paprika. Place a mixture of baking powder in a bag, apply some of the chicken wings, and shake to cover the bag. Remove the wings from the jar, shake off the excess flour, and repeat until the baking powder mixture has covered all the wings.

3. With cooking oil, gently oil the wings, put in the prepared air fryer basket, and cook for twenty minutes, shaking and flipping halfway through the wings. Increase up the temperature to 450 degrees F and bake till crispy, around 5 minutes more. You will have to cook the wings in batches, depending on the capacity of your air fryer.

4. Meanwhile, in a saucepan over medium heat, add 1/4

cup of water, honey, balsamic vinegar, chili sauce, soy sauce and garlic. Carry to a low boil and simmer for around fifteen min until the sauce has diminished. In a shallow cup, mix 1 tsp of water and cornstarch and add into the sauce; swirl until the sauce thickens.

5. In a wide cup, put the crispy wings, mix with sauce, and swirl until well coated.

37. Air Fryer Loaded Greek Fries

Ingredients

- ❖ Cucumber (1/2 small)
- ❖ Salt (1/2 tsp.)
- ❖ Greek yogurt (6 ounces)
- ❖ Lemon juice (1 tbsp.)
- ❖ Freeze-dried dill (2 tsp.)
- ❖ Garlic minced (1 tsp.)
- ❖ Vinegar (1 tsp.)
- ❖ Crumbled feta cheese box (4 ounces)
- ❖ Russet potatoes (4 medium-sized)
- ❖ Olive oil (2 tsp.)
- ❖ Greek seasoning (2 tsp.)
- ❖ Cooking mist

- ❖ 1 tiny red onion, sliced into thin strips
- ❖ Kalamata olives sliced (1/4 cup)
- ❖ Grape tomatoes each, halved (12)

Steps

1. Place the shredded cucumber and sprinkle it with salt in a colander. For ten min, let it drain.

2. Meanwhile, apply the milk, vinegar, dill, garlic, lemon juice and feta to a tiny bowl to prepare the rest of the tzatziki. Stir once mixed equally. Stir in the shredded cucumber when ready to use and put aside.

3. Heat up to 450 degrees F with an air fryer.

4. In a big cup, mix the olive oil, fries, and Greek spices, and stir until uniformly mixed. Using non - stick cooking spray to coat the tray of the air fryer. To the basket, add 1/2 of the fries.

5. Fry for ten min on the air fryer. Flip when baked, perhaps Five minutes longer, to the perfect

crispness. Repeat for the fries that remain.

6. Split the fries into four serving plates. Drizzle over the top of the fries with cucumber sauce. Marinade the olives, Kalamata, red onion strips, and grape tomatoes on each dish.

38. Air Fryer Arancini

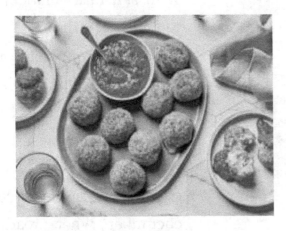

Ingredients

- ❖ Chickens (3 big)
- ❖ Cooked rice (2 1/2 cups)
- ❖ Grated Parmesan cheese (2/3 cup)
- ❖ Sugar, melted (1/3 cup)
- ❖ Italian cheese (1/2 tsp.)
- ❖ Salt (1/2 tsp.)
- ❖ Black pepper (1/4 tsp.)
- ❖ Mozzarella cheese (2 ounces)
- ❖ Breadcrumbs (1 cup)
- ❖ Italian seasoning (1/2 tsp.)
- ❖ Salt (1 pinch)
- ❖ Black pepper (1 pinch)
- ❖ Nonstick cooking mist

Steps

1. Lightly beat 2 eggs in a wide cup. Stir in parmesan cheese, flour, sugar, scatter with garlic, and 1/4 teaspoon of salt and 1/2 teaspoon of pepper; blend to mix. Cover and refrigerate for 22 minutes with the combination.

2. Heat the fryer to 375 degrees F.

3. Mix and roll into 1 1/2-inch round. Press a cube of mozzarella into the middle of each ball and reshape it.

4. In a shallow bowl, combine the Italian seasoning, panko breadcrumbs, salt, and pepper. In a second bowl, whip the remaining egg gently. Dip each rice ball into the egg first, then roll in the mixture of panko. Place the rice balls in the basket of the air fryer and spray them with cooking spray.

5. Cook for 6 minutes in the preheated air fryer. Improve the heat to 450 degrees F

and fry the air for another 3 minutes.

39. Air Fryer Mac and Cheese Ball

Ingredients

- ❖ Water (6 cups)
- ❖ 1 bag of macaroni and cheese (7.12 ounce)
- ❖ Milk (1/4 cup)
- ❖ Margarine (4 tbsp.)
- ❖ Shredded sharp Cheddar cheese (3/4 cup)
- ❖ Nonstick cooking mist
- ❖ Panko breadcrumbs (1/2 cup)
- ❖ Breadcrumbs (1/2 cup)
- ❖ Salt (1/2 tsp.)
- ❖ Powdered garlic (1/2 tbsp.)
- ❖ Two big eggs

Steps

1. Add water in a dish and boil it. Mix in the pasta macaroni from the dinner pack. Cook, occasionally stirring, for 6 - 8 minutes, until soft. Please drain; do not wash. Return to the pot and stir in the cheese sauce, milk and margarine included. Attach the cheddar cheese and stir until the cheese is melted and well mixed.

2. Refrigerate until solid, from 2 hours to midnight, with macaroni and cheese.

3. Scoop the macaroni and cheese into 1/2-inch balls and put them on a baking sheet lined with parchment paper.

4. Heat an air fryer to 355 degrees F. Oil the basket with non - stick cooking spray.

5. In a medium dish, combine the salt, breadcrumbs, panko, and garlic powder. Dip each ball into the pounded eggs and then into the mixture of panko.

6. Put the mac and cheese balls in a single layer in the air fryer basket, make sure they do not touch, if appropriate, and cook in batches.

7. Cook in the preheated air fryer for 8 to 12 minutes. Switch and fry until lightly browned, for three or four more minutes.

40. Air Fryer Fingerling Potatoes with Dip

Ingredients

- ❖ Fingerling potatoes (12 ounces)
- ❖ Olive oil (1 tbsp.)
- ❖ Garlic (1 tsp.)
- ❖ Paprika (1/4 tsp.)
- ❖ Salt and ground black pepper

Sauce dipping:

- ❖ Sour cream (1/3 cup)
- ❖ Mayonnaise (2 ounces)
- ❖ Parmesan cheese finely grated (2 tsp.)
- ❖ Ranch dressing (1 ½ tsp.)
- ❖ White vinegar (1 spoon)
- ❖ New parsley chopped (1 tbsp.)

Steps

1. Heat an air fryer for five min to 395 degrees F.
2. Add the paprika, olive oil, salt, garlic powder and pepper and put the potatoes in a dish. Toss till the potatoes are covered and move them to the basket of the air fryer.
3. Cook in the preheated air fryer, shaking halfway through the basket, 18 to 30 minutes before the potatoes are fried through and crispy.
4. Mix the mayonnaise, sour cream, ranch dressing mix, parmesan cheese and vinegar in a little bowl as the potatoes are frying.
5. Drop the fried potatoes and garnish them with parsley on a tray. Serve directly with sauce for dipping.

41. Air Fryer Taco Soup

Ingredients

- ❖ Corn tortillas (4 inches)
- ❖ Oil
- ❖ Sea salt
- ❖ 1 tiny chopped onion
- ❖ Ground garlic (2 cloves)
- ❖ Ground sirloin (1 1/2 lbs.)
- ❖ Taco seasoning (1)
- ❖ Pinto beans (1 15 oz.)
- ❖ Corn (1 15 oz.)
- ❖ Diced tomatoes (1 15 oz.)
- ❖ Salsa (1 cup)
- ❖ Chicken (3 cups)
- ❖ For serving, sliced cheddar cheese and sour cream

Steps

1. Pour sufficiently of the oil into the pan into a big, non-

stick skillet such that it is around 1/6-inch to 1/4-inch thick. There's a lot of oil you don't use. Over moderate pressure steams the liquid. Place the tortillas gently in the air fryer to fry until it is warmed. Enable them to fry before they start to puff a little and brown slightly. Then turn them over and cook for an additional couple of minutes. Remove the tortillas from a tray lined with paper towels and brush them with sea salt. Continue to cook the tortillas until enough for you.

2. Heat a pot of soup over high-medium heat. One tbsp. of oil is applied. When it is light, mix the garlic and onion and cook for 2 minutes, only until the garlic is fragrant.

3. Apply the seasoning to the taco and cook for around one minute.

4. Then beans, maize, salsa, tomatoes, and broth are included. Bring the soup to a gentle boil and mix properly.

5. Turn low the heat and cover the broth so that it can cook softly. Enable the soup to boil twenty minutes before eating, at least.

6. Serve the soup served with tortillas of freshly fried rice, shredded cheese, and sour cream.

42. Air Fryer Coconut Shrimp

Ingredients

- ❖ Big uncooked shrimp (1/2 pound)
- ❖ Shredded coconut (1/2 cup)
- ❖ Panko breadcrumbs (3 tsp.)
- ❖ 2 big egg whites
- ❖ Salt (1/8 tsp.)
- ❖ Pepper
- ❖ Louisiana-style hot sauce
- ❖ Flour (3 tsp.)

Ingredients for sauce

- ❖ Apricot (1/3 cup)
- ❖ Vinegar (1/2 tsp.)
- ❖ Crushed red pepper flakes

Steps

1. Heat a 380° air fryer. Shrimps peel and finely dice, keeping tails around.

2. Toss the coconut with the breadcrumbs in a small dish. Whisk together the pepper, egg whites, salt, and spicy sauce in another small dish. In a shallow third cup, put flour.

3. Dip the shrimp gently in flour to coat; shake off the residue. Dip in the egg white mixture, then pat in the coconut mixture to help adhere to the coating.

4. In the air-fryer basket, put the shrimp in one layer on the greased plate. Cook for four minutes, switch the shrimp and resume cooking for another four min. Until the coconut is gently golden brown, and the shrimp becomes yellow.

5. Meanwhile, mix the sauce ingredients in a shallow saucepan; cook and stir until the preserves are dissolved over medium-low heat. Serve the shrimp with sauce promptly.

43. Air Fryer Loaded Cheese and Onion Fries

Ingredients

- Cucumber (1/2 small)
- Salt (1/2 tsp.)
- Greek yogurt (6 ounces)
- Lemon juice (1 tbsp.)
- Freeze-dried dill (2 tsp.)
- Onion (6 pieces)
- Garlic minced (1 tsp.)
- Vinegar (1 tsp.)
- Crumbled feta cheese box (4 ounces)
- Russet potatoes (4 medium-sized)
- Olive oil (2 tsp.)
- Greek seasoning (2 tsp.)
- Cooking mist
- 1 tiny red onion, sliced into thin strips
- Kalamata olives sliced (1/4 cup)
- Grape tomatoes each, halved (12)

Steps

1. Place the shredded cucumber and sprinkle it with salt in a colander. For ten min, let it drain.

2. Meanwhile, apply the milk, vinegar, dill, garlic, lemon juice and feta to a tiny bowl to prepare the rest of the tzatziki. Stir once mixed equally. Stir in the shredded

cucumber when ready to use and put aside.

3. Heat up to 450 degrees F with an air fryer.

4. In a big cup, mix the olive oil, fries, and Greek spices, and stir until uniformly mixed. Using non - stick cooking spray to coat the tray of the air fryer. To the basket, add 1/2 of the fries.

5. Fry for ten min on the air fryer. Flip when baked, perhaps Five minutes longer, to the perfect crispness. Repeat for the fries that remain.

6. Split the fries into four serving plates. Drizzle over the top of the fries with cucumber sauce. Marinade the olives, Kalamata, red onion strips, and grape tomatoes on each dish.

44. Air Fryer Paneer Pakoras

Ingredients

- ❖ Sliced cauliflower (2 cups)
- ❖ Potatoes diced (1 cup)
- ❖ Cheese
- ❖ Chickpea flour (1 1/4 cups)
- ❖ Water (3/4 cup)

- ❖ Red onion, chopped (1/2 tbsp.)
- ❖ Salt (1 tbsp.)
- ❖ Garlic (1 clove)
- ❖ Powdered curry (1 tsp.)
- ❖ Cilantro (1 tsp.)
- ❖ Cayenne pepper (1/2 tsp.)
- ❖ Cumin (1/2 tsp.)
- ❖ Cooking spray

Steps

1. In a large bowl, mix the potatoes, curry powder, cauliflower, water, red onion, cilantro, cayenne, cheese, chickpea flour, salt, garlic, and cumin. Put aside for 10 mins to relax.

2. Heat the air-fryer to 180 degrees C.

3. Spray the air-fryer basket with the cooking spray. Fill the basket with 2 tsp of the cauliflower mixture and flatten it. Repeat this without touching the paneer pakoras.

4. Flip and cook 8 minutes. Transfer it to a plate lined with paper towels. Repeat for the batter that remains.

45. Air Fryer Pork Balls

Ingredients

- ❖ Oats for quick cooking (2/3 cup)
- ❖ Ritz crackers (1/2 cup)
- ❖ Beaten eggs (2)
- ❖ Milk (5 ounces)
- ❖ Minced onion (1 tbsp.)
- ❖ Salt (1 tsp.)
- ❖ Garlic (1 tsp.)
- ❖ Cumin ground (1 tsp.)
- ❖ Honey (1 tsp.)
- ❖ Mustard (1/2 tsp.)
- ❖ Pork (2 pounds)

Ingredients for Sauce

- ❖ Brown sugar (1/3 cup)
- ❖ Honey (1/3 cup)
- ❖ Orange marmalade (1/3 cup)
- ❖ Cornstarch (2tsp.)
- ❖ Soy sauce (2 tsp.)
- ❖ Louisiana-style hot sauce (1 -2 tsp.)
- ❖ Worcestershire sauce (1 tbsp.)

Steps

1. Heat the air fryer at 380 °. Mix the first ten ingredients in a wide bowl. Add pork, blend deeply but lightly. Mold to 1-1/4-in balls.

2. In a single layer, arrange the pork balls on a greased tray in an air-fryer basket. Cook for 14-15 minutes, until browned and fully baked. Meanwhile, combine the sauce components in a small saucepan. Cook and stir until it thickens, over medium heat.

46. Air Fryer Crab Cake

Ingredients

- ❖ Lamb crab meat 8 ounces
- ❖ Almond flour ¼ cup
- ❖ Chopped fresh parsley 2 tablespoon
- ❖ Sliced green onion 1
- ❖ Old Bay seasoning ½ teaspoon
- ❖ Salt ½ teaspoon
- ❖ Pepper ¼ teaspoon
- ❖ Egg 1 large
- ❖ Mayonnaise 1 tablespoon
- ❖ Dijon mustard 2 teaspoon
- ❖ Melted butter 2 tablespoon

Steps

1. Break up the crab meat in a wide bowl with a fork. Add the green onion, almond flour, parsley, pepper,

cinnamon, and Old Bay until well mixed.

2. Stir in the mustard, mayo, and egg before the mixture is sufficiently humidified. Using your palms, each about 3/4 inch to 1 inch thick, to shape 4 patties. Put it on a plate lined with waxed paper and cool for at least 30 minutes.

3. Spray the air fryer rack with oil or brush it. Rub melted butter over the crab cakes on both sides and put on the shelf.

4. Air fried for 10 minutes at 350-degree F, turning gently halfway through frying.

5. For the mayo, mix the ingredients in a tiny cup.

47. Homemade Chicharrones (Pork Rind)

Ingredients

- ❖ Pork back fat and skin 3-4 lb.
- ❖ Salt and pepper
- ❖ Cooking oil spray

Steps

1. Place a wire rack over a baking sheet and preheat the oven to 250-degree F.

2. Cut the pork into long strips, around 2 inches across, using a very sharp knife. Every two inches rate the fat on each strip. At one end of the strip, gently place a knife between the skin and the fat and cut a part of the fat.

3. You should keep the skin in one hand until the first section of fat is extracted while you slip the knife down the strip to extract much of the fat. Again, it is okay with a little fat already sticking to the muscle.

4. Cut every strip into 2-inch squares after the fat has been stripped and put, fat-side down, on the wire shelf.

5. Bake for 3 hours, until the skin is completely dry.

6. Meanwhile, if you want to cook your chicharrones with pork fat, put them in a wide saucepan over medium-low heat. Cook gently for around 2 hours, until much of the fat has liquified. Remove any residual solids with a slotted spoon. Dispose of (or feed, they

taste like bacon and they're fantastic for salad).

7. Heat oil/lard to a deep around 1/3 in the pan while baking time is running out. Or you can only get a couple of inches of oil and prepare batches of your pork rinds. Oil is expected to be moderately hot but not bubbling.

8. Add the pork rinds and cook for around 3 to 5 minutes, before they bubble and puff up. Remove and rinse on a tray lined with paper towels. Sprinkle with salt and pepper promptly.

48. Air Fryer Korean Sweet Potatoes

Ingredients

❖ Sweet potato (about 4 ounces)

❖ Purple potato (about 4 ounces)

❖ Olive oil (2 tbsp.)

❖ Salt and black pepper

❖ Red beet (about 6 ounces)

❖ Golden beet (about 6 ounces)

Steps

1. Cut the slices of potatoes into 1/14 inch and wash with water so that white starch comes down and then dry it.

2. After placing the potatoes into a bowl, add oil, salt, and pepper in it.

3. The air fryer is heated to a 3.5-quart air fryer at 350°F. Place the potatoes in the layers and cook until it becomes golden and changes its side after every 8 minutes.

4. After that, place it in another bowl and mix oil, salt, red beat, and pepper till uniformly covered.

5. Add the potato chips and beet chips in a dish and sprinkle salt and mix them. Allow it to cool, and you can store it in a container.

Chapter 5: Snacks and Kebabs

1. Air Fryer Jalapeno Poppers

Ingredients

- ❖ Jalapeno peppers 10
- ❖ Cream cheese 8 oz
- ❖ Parsley 1/4 cup
- ❖ Breadcrumbs ¾ cup

Steps

1. Add 1/2 of the crumbs and the cream cheese together. Add in the parsley until blended.
2. With this combination, stuff each pepper.
3. To build the surface layer, gently push the peppers' tops onto the remaining 1/4c of crumbs.
4. Cook for 6-8 minutes in an air fryer at 370 ° C., OR 20 minutes in a standard oven at 375 degrees F.
5. Let it cool off and Eat.

2. Air Fryer Egg Rolls

Ingredients

- ❖ Sesame oil 2 teaspoons
- ❖ Garlic 1 teaspoon
- ❖ Ginger 1 teaspoon
- ❖ Chicken 1 pound
- ❖ Onions 4
- ❖ Soy sauce 1 tablespoon
- ❖ Rice wine vinegar 1 tablespoon
- ❖ Cabbage 350 g
- ❖ Egg 1
- ❖ Egg roll 12

Steps

1. In a pan, introduce 2 teaspoons of oil and cook the ground chicken until cooked. Then add the garlic and ginger for a full 30 seconds, or until the mixture is fragrant.
2. Using the sliced cabbage and green onions to toss in. Cook until the cabbage, which takes around 4-5 minutes, has turned brown.
3. Drizzle the combination with the soy sauce and vinegar, toss to blend, and then turn the heat off.

Wrap Egg Rolls

1. With one corner pointing toward you, lay the egg roll wrapper out flat.
2. Position about 3 tablespoons of filling just below the egg roll wrapper's middle.
3. To make a triangle, fold two opposite corners together, then fold the sides into them and roll tightly.

4. To secure the closed sides, rub a tiny quantity of the beaten egg.

5. To assemble the rest of the egg rolls, repeat this process.

6. Until frying, brush or spray the remaining oil on each one.

Air Fryer Oven

1. Heat the air fryer to 350F / 180C, then apply a non-stick cooking spray with the basket.

2. Within the air fryer basket, put the egg rolls seam side down in a single sheet, making sure they do not contact.

3. For 10-12 minutes, cook. Switch over halfway into the cooking period for egg rolls.

4. For dipping, serve with soy sauce.

3. Air Fryer Biscuits

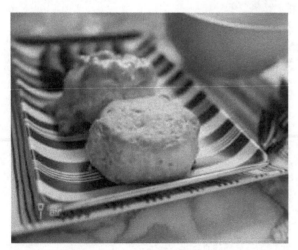

Ingredients

- ❖ Flour 2 cups

- ❖ Brown sugar ½ cup

- ❖ Pie spice 1 ½ teaspoons

- ❖ Baking powder 2 teaspoons

- ❖ Salt ½ teaspoon

- ❖ Unsalted cold butter ½ cup

- ❖ Cream ¼ cup

- ❖ Pumpkin puree ½ cup

- ❖ Vanilla extract 1 teaspoon

Steps

1. In a mixing bowl, mix the sugar, flour, pie spice, butter, baking powder, and salt.

2. Add heavy cream, vanilla extract, and pumpkin purée and pulse until dough develops.

3. On a floured board, roll out the pastry, cut out the biscuits, and spray with milk.

4. Leave an inch for both each, insert to the baking paper lining air fryer, and fry for 11-13 minutes until golden and roasted through.

5. Enable them to be removed, cooled on a cooling rack, and then eaten.

4. Air Fryer Tortilla Chips

Ingredients

- ❖ Corn tortillas 8
- ❖ Olive oil

Steps

1. Heat the air fryer to 350 F / 180 C.

2. Place the corn tortillas on a chopping board and break them into 8 triangles with a sharp blade.

3. Roll them out and brush them with either olive oil or cooking spray.

4. Turn them up, and sprinkle on the second hand.

5. In the air fryer basket, put a few tortillas and fry them for 7-9 minutes, rotating them midway through frying.

6. Stir to combine chips before all is over.

7. Until eating, allow them to settle on a cooling rack when they crisp up once cool.

5. Air Fryer Fried Wontons

Ingredients

❖ Chicken, beef, pork 1 pound

❖ Ginger 1 tablespoon

❖ Garlic 2

❖ Chopped scallions 2 tablespoons

❖ Gluten-free soy sauce 1 tablespoon

❖ gluten-free sweet chili sauce 2 tablespoons

❖ Chopped fresh greens such as kale, brussels sprouts, and cabbage 2 cups

❖ Egg wash (1 egg beaten with 1 tablespoon water)

❖ Oil, for coating (or for frying)

Steps

1. Create the wonton bags, sliced into roughly 3-inch triangles, as per the formula. Put aside the bags. Place the beef, scallion, garlic, soy sauce, ginger, oyster sauce or spicy chili sauce, and greens in a wide bowl and blend well to incorporate. It would be dense and reasonably sticky in the mixture.

2. Placed a wonton wrap straight in the fist to mount the wontons. In the egg wash, drop the free hand's index finger and outline the 4 sides of the coating with the egg wash. To the middle of the wrapper, apply roughly 1 teaspoon of the loading mixture. To seal the filling, insert one corner of the catty-corner wrapper into the opposite side. Tightly close the wrapping around the filling, forcing any air bubbles free.

3. Place the rounded and packed wontons in a single layer in the air fryer's basket and kindly spray or rub with oil on both ends. Put in an air fryer and fry for 4 minutes

at 350 ° F. Remove and shake the basket over it, turning as many wontons as possible around it. Remove the bowl to the air fryer and finish frying for 5-7 minutes, or until all of it is golden brown. For extra sweet chili sauce or soy sauce, eat immediately.

6. Air Fryer Plantains

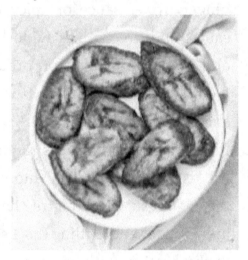

Ingredients

- ❖ Plantain 1
- ❖ Oil 1 teaspoon
- ❖ Salt 1 pinch

Steps

1. Heat the air fryer at 350F /180C.
2. Peel and break the plantain into strips and add it to a dish.
3. Combine the salt and oil softly until the plantains on both ends are covered.
4. Placed each of the plantain strips in a thin layer in the air freezer basket.
5. Cook midway through after 9-10 mins, rotating.
6. Serve it immediately.

7. Air Fryer Pita Bread Cheese Pizza

Ingredients

- ❖ Bread 1
- ❖ Pizza sauce 1 tablespoon
- ❖ Mozzarella cheese ¼ cup
- ❖ Legged trivet 1
- ❖ Olive oil 1 drizzle

Steps

1. Using a tablespoon and sprinkle on the Pita Bread with Pizza Sauce. Insert your favorite cheese and toppings. On top of the slice, apply a very little sprinkling of olive oil.
2. Put a drip pan above Pita Bread in an Air Fryer. Cook for 7 minutes at 350 °. Pull from the Air Fryer cautiously and carve.

8. Air Fryer Apple Chips

Ingredients

- ❖ Apples 6 Medium
- ❖ Extra Virgin Avocado Oil 1 Tbsp
- ❖ Cinnamon_1 Tbsp

Steps

1. Thinly dice the six medium-sized apples using a vegetable slicer (or anything similar). Try to throw sliced apples with oil using favorite balanced oil.

2. Sprinkle the apples with cinnamon after you've applied the oil.

3. Only cook. Load it into an air fryer and fry at 200c/400f for 15 minutes.

4. Dehydrate yourself. Adjust the cooking time to 3-4 hours and heat at 30c/85f but use the air fryer microwave.

9. Air Fryer Sriracha-Honey Chicken Wings

Ingredients

❖ Chicken wings 1 pound

❖ Honey 1/4 cup

❖ Sriracha sauce 2 tablespoons

❖ Soy sauce 1 1/2 tablespoons

❖ Butter 1 tablespoon

❖ juice of 1/2 lime

❖ Cilantro, chives, or scallions for garnish

Steps

1. The air fryer is heated up to 360 ° F. To ensure sure the wings are sufficiently browned, put the wings of chicken to the air fryer bowl and cook for 29-30 minutes, rotating the chicken around every 6-8 minutes with tongs.

2. Insert the sauce components to a medium saucepan as the wings are frying and continue cooking for around 3 minutes.

3. Try to throw them in a bowl only with sauce until thoroughly covered, spray with the garnish when the wings are fried, and served rapidly.

10. Air fryer Baked Thai Peanut Chicken Egg Rolls

Ingredients

❖ Egg roll 4

❖ Chicken 2 cup

❖ Thai peanut sauce ¼ cup

❖ Carrot 1 medium

❖ Onions 3

❖ Red pepper ¼

❖ Oil

Steps

1. Heat the air fryer or oven to 390 ° or 425 °.

2. Try to throw the chicken with Thai peanut sauce in a tiny tub.

3. On a clean, dry board, spread out the egg roll wrappers. Arrange 1/4 of the beet, onions, and bell pepper along the lower quarter of an egg roll wrapper. Spoon over the vegetables with 1/2 cup of the chicken combination.

4. Using water to moisten the outer sides of the packaging. Roll the wrapper's sides into the middle then roll securely.

5. Continue for the wrappers that remain.

6. Spray with nonstick cooking spray on the assembled egg rolls. Switch them over and even spray the sides of the bottom.

7. In the air fryer, put the egg rolls and bake at 390 ° C for-9 minutes or until crispy and lightly browned.

8. Put them on a baking dish sprayed with cooking spray if you bake the egg rolls in an oven. Bake for 15-20 minutes at 425 °).

9. Cut in half and use for dipping with extra Thai Peanut Sauce.

11. Air Fryer Twice Baked Potatoes

Ingredients

- ❖ Yukon Gold potatoes 2 large
- ❖ Broccoli florets 1/2 cup
- ❖ Butter 4 tbsp
- ❖ Cream cheese 1/4 cup
- ❖ Sour cream 2 tbsp
- ❖ Cheese Muenster 1/2 cup
- ❖ Salt 1 tsp
- ❖ Smoked paprika 1/2 tsp
- ❖ Black pepper 1/2 tsp

Steps

1. Bake the potatoes.

2. Allow it to cool for 10 minutes or so. Break them in half with the potatoes. Scoop the interior of the potatoes carefully into a clean tub. Put aside certain skins.

3. Mash the fried potato, butter, sour cream, broccoli, cream cheese, 1/4 of a cup of garlic, cinnamon, pepper, and paprika together.

4. To flatten the sides, pour the potatoes filling thinly onto the skins and gently push down on end.

5. The top half of each twice-baked potato with cheese.

6. In the bowl of air fryer, put the potatoes, loading side up.

7. At 400 degrees F, cook the twice-baked potatoes for around 9-14 minutes till the filler is hot, and the tips are lightly browned.

8. Immediately serve.

12. Air-Fryer Honey Cinnamon Roll-ups

Ingredients

- ❖ Walnut 2 cups

- ❖ Sugar 1/4 cup

- ❖ Cinnamon 2 teaspoons

- ❖ Frozen phyllo dough 12 sheets

- ❖ Butter 1/2 cup

- ❖ Honey 1/2 cup

- ❖ Sugar 1/2 cup

- ❖ Water 1/2 cup

- ❖ Lemon juice 1 tablespoon

Steps

1. Heat up at 325 ° air fryer. Place the walnuts, cinnamon, and sugar together.

2. Place 1 layer on a 15x12-in phyllo dough tray. Bit of waxed paper; butter on a brush. Put on the top of a second phyllo layer, coating this with butter. Sprinkle over 1/4 cup of walnut combination. Tightly roll up the jelly-roll style with waxed paper, beginning on a long hand, extracting paper when you roll. Cut it into four smaller rolls. Rub with butter, with toothpicks, stable. Repeat with 1/4 cup of walnut mixture and the leftover phyllo dough. Put in a thin layer on the greased tray in the air-fryer basket in batches. For 9-11 minutes, cook till light brown, on a wire rack, nice. Cast out toothpicks.

3. Meanwhile, add all the syrup components in a shallow saucepan. Just get it to a simmer. Lower the heat; boil for 5 minutes. 10 minutes to calm. Move the rolls of cinnamon to a serving dish. Sprinkle with the leftover blend of walnuts.

13. Air-Fryer Acorn Squash Slices

Ingredients

- ❖ Acorn squash 2 medium
- ❖ Butter ½ cup
- ❖ Brown sugar 2/3 cup

Steps

1. Heat the 350 ° air fryer. Split the squash lengthwise in half; cut and

discard the seeds. Split sliced lengthwise into 1/2-in each portion. Slices; ends to discard. Organize squash in a thin layer in batches on an oiled tray in an air-fryer bowl. Cook until soft, five minutes on either hand.

2. Combine the butter and sugar, place on the squash. Cook for 3 more minutes.

14. Air-Fryer Beefy Swiss Bundles

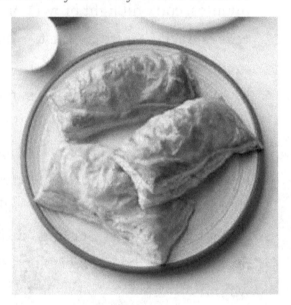

Ingredients

- ❖ Beef 1 pound
- ❖ Sliced fresh mushrooms 1-1/2 cups
- ❖ Onion 1/2 cup
- ❖ Garlic 1-1/2 teaspoons
- ❖ Worcestershire sauce 4 teaspoons
- ❖ Dried rosemary 3/4 teaspoon
- ❖ Paprika 3/4 teaspoon
- ❖ Salt 1/2 teaspoon
- ❖ Pepper 1/4 teaspoon
- ❖ Frozen puff pastry 1 sheet
- ❖ Freeze mashed potatoes 2/3 cup
- ❖ Swiss cheese 1 cup
- ❖ Egg 1 large
- ❖ Water 2 tablespoons

Steps

1. Heat a 375 ° air fryer. 9 Cook the beef, onion, and mushrooms over medium heat in a broad skillet until the meat are no longer pink, and the vegetables are soft, 9-11 minutes. Stir in garlic; simmer for 1 minute longer. Stir in the seasonings and sauce from Worcestershire. Withdraw from the heat; put down.

2. Wrap puff pastry into a 16x12-in on a thinly floured table, with rectangles. Over each rectangle, put around 2 teaspoons of potatoes; extend to within 1 inch from the margins. Cover each with a mixture of 3/4 cup beef; scatter with 1/4 cup cheese.

3. Whip the egg and water; rub some around the sides of the pastry.

Place opposite pastry corners across each bundle; pinch the seams to seal. Rub for the leftover combination of shells. Place the pastries in batches in a thin layer on the tray in the air-fryer bowl; cook for 10-12 minutes until golden brown.

4. Ice unbaked pastries until secure on a cloth-lined baking sheet. Shift to an airtight bag; return to the freezer. -Cook frozen pastries until lightly browned and heated through, growing time to 18-19 minutes, as guided for usage.

15. Mexican Air Fryer Corn on the Cob

Ingredients

❖ Corns 4 ears shucked
❖ Mexican sour cream ½ cup
❖ Cotija cheese ¼ cup
❖ Cilantro 2 tablespoon
❖ Chili powder 2 teaspoon
❖ Olive oil spray
❖ Lime juice

Steps

1. Wash the corn and dry it. Place the corn in a single layer of the Air Fryer bowl and gently spray it with oil.

2. Set the Air Fryer to 400 ° f with a 15-minute timer.

3. Open the basket after 8 minutes, turn the corn over and gently spray it again. Keep cooking.

4. Remove the corn to a dish until the timer is up.

5. Spread on both sides of the corn with Mexican milk. Sprinkle with chili powder, cilantro, and cotija butter. Until eating, pinch it with lime.

16. Air Fryer Asparagus

Ingredients

❖ Asparagus 1 pound
❖ Salt 1/8 teaspoon
❖ Black pepper 1/8 teaspoon
❖ Olive oil 1 tablespoon

Steps

1. Cut the edges of the asparagus from the bottom about an inch away.

2. Put the asparagus on a dish. Drizzle over the asparagus with olive oil. Sprinkle on the top of salt and black pepper and toss to cover the asparagus.

3. Bring the spears into the basket of the air fryer and close them. Turn the fryer to an air temperature of 400 degrees and set it for 7 minutes.

4. Remove the basket until the time is out and represent the asparagus.

17. Air Fryer Zucchini Fries

Ingredients

- ❖ Zucchini 2 medium
- ❖ Egg 1 large
- ❖ Almond flour ½ cup
- ❖ Parmesan cheese ½ cup
- ❖ Italian seasoning 1 teaspoon
- ❖ Garlic powder ½ teaspoon
- ❖ Olive oil spray
- ❖ Salt and pepper 1 pinch

Steps

1. Break the zucchini in half and into around 1/2-inch-thick and 3-4-inch-long sticks.
2. Merge the almond flour, parmesan, the seasoning and a pinch of salt and pepper in a small dish. Blend and mix.
3. Dredge the zucchini in the egg mixture and then the almond flour and put it on a baking sheet or tray. Spray the zucchini generously with cooking spray.
4. Put the zucchini fries in a thin layer in the air fryer, operating in batches. Cook at 400F, or until crispy, for 10 minutes.

18. Air Fryer Banana Bread for Two

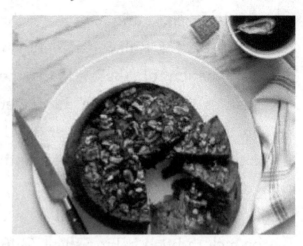

Ingredients

- ❖ Flour 1 cup
- ❖ Baking powder 1 teaspoon
- ❖ Salt ¼ teaspoon
- ❖ Baking soda ¼ teaspoon
- ❖ Ripe bananas 2
- ❖ Sugar 1/3 cup
- ❖ Vegetable oil ¼ cup
- ❖ Egg 1 large
- ❖ Sour cream 2 tablespoons
- ❖ Peanut butter 2 tablespoons
- ❖ Vanilla extract 1 teaspoon
- ❖ Walnuts ¾ cup

Steps

1. Heat the oven to 33⁰F. With nonstick cooking oil, oil the bottom and sides of the nonstick baking dish; set aside.
2. Add the baking powder, flour, salt, baking

soda, and whisk to mix in a medium bowl; set aside.

3. Add the bananas to a wide bowl and mash with a fork.

4. Until blended, add milk, sugar, egg, peanut butter, sour cream, vanilla, and whisk.

5. Apply the mixture of flour and whisk until just mixed.

6. Optionally, add in the chocolate chips or walnuts.

7. Turn the batter into a prepared baking dish and distribute it with a spatula thinly.

8. Place the baking dish carefully in the separate cooking basket and put the bowl into the air fryer.

9. Bake for around 30 to 40 minutes, or until the middle comes out clean with a toothpick inserted.

10. Remove the baking dish from the air fryer, put it on a rack of string, and cool the bread for 10 minutes. Turn the bread on a cutting board and flip it up on the right side.

19. Air Fryer Kale Chips

Ingredients

- ❖ Kale sliced 6 cups
- ❖ Olive oil 2 tablespoons
- ❖ Garlic powder 1 teaspoon
- ❖ Salt ½ teaspoon
- ❖ Onion powder ½ teaspoon
- ❖ Black pepper 1/8 teaspoon

Steps

1. Blend kale and olive oil in a wide bowl before the kale is fully covered.

2. Add cinnamon, garlic powder, pepper, and onion powder to kale.

3. Shift a single sheet of kale leaves to the bowl of an air fryer. Made sure they are spread equally.

4. Cook on 360 ° F for 6 minutes.

5. To pass the leaves around, shake the air fryer bowl, ensuring the leaves are spread equally.

6. Cook for a further 2 minutes at 360 ° F.

7. Move kale chips to a baking sheet to cool without hitting each other.

8. Enjoy it or cause it to cool fully instantly.

20. Crispy Air Fryer Chickpeas

Ingredients

❖ Chickpeas 15 ounce

❖ Vegetable 1 tablespoon

Steps

1. Heat the air fryer for 10 minutes to 390 ° F.

2. Prep the chickpeas: completely dry the chickpeas on a paper towel or a clean kitchen towel. During this stage, discard any skin that falls off the chickpeas.

3. Season the chickpeas: In a bowl, combine the oil and spice mix and whisk to coat. Until sprayed, softly add the chickpeas.

4. Chickpeas air-fried: Move to the hot oven air fryer and fried until crispy for 8 to 10 minutes. Taste one of the chickpeas then proceeds to cook for another 1 to 3 minutes if it's not as crispy as you'd like.

5. Season and serve: Remove, and add more salt, pepper or seasoning of your liking from the basket to a dish. Serve immediately; there would be no crispy chickpeas remaining.

21. Air Fryer Baked Potato

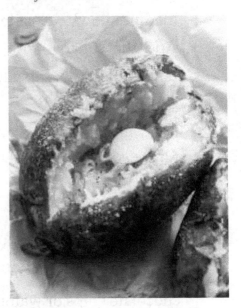

Ingredients

❖ Potatoes 2 large

❖ Peanut oil 1 tablespoon

❖ Sea salt ½ teaspoon

Steps

1. Heat an air fryer at 400 degrees F.

2. Rub the peanut oil with the potatoes and dust them with salt. Put them in the air fryer bowl.

3. Cook the potatoes for around 1 hour, until finished. By poking them with a fork, test for doneness. Until frying, the potatoes may not need to be pierced with a fork or twisted before frying.

22. Air Fryer Olive Fries

Ingredients

❖ Olives

- ❖ Egg 1 large

- ❖ Almond flour ½ cup

- ❖ Parmesan cheese ½ cup

- ❖ Italian seasoning 1 teaspoon

- ❖ Garlic powder ½ teaspoon

- ❖ Olive oil spray

- ❖ Salt and pepper 1 pinch

Steps

1. Merge the olives, almond flour, parmesan, the seasoning and a pinch of salt and pepper in a small dish. Blend and mix.

2. Dredge the zucchini in the egg mixture and then the almond flour and put it on a baking sheet or tray. Spray the zucchini generously with cooking spray.

3. Put the zucchini fries in a thin layer in the air fryer, operating in batches. Cook at 400F, or until crispy, for 10 minutes.

Air Fryer Kebabs

1. Low Country Boil Skewers

Ingredients

- ❖ Red potatoes 6 baby
- ❖ Salt to taste
- ❖ Crab boil seasoning 2 tbsp
- ❖ Corn 1 ear of
- ❖ Butter 4 tbsp
- ❖ Garlic, finely chopped 3 cloves
- ❖ Hot sauce 2 tsp
- ❖ Cider vinegar 1 tsp
- ❖ Shrimp 10 large
- ❖ Smoked pork, sliced into ½ inch thick rounds, 8 oz.
- ❖ Lemon wedges, for serving

Steps

1. In a saucepan, add the potatoes and coat with cold water. Add the salt and 1 tbsp of the seafood seasoning to taste. Bring to a boil, lower down to a simmer, and cook for 10-12 minutes till the potatoes are tender. And, within the last 5 minutes, add in the corn. Let the water drain and cool.

2. In a small skillet on medium heat, melt the butter. Add the sauce and garlic until fragrant, until the butter has fragrance. Stir in the vinegar and the spicy sauce. Then, remove half of the dressing from the heat and reserve it.

3. On the skewers, break and loop the potatoes, sausage, shrimp, and shrimp again. Brush the shrimp with half of the glaze.

4. Put skewers in the appliance using your Air Fryer Oven and use the rotisserie configuration. Air fry the skewers for 10 minutes at 320 ° F. With lemon wedges, serve the skewers and drizzle with the leftover sauce.

2. Greek Chicken Kebabs with Tzatziki Sauce

Ingredients

- ❖ Boneless skinless chicken breasts, diced into 1 ¼ inch cubes, 1 ¾ lb.
- ❖ Olive oil ¼ cup + 2 tbsp
- ❖ Lemon juice 3 tbsp
- ❖ Red wine vinegar 1 tbsp
- ❖ Garlic 3 cloves
- ❖ Dried oregano 2 tsp
- ❖ Dried basil ½ tsp
- ❖ Dried thyme ½ tsp
- ❖ Dried coriander ½ tsp

- ❖ Salt and pepper to taste
- ❖ Red bell peppers 2 large
- ❖ Zucchini sliced 3 smalls
- ❖ Red onion 1 large

Tzatziki Sauce:

- ❖ Cucumber 1 medium
- ❖ Salt 1 tsp
- ❖ Greek yogurt 2 – 5.3 oz. containers
- ❖ Garlic 1 clove
- ❖ Lemon juice 1 tbsp
- ❖ Fresh parsley 1 tbsp
- ❖ Fresh dill 1 tbsp

Steps

1. Merge lemon juice, 1/4 cup of olive oil, vinegar, oregano, garlic, basil, cilantro, thyme, and season to taste with salt and pepper in a dish. Blend and mix.

2. In a Ziploc container, put the chicken and pour the olive oil combination over the chicken and force it into the marinade. For 30-45 minutes, refrigerate. Drizzle and toss the vegetables with the 2 teaspoons of left olive oil. With salt, season gently.

3. Thread each skewer with red bell pepper, red onion, zucchini, and 2 chicken parts and repeat twice.

Repeat until you have the skewers complete.

4. Put your skewers in the appliance using your Air Fryer Oven and use the rotisserie configuration. Air fried the skewers for 10 minutes at 400 ° F.

5. Prepare your Tzatziki sauce as you are waiting for your skewers to cook. Sprinkle with salt, toss uniformly to cover and enable to rest for 25-30 minutes at room temperature. Begin by putting your diced cucumber in a mesh strainer.

6. Squeeze out some of the remaining moisture from the cucumbers and clean the cucumbers. In a blender, put the cucumbers and pulse finely to chop. Then, in a mixing cup, dump the cucumbers and apply the remaining sauce components, whisking to blend.

7. Store the sauce in the fridge until it is fit for serving.

3. Spicy Cumin Lamb Skewers

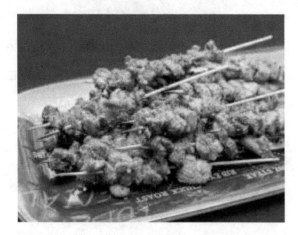

Ingredients

- ❖ Red chili flakes 1 tbsp
- ❖ Cumin seed 1 tbsp
- ❖ Fennel seed 2 tsp
- ❖ Kosher salt 1 tsp
- ❖ Granulated garlic 2 tsp
- ❖ Lamb's shoulder chops 1 ¼ lb.
- ❖ Vegetable oil 1 tbsp
- ❖ Pale, dry sherry 2 tsp

Steps

1. Coarsely ground the chili powder, cumin and fennel in a mortar and pestle grinder. To split into smaller bits, add the garlic and salt and briefly grind. Combine the products thoroughly.

2. In a shallow bowl, reserve 1 tablespoon of the spice blend. Add the lamb slices to a wide bowl and toss them thoroughly with the remaining spice blend, oil, and vinegar.

3. Place the skewers with the seasoned lamb slices and place them in the Air Fryer Oven. Air fry the skewers for 10 minutes at 340 ° F using the Rotisserie configuration.

4. Spray the reserved spice mix (optional) on them when the skewers are almost cooked through and let them finish frying.

5. Remove the oven skewers and eat immediately.

4. Italian Chicken Skewers

Ingredients

- ❖ Skinless and boneless chicken breasts 1 lb.
- ❖ Salt and pepper to taste
- ❖ Tomato paste 2 tbsp
- ❖ Olive oil ¼ cup
- ❖ Garlic 3 cloves, minced
- ❖ Fresh Italian parsley 1 tbsp
- ❖ 1 French baguette, cut into cubes

Steps

1. Season the chicken with salt and, to taste, pepper.

2. Merge the olive oil, tomato paste, garlic cloves and sliced parsley in

a medium-sized bowl to create the marinade. In a Ziploc jar, add the chicken and marinade and flip to cover entirely. For 30 minutes, refrigerate it.

3. Skewer the bread and chicken. Drizzle with olive oil and apply salt and pepper to taste. Put your skewers in the appliance using Air Fryer Oven and use the rotisserie configuration. Air fried the skewers for 10 minutes at 400 ° F.

4. Garnish and eat the parmesan and parsley.

5. Air Fryer Kofta Kabab

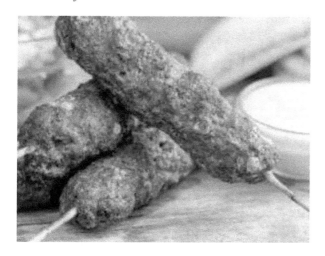

Ingredients

- ❖ Oil 1 tablespoon
- ❖ Lean Ground Beef 1 pound
- ❖ Chopped Parsley ¼ cup
- ❖ Minced Garlic 1 tablespoon

- ❖ Kofta kabab spice mix 2 tablespoons
- ❖ Kosher Salt 1 teaspoon

Steps

1. Blend all ingredients using a stand mixer. Let the mixture stay for 30 minutes in the fridge.

2. Make balls. While I have done this with and without skewers, the result just makes no difference.

3. Heat the air fryer at 375 degrees F.

4. Spread a foil in a baking pan and put a rack within the pan. Kebabs should be placed on the rack till the fat drips down. Cook and serve.

6. Air Fryer Chapli Kebab

Ingredients

- ❖ Minced chicken thighs 2 lbs.
- ❖ 1 large onion, chopped
- ❖ Tomato slices for decorating
- ❖ Chickpea flour or maize flour 2 tbsp
- ❖ 2-3 green chilies, finely chopped
- ❖ Oil for cooking
- ❖ Dry Spices
- ❖ coriander seeds 1 tbsp

- ❖ pomegranate seeds 2 tbsp
- ❖ cumin seeds 1 tbsp
- ❖ red chili powder 1/2 tsp
- ❖ chili flakes 1 tsp
- ❖ Salt to taste

Steps

1. In a coffee grinder, put the cumin seeds, coriander, and pomegranate seeds and loosely grind, not powder.

2. With the chopped onion, green chili, salt, chili flakes, flour of your choice, combine the roughly crushed spices. Apply this to the chicken. When evenly incorporated, blend with your hands. Make the kebabs.

3. Glove your hand in a Ziploc bag. Wet your other hand and spread it on your gloved palm, take a handful of the chicken mixture and form any shape of kebabs you like (e.g., round).

4. Through the kebab, hold 1 tomato slice.

5. Place the patty tenderly with tomato side down in the air fryer bowl. Repeat the procedure for 4-5 patties and put it in the container. Rub the top with oil on each of the patties. Set the temperature to 350 ° F and fry for 7 to 8 minutes on each side until brown and crispy.

6. Transfer to a serving dish until cooked and finish producing more kebabs.

Chapter 6: Dinner

1. Crispy Chicken Leg Piece

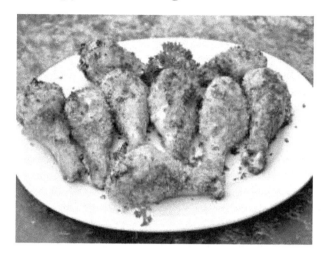

Ingredients

- 6 legs of the chicken
- 1 tsp of olive oil
- 1 tsp of Creole spice or your preferred combination of spices
- Salt

Sriracha mayo:

- 1/2 cup sriracha sauce (120 ml)
- 1/2 cup of mayonnaise (120 ml)
- 1 clove of minced garlic
- Juice of a lemon (1 ½ Tbsp)
- Sea salt powder for flavoring

Steps

1. Preheat the 400F/200C air fryer.

2. To make a paste-like combination, mix oil, spices, and salt together if necessary.

3. Add in the legs of the chicken to coat with spices.

4. In the air fryer, put the chicken legs and roast for 16-20 mins.

5. Nearly halfway through, turn out the chicken to ensure that both sides cook uniformly.

6. Test the thickest section of the leg piece for the temp of the chicken.

7. A minimum of 165°F/75°C should be achieved with chicken.

8. Serve immediately with your favorite hot mayo sauce or any other sauce.

INSTRUCTIONS FOR THE SPICY MAYO SAUCE:

1. Place the mayo and sriracha sauce together in a dish

2. Add chopped garlic and lemon juice to mix.

3. To test, add salt and swirl to mix.

2. Sliced Air Fryer Pork

Ingredients

- ❖ 2 pieces of boneless pork chops (weigh 0.5 lbs.)

- ❖ Almond powder (35 g)

- ❖ Sliced parmesan cheese (3tbsp)

- ❖ Paprika (1 tsp)

- ❖ Herbs of Corsica or blended dried herbs (1tsp)

- ❖ Cajun (1 tsp)

- ❖ Spray for cooking

Steps

1. Heat the air fryer to about 180°C or 350°F.
2. Almond powder, grated parmesan, paprika, herbs of Corsica, Cajun or other spices are blended.
3. Calorie cooking spray is sprinkled on all sides of the pork chops or ru b with olive oil if not adopting a ca lorie-controlled diet.
4. Add the coating mixture on all sides of the pork chops and put the chops in the air fryer's basket. Be ensure they are not contacting the pork chops depending on the size of pork chops cooking will take 8-12 minutes at any stage.
5. My pork chops took eight minutes. I suggest beginning with 8 minute s while

6. cooking for the first time and then testing for density.

3. Air Fryer Shrimp

Ingredients

- ❖ Shrimp 1 lb. (detach tail and shell if needed)

- ❖ Olive oil (1 ½ tsp)

- ❖ Lemon juice (1 ½ tsp)

- ❖ Honey (1 ½ tsp)

- ❖ Minced garlic (2 pieces)

- ❖ Salt (1/8 tsp)

For garnishing

- ❖ Wedge slime lime wedges

- ❖ Cilantro

Steps

1. Whisk together all the ingredients such as lime juice, olive oil, garlic, honey, and salt in a large dish.
2. For 25-30 minutes, add the shrimp and blend.
3. Heat the air fryer to a temperature of 395° F/200 ° C.
4. Shake off the shrimp's extra sauces and place the whole sample in the air fryer.
5. Give the basket a gentle shake, cook over medium heat, and

transfer to the air fryer. Cook for 3-4 more minutes, till the shrimp, is pink and cooked completely.

6. Eat and enjoy with lime slices and cilantro to eat.

4. Air Fryer Loaded Pork Burritos

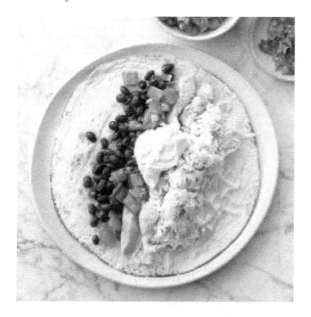

Ingredients

* ❖ Limeade concentrate thawed (3/4 cup)
* ❖ Olive oil (1 tbsp.)
* ❖ Salt (2 tsp)
* ❖ Pepper (1 1/2 tsp.)
* ❖ Boneless loin of pork sliced into thin pieces (1-1/2 lbs.)
* ❖ Seeded diced fresh tomatoes (1 cup)
* ❖ Green pepper, diced (1 small)
* ❖ Chopped onion (1 small)
* ❖ Fresh cilantro minced (1/4 cup)
* ❖ Seeded and diced jalapeno pepper (1 small)
* ❖ Juice of a lime (1 tsp.)
* ❖ Garlic powder (1/4 tsp.)
* ❖ Raw long grain of rice (1 cup)
* ❖ Monterey Jack cheese (3 cups shredded)
* ❖ 6 tortillas of flour (12 inches)
* ❖ Rinsed and drained black beans, 1 can (15 ounces)
* ❖ Whipped cream (1-1/2 cups)
* ❖ Cooking mist

Steps

1. Mix the oil, limeade, salt, and pepper in a big shallow dish; add the pork. Turn to coat; cover for at least 20 minutes, then put in the fridge.

2. Mix the peppers, green pepper, onion, lime juice, cilantro, jalapeno, garlic powder and the remaining salt and pepper for the salsa in a shallow dish.

3. Cook rice according to box instructions. Mix the remaining coriander.

4. Rinsed the pork and discarded the marinade.

Heat the fryer to 355 degrees. Place the pork in batches in a single layer on the oiled tray in the air-fryer basket, sprinkle with the cooking mist. Cook for 8-10 minutes, rotating halfway through until the pork is no longer pink.

5. Sprinkle on each tortilla with 1/3 cup cheese. Cover each with salsa, rice blend, black beans, and sour cream and with pork. Bend the sides, and the filling ends. Serve and enjoy with the leftover salsa.

5. Air Fryer Sweet and Sour Pineapple Pork

Ingredients

- ❖ Smashed unsweetened pineapple (8 ounces or 1 can)
- ❖ Vinegar (1 cup)
- ❖ Sugar (1/2 cup)
- ❖ Packed dark brown sugar (1/2 cup)
- ❖ Ketchup (1/2 cup)
- ❖ Soy sauce (2 cups)
- ❖ Mustard Dijon (1 tbsp.)
- ❖ Garlic (1 tsp.)

- ❖ 2 tenderloins of pork (3/4 pounds each)
- ❖ Salt (1/4 tsp.)
- ❖ Pepper (1/4 tsp.)
- ❖ Diced onions

Steps

1. Mix the first 8 ingredients in a broad frying pan and boiled it at a lower flame. Stir it periodically and exposed, for 15-20 minutes until thickened.

2. Preheat the air fryer at 350 °. Add salt and pepper to the pork. Put the pork in an air-fryer bowl on a greased plate. Cook for 7-8 minutes before the pork starts to brown around the edges. Mix the top of the pork with sauce. Cook until at least 146 ° C for 8-10 min. Let the pork stay before slicing for 5 minutes. Serve with the spicy sauce. Top with chopped green onions if needed.

6. Air Fryer Green Tomato BLT

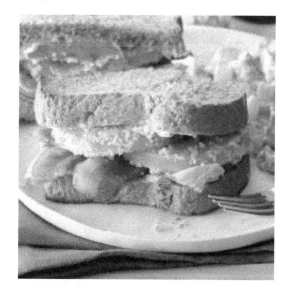

Ingredients

- ❖ Green tomatoes (10 ounces)
- ❖ Salt (1/2 tsp.)
- ❖ Pepper (1/4 tsp.)
- ❖ Large egg (1 beaten)
- ❖ Flour (1/4 cup)
- ❖ Crumbs of panko bread (1 cup)
- ❖ Cooking mist
- ❖ Mayonnaise (1/2 cup)
- ❖ Diced green onions (2)
- ❖ Fresh sliced dill (1 tsp.)
- ❖ Wheat bread slices (8 slices)
- ❖ Cooked pork strips (8 slices)
- ❖ Chopped lettuce (4 leaves)

Steps

1. Preheat the air fryer at 350 °C. Sliced each tomato crosswise in 4 pieces. Salt and pepper were added. In a different shallow container, egg, flour, and breadcrumbs were added. Drop tomato pieces in flour, shake off the residue, and then drop into the egg and eventually into the bread crumb mixture.

2. Arrange tomato slices in batches on a greased tray in the air-fryer basket in a single layer, sprinkle with cooking spray. Cook for 5-6 minutes before its golden brown.

3. Meanwhile, blend the mayonnaise, dill, and green onions. Lay each of the 4 bread slices with 2 slices of bacon, 1 leaf of lettuce and 2 pieces of tomato. Apply the mixture of mayonnaise over the leftover bread slices and serve it.

7. Air fryer roasted green beans

Ingredients

- ❖ Fresh green beans (1 lb.)
- ❖ Mushrooms (1/2 pound)
- ❖ Finely chopped onion (1 small)
- ❖ Olive oil (2 tsp.)
- ❖ Italian seasoning (1 tsp.)

❖ Salt (1/4 tsp.)

❖ Mustard (1/8 tsp.)

Steps

1. Preheat the air fryer at 375 ° Mix all the ingredients in a wide bowl.

2. Organize vegetables in air-fryer buckets on a greased plate. Cook for 10-12 minutes until just soft. Change the side and cook until browned for 10-12 minutes longer.

8. Spicy air fryer chicken breasts

Ingredients

❖ Buttermilk (2 cups)

❖ Mustard Dijon (2 tbsp.)

❖ Salt (2 tsp.)

❖ Hot pepper sauce (2 tsp.)

❖ Garlic powder (1-1/2 teaspoons)

❖ 8 chicken breast pieces (8 ounces each)

❖ Breadcrumbs (2 cups)

❖ Corn flour (1 cup)

❖ Canola oil (2 tsp.)

❖ Seasoning for poultry (1/2 teaspoon)

❖ Mustard (1/2 tsp.)

❖ Paprika (1/2 tsp.)

❖ Cayenne pepper (1/2 tsp.)

❖ Oregano (1/4 tsp.)

❖ Dry flakes of parsley (1/4 tsp.)

Steps

1. Preheat air fryer at 375 ° C. Combine the first 5 ingredients in a wide dish. Mix with the chicken and then change the coat over. Refrigerate, sealed, overnight or for 60 minutes

2. Discard sauces from the chicken. In a deep bowl, mix the remaining ingredients and swirl to blend. Marinate chicken too with the mixture (1 piece at a time) with the brush. In the air-fryer basket, place it in a single layer on a greased plate. Cook for about 25minutes before the thermometer measures 170 °, rotating halfway through cooking. Transfer all the chicken to the air fryer and cook for 3-4 minutes longer, until heated.

9. Air fryer Reuben Calzones

Ingredients

❖ Refrigerated pizza crust (13.8 ounces)

- Swiss cheese pieces (4)

- Sauerkraut (1 cup)

- Cooked corned beef (1/2 lb.)

- Thousand Island dressing for the salad

Steps

1. Preheat air fryer at 400 °C. Unroll the pizza crust on a gently floured area and press it into a 14-inch square. Slice into 4 blocks. Layer 1 diagonally over half of each piece slice of cheese and a fourth of the bratwurst and corned beef within 1/2 in an inch of edges. Fold 1 corner to the opposite corner, creating a triangle over the filling; force the edges to close with a fork. In an air-fryer basket, put two calzones in a thin layer on a greased plate.

2. Cook, 10-12 minutes, until golden brown, turning halfway through cooking. Serve with sauce and the salad.

10. Teriyaki Salmon Fillets with Broccoli

Ingredients

- Tiny cloves of broccoli (2 cups)

- Vegetable oil (2 tsp.)

- Salt and black pepper (as needed)

- Soy sauce (1 tbsp.)

- Sugar (1 tsp.)

- Vinegar (1 tsp.)

- Cornstarch (1/4 teaspoon)

- Diced ginger (1 1/2-inch)

- 2 salmon fillets (6 ounces each)

- Scallion (1 slice)

- White rice (cooked) for serving

Steps

1. Mix the broccoli in a bowl of 1 tsp of the oil. Sprinkle with the salt and pepper. At a 3.5-quart air fryer, shift the broccoli.

2. In a small bowl, mix the sugar, soy sauce, vinegar, cornstarch, and ginger. While the remaining 1 tbsp of oil spray to salmon fillets on both sides, then with the sauce. Organize the skin-side down salmon on top of the broccoli.

3. Cook at 390 degrees F till the broccoli is soft, and the salmon is baked within, depending on the thickness of the fillets 8 to 10 minutes for medium to well finish. Sprinkle with the

scallion slices, move to serve plates, and top with rice.

11. Air fryer steak with garlic herb butter

Ingredients

- ❖ Steak of sirloin (1-pound)
- ❖ Salt and black pepper
- ❖ Butter (4 tsp.)
- ❖ Parsley thinly sliced (1sp.)
- ❖ Chives (1 tbsp.)
- ❖ Garlic clove (1 clove)
- ❖ Crushed flakes of red pepper (1 tbsp.)

Steps

1. Before baking, allow the steak to stay at room temperature for 35 minutes.

2. To 405 degrees F, preheat a 3.5-quart air fryer. Season the steak with a generous grain of salt and a couple of black pepper piles on both sides. Place pieces of steak in the middle of the air fryer bowl and cook until needed, around 12 minutes for moderate-rare. Shift the steak to a cutting board and let it sit for about 10 minutes.

3. Meanwhile, in a small bowl, stir together the parsley, butter, chives, garlic and crushed red pepper until blended. Cut the steak into ¼ inch bits against the grain. Apply the garlic-herb butter to the top.

12. Air fryer fried rice with sesame sriracha sauce

Ingredients

- ❖ White cooked rice (2 cups)
- ❖ Oil (1 tbsp.)
- ❖ Sesame oil toasted (2 tsp.)
- ❖ Salt and black pepper (as needed)
- ❖ Sriracha (1 tsp.)
- ❖ Soya sauce (1 tsp.)
- ❖ Sesame seeds (1/2 tsp.)
- ❖ Big egg (1)
- ❖ Peas and carrots (1 cup)

Steps

1. In a cup, mix the vegetable oil, rice, sesame oil and 1 tbsp of water. Use salt and pepper to taste and swirl to cover the rice. Shift to a metal cake pan or foil pan for a 7-inch circular air fryer.

2. Place the pan in a 5.3-quart air fryer and cook for around 14minutes at 350 degrees F,

stirring halfway thru, until the rice is lightly baked and crunchy.

3. Meanwhile, in a shallow cup, add the sriracha, sesame seeds, soya sauce, and the remaining 1 teaspoon of sesame oil.

4. Open an air-fryer and place the rice over the egg. Cover it and cook for another 4 minutes before the egg is cooked clean. To spread the potato, open again, introduce the peas and carrots and mix into the rice. To heat the peas and carrots, close them and cookfor2 minutes more.

5. Place in dishes and drizzle with some of the sauce.

13. Air fryer Roast Chicken

Ingredients

- ❖ Nonstick spray (for frying)
- ❖ Chicken (3 to 3 1/2 pounds)
- ❖ Olive oil (1 tbsp.)
- ❖ Salt and black pepper
- ❖ New rosemary
- ❖ Garlic (8-12 cloves)
- ❖ Lemon (1/2 tsp.)

Steps

1. Preheat a 3.5-quart air fryer to 375 ° F and sprinkle nonstick frying spray on the dish.

2. Use the olive oil to smooth the exterior of the chicken.

3. 1 tsp salt and several punches of pepper are sprayed on the chicken inside and outside. Use spices, garlic, and lemon to fill the gap. Place the chicken up in the breast-side bowl, forcing it down to not contact the fryer top.

4. Roast the chicken in the thickest section of the thigh till it is crispy and gold at160 ° in 65 minutes.

14. Air Fryer Mini Swedish Meatballs

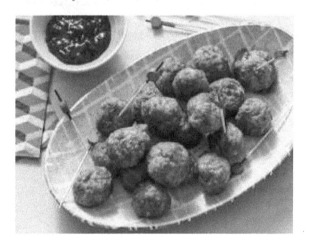

Ingredients

- ❖ White bread (2 slices)
- ❖ Milk (1/2 cup)
- ❖ Beef (8 ounces)

❖ Pork (8 ounces)

❖ Chopped Onion (¼ inches)

❖ All spices (3/4 tsp.)

❖ Egg (1 large)

❖ 1 large egg

❖ Salt and black pepper

❖ Nonstick cooking spray (for the tray)

❖ Lingonberry jam

Steps

1. For almost 6 minutes, immerse the pieces of bread in the milk and pour out the extra milk. Add the pork, onion, beef, egg, salt, spices, and pepper into the bread. Make small balls of ingredients added.

2. Spray the vegetable oil in the air fryer's basket and maintain the temperature up to 360° F. heat until the balls become golden brown and serve with the jam.

15. Air Fryer Fried Shrimp

Ingredients

❖ Cooking Spray (Non-stick)

❖ 16-20 shrimps (1 pound)

❖ Salt and black pepper

❖ Rice (½ cup)

❖ Eggs (2 oversized)

❖ Breadcrumbs for panko (1 cup)

❖ Sauce with Fiery Remoulade:

❖ Mayonnaise (1/2 cup)

❖ Diced jalapenos (2 tsp.)

❖ Mustard (2 tsp.)

❖ Ketchup (tbsp.)

❖ Sauce (1 tablespoon)

❖ Scallion (1 piece)

Steps

1. For fried shrimp: Coat the basket with spray on a 3.5-quart air fryer and put aside. With a few paper towels, press the shrimp dry, then season with a pinch of salt and a few squeezes of black pepper.

2. In a small bowl, whisk the flour with salt and a few mounds of pepper. In another small cup, whisk the eggs with a bit of salt. To a third small bowl, apply the panko. In the flour mixture, dip the shrimp, shake off any residue, then dip in the beaten eggs, dredge in the panko and transform until

finely covered. Move and repeat with the remaining shrimp to a wide plate or a rimmed baking sheet.

3. The air fryer should be preheated to 420 degrees. Working in groups, put some of the shrimp in the fryer basket in a single sheet, then gently spray with more non - stick cooking spray. Cook for about ten min until the shrimp is golden brown and cooked thru, turning halfway.

4. Besides that, stir together all the mayo, pickled jalapeños, mustard, ketchup, chili sauce and scallion in a small bowl until smooth. Serve the sauce with the fried shrimp.

16. Air Fryer Bread

Ingredients

- ❖ Unsalted butter (2 tbsp.)
- ❖ Dry yeast (1 1/2 tsp.)
- ❖ Sugar (1 1/2 tsp.)
- ❖ Salt (1 1/2 tsp.)
- ❖ Flour (2 2/3 cups)

Steps

1. Place butter in a small 6-by-3-inch pan and put it aside.

2. In a stand mixer equipped with a dough hook extension, add the butter, yeast, salt, sugar and 1 cup warm water. Add flour at a time with the mixer on a low level, waiting for each addition to be completely blended before adding more. When all the flour has been applied, knead for 8 minutes at medium pressure.

3. Move the dough to the prepared plate, cover it, and let it grow for around 60 hours before it doubles in size.

4. Connect the pan to a 3.5-quart air fryer with the dough and adjust it to 380 degrees F. Cook for around 20 minutes, till the bread is brownish and the internal temperature is 201 degrees F. In the pan, leave to cool for five min, then switch on a shelf to cool fully.

17. Air Fryer Thanksgiving Turkey

Ingredients

- ❖ Salt (1 tsp.)
- ❖ Dried thyme (1 tsp.)
- ❖ Rosemary (1 tsp.)

- ❖ Black pepper (1/2 tsp.)
- ❖ Dried sage (1/2 tsp.)
- ❖ Garlic powder (1/2 tsp.)
- ❖ Paprika (1/2 tsp.)
- ❖ Brown sugar (1/2 tsp.)
- ❖ Turkey breast with skin (approx. 2 1/2 pounds)
- ❖ Olive oil

Steps

1. In a tiny cup, blend the cinnamon, rosemary, thyme, pepper, garlic powder, sage, brown sugar and paprika together.
2. Cover the turkey breast with olive oil and brush with the dry buff mixture on both sides, meaning that it gets under the skin wherever possible. Place the turkey skin-side down in a 3.5-quart air fryer basket and roast for 20 minutes at 365 degrees F.
3. Open the air fryer gently and turn the turkey over so that it is skin-side-up. Cover the air fryer and

roast before 165 degrees F is inserted into the meat's thickest portion with an instant-read thermometer, around an extra 15 minutes. Let it cool for 10 minutes or more, then cut and serve.

18. Air Fryer Frozen Chicken Breast

Recipe ingredients

- ❖ Nonstick spray
- ❖ Frozen boneless chicken breast (about 6 ounces)
- ❖ Olive oil (1 tsp.)
- ❖ Salt and black pepper

Steps

1. Preheat a 3.5-quart air fryer to 370 degrees F and sprinkle nonstick oil on the basket.
2. Sprinkle the olive oil with the chicken breast. Sprinkle on both sides of salt and a few mounds of pepper. Place the chicken in the air fryer's basket and cook at 365 degrees F for 20 to 24 minutes.

19. Air Fryer Banana Bread

Ingredients

- ❖ Rice (½ cup)

- ❖ Wheat germ or flour (1/4 cup)

- ❖ Salt (1/2 tsp.)

- ❖ Soda for baking (1/4 teaspoon)

- ❖ Bananas (2)

- ❖ Sugar (1/2 cup)

- ❖ Oil for vegetables (1/4 cup)

- ❖ Yogurt (1/4 cup)

- ❖ Extract of pure vanilla (1/2 tsp.)

- ❖ Egg (1)

- ❖ Turbinado sugar (1 to 2 tsp.)

Steps

1. Use non - stick spray to coat on a 7-inch diameter air-fryer plate, metal cake tray or foil sheet.

2. In a medium dish, whisk together the rice, nutritional yeast, salt, and baking soda. In a separate medium cup, mash the bananas until very creamy. Cover the banana with the granulated sugar, cream, milk, vanilla and egg and whisk until smooth. Sift the dry ingredients over the moist one and fold together until just blended with a spoon. Through the prepared plate, scrape the mixture and smooth the surface. For a crunchy, soft coating, spray the top of the batter with the turbinado sugar if needed.

3. Place the pan in an air fryer and cook at 315 degrees F, rotating the pan halfway through before it comes out clean, 15 to 30 minutes, with a toothpick inserted in the center of the loaf. To cool for ten min, move the pan to a shelf. Knead the dough of the banana bread from the pan before slicing into slices to eat to let it cool entirely on the shelf.

20. Air Fryer Veggie Chip Medley

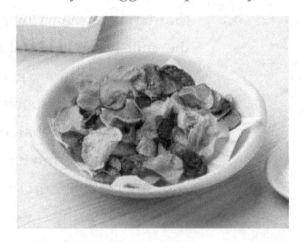

Ingredients

- ❖ Sweet potato (about 4 ounces)

- ❖ Purple potato (about 4 ounces)

- ❖ Olive oil (2 tbsp.)

- ❖ Salt and black pepper

- ❖ Red beet (about 6 ounces)

- ❖ Golden beet (about 6 ounces)

Steps

6. Cut the slices of potatoes into 1/14 inch and wash with water so that white starch comes down and then dry it.

7. After placing the potatoes into a bowl, add oil, salt, and pepper in it.

8. The air fryer is heated to a 3.5-quart air fryer at 350ºF. Place the potatoes in the layers and cook until it becomes golden and changes its side after every 8 minutes.

9. After that, place it in another bowl and mix oil, salt, red beat, and pepper till uniformly covered.

10. Add the potato chips and beet chips in a dish and sprinkle salt and mix them. Allow it to cool, and you can store it in a container.

21. Air Fryer Spareribs

Ingredients

- ❖ Salt and black pepper

- ❖ Paprika (3 tsp.)

- ❖ Pork ribs (2 1/2 to 3 pounds)

- ❖ Ketchup (2 cups)

- ❖ Vinegar (1/3 cup)

- ❖ White vinegar (1/3 cup)

- ❖ Dark brown sugar (1/3 of a cup)

- ❖ Sauce from Worcestershire (2 tsp.)

- ❖ Sweet sauce (1 or 2 tsp.)

Steps

1. In a big cup, whisk together a pinch of salt, two tbsp of pepper and 1 tsp of paprika till just mixed. Attach the ribs and swirl to cover,

squeezing each rib with the spices.

2. To 325 degrees, preheat a 3.5-quart air fryer. Move the ribs to the fryer basket and cook for around 45 minutes until the ribs are crispy and golden brown.

3. Meanwhile, in a medium saucepan, mix the vinegar, ketchup, white vinegar, Worcestershire, brown sugar, chili sauce, 2 tbsp of salt, 2 tsp of pepper, 3 cups of water and the other 2 tbsp of paprika. Cook over medium heat, constantly stirring, for around 2 minutes, until the sugar is dissolved, and the sauce is cooked through. Cover and put it over low heat.

4. Dip each one into the sauce until the ribs are fried, allowing the surplus runoff. Serve with the leftover sauce.

22. Homemade Italian meatball air fryer

Ingredients

- ❖ Ground beef (2 lb.)
- ❖ eggs (2 large)
- ❖ Breadcrumbs (1-1/4 cup)
- ❖ parsley chopped (1/4 cup)
- ❖ Dried oregano (1 tsp.)
- ❖ Parmigiano Reggiano (1/4 cup)
- ❖ Diced garlic clove (1 tiny)
- ❖ Salt and pepper

Steps

1. 1 teaspoon of light oil is squirted on a soft cloth to cover an air fryer's basket.

2. Put the meat in a broad mixing bowl with all the spices.

3. Mix all the products and with your hands together. To start the mixing phase, you may use a wooden spoon, but using your hands is the easiest way to combine it. Only mix the ingredients, so everything is well mixed.

4. Gobble up a little handful of meat and roll up to your perfect size meatball (approximately 6 mm round) in the palm of your side. Or you can use a cookie

scoop that will send you meatballs of the same amount.

5. As per the manufacturer's directions, ready the Air Fryer. I cover the basket loosely with a paper towel and sprinkle avocado oil on it.

6. Cook them until gently browned at 350 degrees for 10-13 minutes. Switch the oven over and cook for 4-5 more minutes. Place it on a tray while it's cooked.

7. To continue cooking, put them in the tomato sauce when ready.

8. Serve with your choice noodles.

23. Twice Air Fried Vegan Stuffed Idaho Potatoes

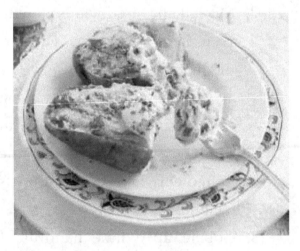

Ingredients

- ❖ Potatoes (2 big)

- ❖ Olive oil (1 to 2 tsp.)

- ❖ Vegan yogurt unsweetened (1/4 cup)

- ❖ Milk (1/4 cup)

- ❖ Nutritional yeast (2 tsp.)

- ❖ Salt (1/2 tsp.)

- ❖ Pepper (1/4 tsp.)

- ❖ Minced spinach (1 cup)

Optional Ingredients for Topping

- ❖ Vegan yogurt unsweetened (1/4 cup)

- ❖ Smoked salt and pepper

- ❖ Chopped parsley chives

Steps

1. On both sides, spray each potato with oil.

2. Preheat your air fryer to 380 °. Add the potatoes to your air-fryer basket until it's warmed.

3. Adjust the cooking time to 40 minutes, change the potatoes over when the time is finished, and steam for 30 more minutes.

4. Note: You may need to cook an extra 15 - 20 minutes, based on your potatoes' size.

5. Let the potatoes cool so that without burning yourself, you may hold them.

6. Lengthwise, split each potato in half and carefully scoop out the center of the potato, leaving enough to create a stable potato skin shell and a thin layer of the white part.

7. Smoothly mash the scooped potato, organic tofu, honey, natural yeast, salt, and pepper.

8. Mix in the diced spinach, and the mixture can cover the potato shells.

9. Heat for 5 minutes at 325 ° (or near as the air fryer can be mounted to that).

10. Serve and enjoy with the topping of your selection.

24. Air Fryer Beef Empanadas

Ingredients

❖ 8 Goya empanada discs

❖ Picadillo (1 cup)

❖ Egg (1 white)

❖ Water (1 tsp.)

Steps

1. For 8 minutes, preheat the air fryer to 325F. With cooking oil, cover the basket gently.

2. Place 2 teaspoons of picadillo in the middle of each disc. Fold it in half and seal the edges with a fork. With the leftover dough, repeat.

3. Add water onto the egg whites, then rub the edges of the empanadas.

4. Cook two or three in an air fryer for 8 mins at a time, until it's golden. Turn off the heat and repeat for the empanadas left.

25. Healthy Fish Finger Sandwich & Optimum Healthy Air Fry

Ingredients

❖ Cod fillets (4 tinies)

❖ Salt and pepper

❖ Flour (2 tbsp.)

❖ Dry breadcrumbs (40 g)

❖ Oil spray

❖ Frozen peas (250 g)

❖ Crème Fraiche (1 tbsp.)

- ❖ Capers (10–12)
- ❖ Lemon juice
- ❖ Bread rolls (4)

Steps

1. Pre-heat the Healthy Fry Ultimate Air Fryer.
2. Take each of the fillets of cod, add salt and pepper, and sprinkle the flour gently. Then roll in the breadcrumbs fast. The aim is to have a thin covering of the fish rather than a dense film of breadcrumbs. Repeat with each fillet of cod.
3. To the edge of the fryer basket, apply a pair of sprays of oil mist. Put the fillets of cod on top and cook for 15 mins on the fish setting (200c).
4. Cook the peas in boiling water for a few minutes on the burner or in the oven while the fish is frying. Drain, then apply the creme fraiche, capers, and lemon juice to a mixer to taste. Blitz once mixed.
5. Remove it from the Healthy Fry Air Fryer until the fish has cooked and start layering the toast, fish, and pea puree with your sandwich. Lettuce, tartar sauce and all other of your favorite toppings may also be included.

26. Quinoa Burgers – Air fryer

Ingredients

- ❖ Crimson (1 cup)
- ❖ Water (11/2 cups)
- ❖ Salt (1 tsp.)
- ❖ Black pepper
- ❖ Rolled oats (11/2 cups)
- ❖ Eggs (3)
- ❖ White onion (1/4 cup)
- ❖ Feta cheese crumbled (1/2 cup)
- ❖ Fresh chives chopped (1/4 cup)
- ❖ Salt and black pepper
- ❖ Palm oil
- ❖ Hamburgers (4 whole-wheat buns)
- ❖ Arugulas (4)
- ❖ Sliced tomato (4 slices)

Yogurt dill sauce with cucumber

- ❖ Diced cucumber (1 cup)

- ❖ Greek yogurt (1 cup)

- ❖ Lemon extract (2 tbsp.)

- ❖ Salt (1/4 tsp)

- ❖ Black pepper

- ❖ Minced fresh dill (1 tbsp.)

- ❖ Olive oil (1 tbsp.)

Steps

1. Make the quinoa: In a saucepan, clean the quinoa in cool water and stir it with your hand until some dried husks hit the top. Drain as much as you can the quinoa and then place the saucepan on the burner. Switch the heat to medium-high and on the stovetop, dry the quinoa, shake the pan periodically until the quinoa shifts quickly, and you can hear the seeds shifting in the pan. Incorporate the water, salt, and pepper. Bring the mixture to a boil and then to a moderate or medium-low heat reduction. You just need to see a pair of bubbles, not a boil. Cover it with a lid, keep it askew (or only place the lid on the pot if you have spouts) and boil for 20 minutes. Switch off the fire and use a fork to fluff the quinoa. If the pot's bottom has some liquid remaining, put it back on the flame for another 3 minutes or so. On a sheet plate, spread the cooked quinoa out to cool.

2. In a wide cup, mix the room temperature quinoa with oats, eggs, onion, cheese, and spices. Season with pepper and salt and blend properly. Shape 4 patties into the mixture. To get the mixture the correct consistency for creating patties, apply a little water or a couple more rolled oats.

3. Spray all edges of the patties appropriately with oil and pass them in

one sheet to the air fryer basket (depending on the air fryer's capacity, you may have to cook these burgers in batches). For 10 minutes, air-fry each batch at 400oF, flipping the burgers around halfway through the heating time.

4. Make the cucumber yogurt dill sauce when the burgers are frying, combining all the ingredients in a cup.

5. Make your burger with arugula, onion, and cucumber yogurt dill sauce on the full-wheat hamburger buns.

27. Air Fryer Pepperoni Pizza

Ingredients

- ❖ Pita wheat (1)

- ❖ Marinara or pizza sauce (2 tbsp.)

- ❖ sliced mozzarella cheese (1/8th cup)

- ❖ Cheddar cheese (1/8th cup)

- ❖ Mozzarella cheese (1/4th cup)

- ❖ Pepperoni slices (8)

- ❖ Spray with olive oil

- ❖ Chopped parsley (1 tbsp.)

Steps

1. On top of the pita bread, dribble the sauce, then load the pepperoni and shredded cheese on top.

2. Using olive oil spray to cover the surface of the pizza.

3. Place it at 400 ° in the Air Fryer for 10 min. At the 6-7-minute point, check-in on the pizza and make sure it does not overcook.

4. Remove the Air Fryer pizza.

Before serving Instructions

1. Spray one side of the pita bread with olive oil for a crisper crust. Place it at 400 ° in the Air Fryer for four minutes. It will make it easier to crisp the pita on one edge.

2. Remove the Air Fryer pita bread. Shift the pita over to the less crisp side. It should have been the hand of the Air Fryer that was face-down.

3. Drizzle the sauce all over and finish it with the pepperoni and sliced cheese.

4. Till the cheese has melted, put the pizza back in the Air Fryer for 3-4 minutes. To achieve the perfect texture, you can need to allow the pizza to cook for an extra couple of minutes.

5. Remove the Air Fryer pizza. I've been using a spoon. Serve and enjoy.

28. Crispy air fryer Tofu with sticky orange sauce

Ingredients

- ❖ Extra-firm tofu (1 pound)
- ❖ Tamari (1 tbsp.)
- ❖ Cornstarch (1 Tbsp.)

For the sauce

- ❖ Orange zest (1 tsp.)
- ❖ Orange juice (1/3 cup)
- ❖ Water (1/2 cup)
- ❖ Cornstarch (2 tsp.)
- ❖ Smashed flakes of red pepper (1/4 tsp.)
- ❖ Minced ginger (1 tsp.)
- ❖ Minced garlic (1 tsp.)
- ❖ maple syrup (1 spoon)

Steps

1. Slice the cubed tofu.

2. Insert a quart-size plastic storage bag with the tofu cubes. Add the tamari to the container and close it. Shake the bag until the tamari is covered with all the tofu.

3. Cover the container with a tablespoon of cornflower. Shake again until it is covered with the tofu. Put aside the tofu for at least 15 minutes to marinate.

4. Meanwhile, mix a tiny bowl of all the sauce ingredients and combine with a spoon.

5. Place the tofu in a single layer in an air fryer.

6. Cook the tofu for 10 minutes at 390 degrees, shaking after 5 min.

7. After the batches of tofu have been prepared, apply everything to a skillet over medium-high heat. Offer a swirl to the sauce and spill it over the tofu. Stir the sauce and

tofu until the sauce is thickened and the tofu is cooked.

8. Serve immediately with, if needed, rice and steamed vegetables.

29. Bourbon Bacon Burger

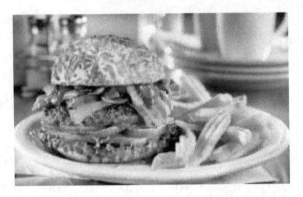

Ingredients

❖ Whiskey (1 tbsp.)

❖ Brown sugar (2 tbsp.)

❖ Maple bacon strips sliced in half (3)

❖ Ground beef 80% (3/4 pound)

❖ Minced onion (1 tbsp.)

❖ BBQ sauce (2 tsp.)

❖ Salt (1/2 tsp.)

❖ Black pepper

❖ Colby Jack or Monterey Jack cheese (2 slices)

❖ Kaiser rolls (2)

❖ Tomato and lettuce for serving

Zesty Sauce for Burger

❖ BBQ sauce (2 tsp.)

❖ Mayonnaise (2 tsp.)

❖ Paprika field (1/4 tsp.)

❖ Black pepper

Steps

1. Heat the air fryer at 390ºF and add a little water into the tray at the bottom of the air fryer. (This would help to stop burning and smoking the grease that drips through the bottom drawer.)

2. In a shallow cup, mix the whiskey with the brown sugar. In the air-fryer bowl, put the bacon strips and rub them with the brown sugar combination. Air-fry it for four hours at 390ºF. Rub with more brown sugar, turn the bacon over and air-fry at 390ºF for an extra four minutes before crispy.

3. Make the burger patties when the bacon is frying. In a large bowl, combine the ground beef, BBQ sauce, cabbage, pepper, and salt. Mix your hands thoroughly

and form the beef into 2 buns.

4. Depending on how you want your burger fried (fifteen min for rare to medium-rare), move the burger patties to the air fryer basket and fry the burgers at 370°F for 20 minutes. Halfway into the cooking process, turn the burgers over.

5. Mix the mayonnaise, BBQ sauce, black pepper, and paprika according to taste in a bowl to produce the burger sauce.

6. Cover each patty with a slice of Colby Jack cheese and air-fry for an extra minute until the burgers are fried to your taste, only to melt the cheese. Sprinkle the sauce on the rolls, put the burgers on these rolls, cover with the lettuce, bourbon bacon, and tomato and enjoy.

30. Leftover Greek Spanakopita Pie in The Air Fryer

Ingredients

- ❖ Leftover from Turkey Shredded Brown Meat
- ❖ Pastry
- ❖ Eggs (2 Large)
- ❖ 1 Tiny Egg (brushing pastries)
- ❖ Spinach (200 g)
- ❖ Onion (1 Large)
- ❖ Eggs (2 Large)
- ❖ Cream Cheese (250 g)
- ❖ Feta Cheese (100 g)
- ❖ Basil (1 Tsp.)
- ❖ Oregano (1 Tbsp.)
- ❖ Thyme (1 Tbsp.)
- ❖ Salt & Pepper

Steps

1. Let the remaining vegetables out of the refrigerator and season with salt and pepper properly.

2. Within a tea towel, put your veggies, and drop out any extra liquid. Put them with your spices and your feta cheese in a mixing dish.

3. Mix the egg and soft cheese until it got a beautiful fluffy combination.

4. Place and apply the mixture to a dish of filo pastry so that it is 3⁄4 complete. Cover most of the pastry and

sprinkle it with the beaten egg.

5. Air fry on 180c for about 20 minutes.

31. Tandoori chicken

Ingredients

- ❖ Chicken with Thighs (4 Legs)

Steps for the first margination

- ❖ Salt (1 Tsp.)
- ❖ Lemon Extract (2 tsp)
- ❖ Ginger Garlic Paste (2 tsp)
- ❖ Red Chili Powder (1 tsp)

For the second margination

- ❖ Curd (2 tbsp.)
- ❖ Ginger Garlic (1 tsp.)
- ❖ Red Chili Powder (1 tsp.)
- ❖ Black Pepper Powder (1/2 tsp.)
- ❖ Turmeric Powder (1/2 Tsp.)
- ❖ Powder of Cumin (1/2 Tsp.)
- ❖ Powdered coriander (1 tsp.)
- ❖ Mustard oil (2 tbsp.)
- ❖ Lemon Juice
- ❖ Cream (2 tsp.)

Steps

1. Wash the chicken and use a sharp knife to cut 3-4 tiny holes on every slice.
2. For the first marinade, mix the ingredients and add it gently on the chicken legs.
3. Cover the pan and allow for 5-6 hours to refrigerate.
4. In a dish, apply the ingredients for the second marinade and cover the chicken.
5. Cover and refrigerate the bowl for an extra 4-5 hours.
6. Preheat the oven to 178 degrees c.
7. Place the dripping plate on the bottom half of the air fryer oven.
8. Set a rack of wire over the dripping tray.
9. Organize the chicken for 20 minutes on a wire rack and barbecue.
10. Switch the legs of the chicken and grill for 15-20 minutes again, until they are cooked.
11. When grilling, baste the chicken with butter.
12. Remove and clean from the air fryer oven.
13. Serve and enjoy with lemons.

32. Air Fryer Chicken Nuggets

Ingredients

- ❖ Skinless chicken (1 boneless breast)
- ❖ Salt (1/4 tsp.)
- ❖ Black pepper (1/8 tsp.)
- ❖ Melted unsalted butter (1/2 cup)
- ❖ Breadcrumbs (1/2 cup)
- ❖ Grated parmesan (2 tsp.)

Steps

1. Preheat the air-fryer for 4 min. to 395 degrees.
2. Cut some chicken breast fat, slice into thick 1 1/2-inch pieces, then cut into 2 to 3 nuggets each. Mix the salt and pepper with the chicken bits.
3. In a small bowl, put the melted butter and the breadcrumbs (with parmesan, if used) in another small bowl.
4. Dip each chicken piece in butter, then apply some breadcrumbs.
5. Put a single layer in the basket of the air fryer. You can need to bake in 2 phases or more, based on your air fryer's size.
6. Set the timer for 8 minutes.
7. When done, verify whether the chicken nuggets have an internal temperature of at least 165 °F. Remove nuggets with chopsticks from the basket and cool on a pan.

33. Air Fryer Ranch Chicken Tenders

Ingredients

- ❖ Eight chicken tenders
- ❖ Spray canola

For Dredge

- ❖ Breadcrumbs (1 cup)
- ❖ Egg (1)
- ❖ Water (2 tbsp.)

For the Seasoning of Ranch Chicken

- ❖ Salt (1/2 tsp.)
- ❖ Black pepper (1/4 tsp.)
- ❖ Garlic powder (1/2 tsp.)
- ❖ Onion powder (1/2 tsp.)
- ❖ Paprika (1/4 tsp.)
- ❖ Parsley (1 tsp.)

Steps

1. Make the Air Fryer heat it. Heat an air fryer for five min by setting it to 375 ° F. Enable it to run about in the basket without any food.

2. Put up a station for dredging. In a small dish, mix the water and egg. In another shallow bowl, mix in the panko breadcrumbs.

3. Prepare the Spice for the Ranch. Combine all the spices for the ranch in a tiny bowl.

4. For the Chicken sauce, sprinkle the ranch spice with the chicken tenders, rotating to cover all ends.

5. In the egg wash, dip the chicken tenders and then press them onto the panko. Switch all sides to coat.

6. Load the basket for the fryer. In the fry basket, bring the breaded tenders in. With the remaining bids, repeat. In batches, you may need to fry.

7. Into the Power Air Fryer, place the Fry Basket. Spray a light coat of non-fat cooking spray of canola oil over the panko. Click the M. Scroll button down to the (415 degrees F) the Control Button is pushed. At 415 degrees, change the cooking time to 12 minutes. Flip the tenders over, halfway through frying, to brown the other hand. The tenders are rendered when 165 degrees F in the middle of the fattest portion of the tender, the meat is no longer pink, and the juices flow pure.

34. Air fryer Beef

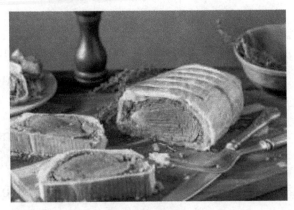

Ingredients

- ❖ Air fryer
- ❖ Grill Pan Air fryer
- ❖ Knife
- ❖ Cling Film
- ❖ Chicken Liver Pate Homemade
- ❖ Homemade Pastry for Short crust
- ❖ Beef Fillet
- ❖ Egg (1 Medium)
- ❖ Salt and Pepper

Steps

1. Take your piece of beef, make it a clean one, cut some noticeable fat, sprinkle with salt and pepper, then seal it with film sticking and put it for an hr. in the fridge.
2. Make chicken liver pate and homemade buttercream pastry with your batch.
3. To further keep it moist for wrapping, spread out the short crust pastry and use a pastry brush with beaten egg all over the sides.
4. Then put a thin layer of the homemade pate within the outer egg line, and you'll no more see the white sausage.

5. Remove the plastic wrap from the meat and place the meat on top of the pate in the core and push it down a bit.
6. Seal the meat and the pate with the pastry around it.
7. Rate the pastry top enough that there is an opportunity for the meat to flourish.
8. Place the Air fryer on the Air fryer Grill Pan and cook at 165 °c/325°F for 30 minutes.
9. Leave for a few minutes to relax, slice, and serve with roast potatoes.

35. Air Fryer Falafel

Ingredients

- ❖ Chickpeas (15.5 ounces)
- ❖ Onion (1 tiny)
- ❖ Garlic cloves (3)
- ❖ Parsley (1/3 cup)
- ❖ Cilantro (1/3 cup)
- ❖ Scallions (1/3 cup)
- ❖ Cumin (1 tsp.)
- ❖ Salt (1/2 tsp.)
- ❖ Crushed flakes of red pepper (1/8 tsp.)

- ❖ Powder for baking (1 teaspoon)
- ❖ Flour (4 tsp.)
- ❖ Olive oil

Steps

1. On paper towels, rinse the chickpeas.
2. In the bowl of a food processor equipped with a steel blade, placed the onions and garlic. Add the flakes of parsley, scallions, coriander, cumin, garlic, and red pepper.
3. Process for 30-60 seconds until mixed, then insert the chickpeas and pulse 3-4 times until mixed but not pureed.
4. Spray with baking powder and flour, mix with a spatula on the dish's sides, and pulse 2 or 3 times.
5. Transfer to a bowl and cool, covered, for 3 to 4 hours.
6. If it is too sticky, mix some flour to your fingers and your cutting board to form the falafel mixture into 12 balls.
7. Preheat the 352-degree F Air Fryer.

8. Sprinkle the falafel with oil. Cook in batches for 14 min until golden brown, turning midway thru.

36. Air Fryer Bacon Burger Bites

Ingredients

- ❖ Cattle (2 lbs.)
- ❖ Raw bacon (4 oz.)
- ❖ Mustard (2 tsp.)
- ❖ Salt (1/2 tsp.)
- ❖ Powder of onion (1/2 tsp)
- ❖ Black pepper (1/4 tsp.)
- ❖ Butter lettuce (1)
- ❖ Tomatoes (30)
- ❖ Jalapeño (30 thin slices)
- ❖ Slices of dill pickle (30 slices)
- ❖ Ketchup, mayo, and yellow mustard (for frying)

Steps

5. Gently blend the meat, pork, mustard, cinnamon, onion powder and pepper together with your fingers.
6. Shaped into 30 balls (tennis ball size).
7. Preheat the 400F Air Fryer. Burgers are arranged in a

single layer by operating in batches.

8. Cook, flipping halfway to your target dosage, for mild, 10 to 15 minutes.

9. Put any burger with lettuce, pickles and tomatoes on a skewer and serve with sauces.

37. Air Fryer Bacon Wrapped Scallops

Ingredients

- ❖ Sea scallops (16 big)
- ❖ Centrally sliced bacon (8 slices)
- ❖ 16 toothpicks
- ❖ Olive oil
- ❖ Black pepper

Steps

1. Preheat an air fryer for three minutes to 402-degree F.

2. To partly cook for three minutes, put the bacon in the air fryer, turning halfway. Remove and leave to cool on a paper towel.

3. On the scallops, eliminate any side muscles. It is necessary to pat the scallops dry with paper towels to eliminate all moisture.

4. Each scallop is wrapped in a bacon slice and fixed with a toothpick.

5. Season lightly with black pepper and brush with olive oil over the scallops.

6. Arrange scallops in the air fryer in a single layer, roast, switch halfway in batches for 8 minutes before the scallop is soft and translucent, and pork is fried through.

38. Air Fryer Chicken Milanese With Arugula

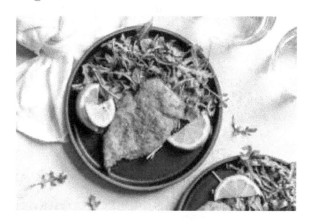

Ingredients

- ❖ Boneless, skinless breasts of chicken (16 oz. Total)
- ❖ Salt (3/4 tsp.)
- ❖ Black pepper
- ❖ (wheat or gluten-free) seasoned whole wheat breadcrumbs (1/2 cup)
- ❖ Parmesan cheese (2 tsp.)
- ❖ Egg (1)
- ❖ Spray with olive oil

- ❖ Arugula cups (6 infants)

- ❖ 3 lemons (sliced into wedges)

Steps

1. Slice the chicken into 4 fillets, put the fillets between 2 sheets of plastic wrap or paper towel and pound out to a thick 1/2-inch.

2. Spray salt and pepper on both ends.

3. Beat the egg and 1 tsp of water together in a shallow bowl.

4. In a small dish, mix the breadcrumbs with the parmesan cheese.

5. Dip the chicken, then the breadcrumb mixture into the egg. Place it on a working surface and spray olive oil on both sides.

6. Preheat the fryer to 402-degree F for air.

7. Switch to the air fryer basket in batches and cook for 8 minutes, turning halfway to golden and cooked thru.

8. With 1½ cups of arugula, serve the chicken and cover with a generous quantity of lemon juice.

39. Air Fryer Asian Glazed Boneless Chicken Thighs

Ingredients

- ❖ 8 boneless chicken thighs (32 ounces)

- ❖ Sodium soy sauce (1/4 cup)

- ❖ Balsamic vinegar (2 1/2 tsp.)

- ❖ Honey (1 tablespoon)

- ❖ Garlic (3 cloves)

- ❖ Sriracha sauce (1 tsp.)

- ❖ Freshly grated ginger (1 tsp.)

- ❖ 1 scallion (sliced green just for garnish)

Steps

1. Combine the balsamic wine, soy sauce, sugar, garlic, sriracha and ginger in a small bowl and blend well.

2. Pour half (1/4 cup) of the marinade into a large chicken dish, cover all the meat, and marinate for at least two hours or if overnight.

3. For later, save the leftover sauce.

4. Preheat the fryer to 400-degree F for air.

5. From the marinade, Take the chicken and shift it to the basket of the air fryer.

6. Cook in batches for 15 min, rotating halfway in the middle before cooked through.

7. Meanwhile, in a small pot, put the remaining sauce and simmer over medium-low heat until slightly reduced and thickened, for around 2 minutes.

8. To eat, over the chicken, drizzle the sauce and finish with scallions.

40. Air Fryer Cajun Shrimp Dinner

Ingredients

- ❖ Cajun or Creole (1 tbsp.)
- ❖ 24 extra jumbo shrimps (1 pound)
- ❖ 6 ounces of Turkey
- ❖ Zucchini (1 medium)
- ❖ Yellow medium squash (8 ounces)
- ❖ Red bell pepper (1 big)
- ❖ Salt (1/4 tsp.)
- ❖ Olive oil (2 tsp.)

Steps

1. Mix the Cajun seasoning and shrimp in a wide bowl, swirl to cover.

2. Add the bacon, zucchini, squash, salt, and bell peppers and mix with the oil.

3. Preheat the 402-degree F Air Fryer.

4. Shift the shrimp and vegetables to the air-fryer basket in two rounds (for smaller baskets) and cook for 10 min, rotating the basket 3 to 4 times.

5. Put back, repeat with the shrimp and vegetables left.

6. Return the first batch to the air fryer when all batches are cooked and cook for 1 minute.

41. Easy Garlic Knots

Ingredients

- ❖ Spray with olive oil
- ❖ White whole wheat flour (1 cup)
- ❖ Salt (3/4 tsp.)
- ❖ Baking powder (2 tbsp.)
- ❖ Greek Yogurt (1 cup)
- ❖ Butter (2 tbsp.)
- ❖ Garlic (3 cloves)

❖ Grated parmesan cheese (1 tbsp.)

❖ Parsley (1 tbsp.)

Steps

1. Preheat the oven to 400 degrees F. With a silicone lining or Silpat cover a studded baking sheet.

2. Mix the rice, baking powder and salt in a big bowl and stir well. Mix the yogurt, then blend when incorporated with a spoon. Using your dried hands then and knead about fifteen times. You should apply a little extra flour if it is too messy. Roll it into a ball.

3. Divide the dough into 8 equal parts, then roll each slice, about Nine inches long, into worm-like pieces.

4. Form each breadstick into a "knot-like" ball; put on the baking tray that has been prepared.

5. Bake for around 20 mins in the top third of the oven until golden. Let it cool for five min.

6. Meanwhile, melt the butter in a medium, nonstick skillet, add the garlic and simmer for 2 minutes until golden.

7. With the melting butter and garlic, throw the knots in the pan or use a brush to coat the garlic's knots.

8. Offer them another mist of olive oil if the knots are too dry. Using parmesan cheese and sliced parsley to scatter.

42. Tostones (Twice air-fried plantains)

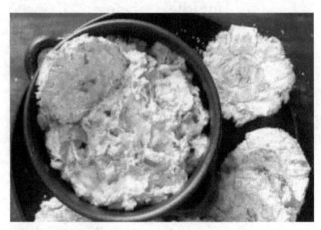

Ingredients

❖ Green plantain (6 oz.)

❖ Spray olive oil

❖ Water (1 cup)

❖ Salt (1 tsp.)

❖ Garlic (3/4 tsp.)

Steps

1. Break the plantain into pieces of 1 inch, Eight total.

2. Mix the water with salt and garlic powder in a shallow cup.

3. Preheat the fryer to 400-degree F for air.

4. If you're able to spray the plantain with olive oil and cook for six minutes, you

will need to do this in two rounds.

5. Remove from the air fryer and measuring cup for flattening when they are sweet.

6. Soak them and put them aside in seasoned water.

7. Preheat the air fryer again to 400degree F and cook five minutes on either side in rounds, spraying olive oil on both sides of the plantains.

8. Send them another spritz of oil when finished and season with salt. Eat straight away.

43. Stuffed Bagel Balls

Ingredients

- ❖ Rice (1 cup)

- ❖ Baking powder (2 tsp.)

- ❖ Salt (3/4 tsp.)

- ❖ Yogurt (1 cup)

- ❖ Fat cream cheese box, sliced into 8 cubes (4 tsp., 4 ounces)

- ❖ 1 egg white (beaten)

Optional toppings: all bagel seasoning, sesame seeds, poppy seeds, flakes of dried garlic, dried onion flakes.

Steps

1. To prevent sticking, spray the basket.

2. Preheat the 320-degree F Air Fryer. Move to non-overcrowded batches and bake for 9 to 10 minutes or until golden.

3. No reason to take turns. Before consuming, let it cool for at least ten

44. Za'atar lamb chops

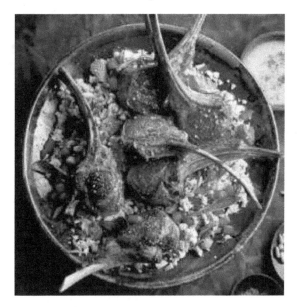

Ingredients

- ❖ 8 lamb loin chops trimmed (each bone-in is around 3.5 oz.))

- ❖ crushed garlic (3 cloves)

- ❖ Extra-virgin olive oil (1 tsp.)

- ❖ Lemon (½ tsp.)

- ❖ Salt (1 ¼ tsp.)

- ❖ za'atar's (1 tbsp.)

❖ Ground pepper

Steps

1. Use oil and garlic to rub the lamb chops.
2. On both ends, pinch the lemon and sprinkle with salt, zaatar, and black pepper.
3. Preheat the fryer to 402-degree F for air. Cook to the desired taste, around four to five minutes on either side, in batches in an even sheet.
4. My pieces had 1 ½ -2 oz. of raw meat on each bone, based on nutritional facts

45. Air Fryer Meatballs

Ingredients

❖ Ground leaf 16 ounces

❖ Ground pork 4 ounces

❖ Italian seasoning 1 teaspoon

❖ Salt ½ teaspoon

❖ Garlic 2 cloves

❖ Parmesan cheese ½ cup

❖ Egg 1

❖ Italian seasoned breadcrumbs 1/3 cup

Steps

1. Heat an air fryer at 350-degree F.

2. Mix all the ingredients in a big bowl and make 16 sized meatballs using an ice cream scoop.
3. Put ½ of the meatballs in the air fryer and heat up for 8 mins. Move the bowl and cook for another 2 mins. Switch it to another tray and repeat for other meatballs the same procedure.

46. Air Fryer Salmon Patties

Ingredients

❖ Mayonnaise ½ cup

❖ Minced garlic 1 teaspoon

❖ Lemon ½ teaspoon

❖ Cajun seasoning 2 pinches

Patties

❖ Salmon 12 ounces

❖ Fresh chives 1 tablespoon

❖ Dried parsley 1 teaspoon

❖ Salt ½ teaspoon

❖ Minced garlic ½ teaspoon

❖ Flour 1 tablespoon

❖ Cooking spray

❖ Lemon 1

Steps

1. In a small cup, mix the garlic, mayonnaise, Cajun

seasoning, and lemon juice and dip the sauce in the fridge until desired.

2. In a medium dish, add the chives, salmon, garlic, parsley, and salt and blend well. Remove the flour and blend well. Divide into four equal parts: form into patties.

3. Heat the air-fryer to 175 degrees C. Break the lemon into four slices.

4. Put lemon slices in the bottom of the air fryer's bowl and cover them with salmon patties. Sprinkle the patties loosely with cooking spray.

5. Put the bowl in the fryer that is preheated and lower the temperature to 135 degrees C.

6. In the air fryer, cook before a thermometer inserted into the middle of a patty reads 10 to 15 minutes, 145 degrees F (63 degrees C). Serve with the sauce.

47. Air Fryer Salmon

Ingredients

❖ Salmon fillets 2

❖ Salt and black pepper to taste

❖ Olive oil 2 teaspoon

❖ Whole grain mustard 2 tablespoon

❖ Brown sugar 1 tablespoon

❖ Minced garlic 1 clove

❖ Thyme leaves ½ teaspoon

Steps

1. Powder the salmon with pepper and salt all over. Whisk the mustard, oil, sugar, thyme, and garlic together in a tiny dish. Spread the salmon on the surface.

2. Organize a bowl of salmon in an air fryer. Set the air fryer to 400 degrees, then cook for 9-10 minutes.

48. Crispy Parmesan Crusted Chicken Breasts

Ingredients

❖ Cooking spray

❖ Panko breadcrumbs ½ cup

❖ Parmesan cheese ⅓ cup

❖ Paprika ¼ teaspoon

❖ Salt ¼ teaspoon

❖ Ground black pepper ¼ teaspoon

❖ Melted butter 3 tablespoons

❖ White wine 2 teaspoons

❖ Dijon mustard 1 teaspoon

❖ 1 clove garlic

Steps

1. Heat the air fryer oven to 200 degrees C. Line an aluminum foil baking sheet and rub with a cooking spray.

2. In a small dish, whisk together the parmesan cheese, breadcrumbs, paprika, salt, and black pepper. In another cup, stir the sugar, white wine, garlic, and mustard together.

3. Dip half of each chicken breast into a melted butter mixture; push to cover uniformly in a bread crumb mixture. Position a single layer of breaded chicken on the prepared baking sheet. Pat the chicken breasts with any remaining bread crumb mixture.

4. In the preheated oven, bake the chicken until the middle is no longer pink and the juices run free for about 20 minutes.

Chapter 7: Desserts

1. Air-Fryer Peppermint Lava Cakes

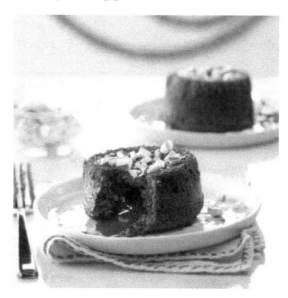

Ingredients

- ❖ Chocolate chips 2/3 cup
- ❖ Butter ½ cup
- ❖ Sugar 1 cup
- ❖ Eggs 2 large
- ❖ Egg yolks 2 large
- ❖ Peppermint extract 1 teaspoon
- ❖ Flour 6 tablespoons

Steps

1. Heat up at 375 ° air fryer. Melt the butter and chocolate chips for 30 seconds in a microwave-proof bowl; stir unless smooth. Whisk the egg yolks, butter and extract into the confectionery when combined. Pull the flour in.

2. Four 4-oz appropriately flour and grease. The ramekins; fill the ramekins with the batter. Don't overfill them. In the air-fryer basket, put the ramekins on the tray; cook unless a thermometer reaches 160 ° and the edges of the cakes are fixed, 10-12 minutes. Should not overcook anymore.

3. Delete from the basket; stop to stand for five minutes. To remove the cake, gently loop a knife multiple times across the sides of ramekins, invert on dessert bowls. Sprinkle the candies with smashed ones. Immediately serve.

2. Air-Fryer Chocolate Chip Oatmeal Cookies

Ingredients

- ❖ Butter 1 cup
- ❖ Sugar ¾ cup
- ❖ Brown sugar ¾ cup
- ❖ Eggs 2 large
- ❖ Vanilla extract 1 teaspoon
- ❖ Oats 3 cup
- ❖ Flour 1-1/2 cup
- ❖ Vanilla pudding 1 package
- ❖ Baking soda 1 teaspoon
- ❖ Salt 1 teaspoon

❖ Chocolate chips 2 cups

❖ Nuts 1 cup

Steps

1. Heat the fryer to 325 °. Sugar and cream butter in a big tub, till smooth, for 6-8 minutes. Whisk in the vanilla and chickens. Whisk the wheat, dry pudding mixture, rice, salt, and baking soda. In another bowl, progressively whisk into the fluffy mixture. Stir in the almonds and chocolate chips.

2. Fall into baking sheets with tablespoonfuls of dough; flatten significantly. For batches, bring 1 inch in the air-fryer basket, and on the greased sheet. For 8-10 minutes, cook till lightly browned. Attach to cool wire tables.

3. Air Fryer Apple Pies

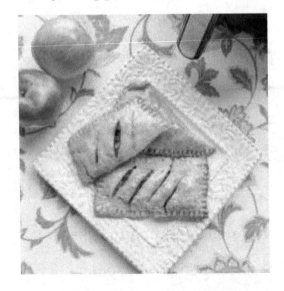

Ingredients

❖ Butter 4 tablespoon

❖ Brown sugar 6 tablespoon

❖ Cinnamon 1 teaspoon

❖ Granny Smith apples 2 medium size

❖ Cornstarch 1 teaspoon

❖ Ice water 2 teaspoons

❖ Pastry ½ package

❖ Cooking spray

❖ Grapeseed oil ½ tablespoon

❖ Powdered sugar ¼ cup

❖ Milk 1 teaspoon

Steps

1. In a non-stick skillet, combine the butter, sugar, apples, and cinnamon.

2. Cook until the apples have softened, around 5 minutes, over medium heat.

3. In cool water, extract the cornstarch. Stir in the apple mixture and boil for around 1 minute before the sauce thickens. Remove the apple pie from the heat and put aside to cool while the crust is being made.

4. On a finely floured board, unroll the pie crust and roll out gently to smooth the pastry's board. Break

the dough into tiny enough rectangles such that 2 will work at one time in your air fryer. Repeat with the leftover crust until you have 8 fair rectangles and, if necessary, re-roll any of the dough scraps.

5. Wet 4 rectangular outer edges with water and put some apple filling around 1/2-inch from the edges in the middle. The remaining four rectangles are carried out, such that they are marginally wider than the filled ones. On top of the filling, position these rectangles; tighten the sides with a fork to cover. Break the tops of the pies through 4 narrow slits.

6. Spray with cooking spray on the bowl of an air fryer. Brush the 2-pie tops with grapeseed oil and use a spatula to move the pies to the air fryer bowl.

7. Place the basket inside and adjust the temperature to 195 degrees C (385 degrees F). Bake for approximately 8 minutes, until golden brown. Remove the pies and repeat with 2 pies remaining in the basket.

8. In a small bowl, mix the powdered sugar and milk. Brush the glaze and allow it to dry on warm pies. Serve hot pies.

4. Air Fryer Oreos

Ingredients

- ❖ Pancake ½ cup
- ❖ Water 1/3 cup
- ❖ Cooking spray
- ❖ Chocolate cookies 9
- ❖ Sugar 1 tablespoon

Steps

1. Mix the combination of pancakes and water till it's blended.

2. Line a bowl of air fryers of parchment sheets. In the pancake combination, dip each cookie and put it in the bowl. Make sure they don't hit them; if possible, cook in batches.

3. Heat up to 400 degrees F for the air fryer. Add the bowl and cook for 5-6minutes; switch and cook 2 to 3 more minutes till lightly browned. Sprinkle of sugar from confectioners.

5. Air Fryer Roasted Bananas

Ingredients

- ❖ 1/8-inch sliced banana
- ❖ Cooking spray

Steps

1. Heat the 375 degrees F of an air fryer.
2. Place slices of banana in the basket to ensure they do not touch; if appropriate, cook in batches. Mist the slices of the banana with avocado oil.
3. In an air fryer, cook for 5 minutes. Carefully cut the basket and rotate the banana slices till soft. Cook for an estimated 2 or 3 minutes before the banana slices are browned and caramelized. Remove it gently from the basket.

6. Air Fryer Beignets

Ingredients

- ❖ Flour ½ cup
- ❖ Cooking spray
- ❖ Water 1/8 cup
- ❖ Sugar ¼ cup
- ❖ Egg 1 large
- ❖ Butter 1 ½ teaspoons
- ❖ Baking powder ½ teaspoon
- ❖ Vanilla extract ½ teaspoon
- ❖ Salt 1 pinch
- ❖ Sugar 2 tablespoons

Steps

1. Heat the air-freezer to 185 degrees C.
2. In a big cup, whisk together the egg yolk, flour, water, sugar, baking powder, butter, salt, and vanilla extract. Stir to blend.
3. Using an electronic hand mixer to beat the white egg in a small bowl at medium speed till soft peaks develop. Fold the batter under. Using a tiny hinged ice cream scoop, apply batter to the filled pot.
4. Place the filled silicone in the air fryer's basket.
5. Fry for 10 minutes in the hot oven air fryer. Carefully extract the mold from the bowl; take out the beignets and turn over a parchment paper ring.
6. Put the circular parchment with beignets directly into the bowl of the air fryer. For an extra 4 minutes, cook. Remove the beignets from the bowl of the air fryer and sprinkle with sugar from the confectioners.

7. Air-Fried Butter Cake

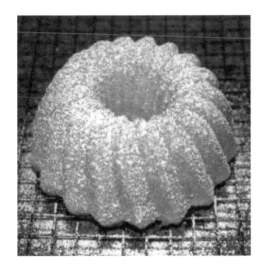

Ingredients

- ❖ Butter 7 tablespoons
- ❖ Cooking spray
- ❖ Sugar ¼ cup
- ❖ White sugar 2 tablespoons
- ❖ Egg 1 large
- ❖ Flour 1 2/3 cup
- ❖ Milk 6 tablespoons
- ❖ Salt 1 pinch

Steps

1. Heat up to 350 degrees F with an air fryer. Using cooking spray to spray a tiny fluted tube plate.

2. Using an electronic mixer to pound the butter and 1/4 cup 2 tablespoons of sugar together under a bowl until light and smooth. Connect the egg and combine until soft and creamy. Stir in the salt and starch. Add milk and completely combine the batter. Shift the batter to the pan and cook; level the surface using the back of a spoon.

3. Put the pan in the basket of an air fryer. Set a 15-minute timer. Bake until the cake turns out clear with a toothpick added.

4. Turn the cake out of the pan and give around 5 minutes to cool.

8. House Gluten-Free Fresh Cherry Crumble

Ingredients

- ❖ Butter 1/3 cup
- ❖ Cherries 3 cups
- ❖ White sugar 10 tablespoons
- ❖ Lemon 2 teaspoons
- ❖ Flour 1 cup
- ❖ Vanilla powder 1 teaspoon
- ❖ Nutmeg 1 teaspoon
- ❖ Cinnamon 1 teaspoon

Steps

1. Heat the air-freezer to 165 degrees C.

2. In a cup, blend the bruised cherries, lemon juice and 2 tbs of sugar; combine well. Apply the cherry mixture to the baking bowl.

3. In a cup, combine the 6 tbsp of sugar and flour. Use fingertips to crack the butter until the flakes are pea-size. Transfer from over cherries and gently force back.

4. In a cup, mix 2 teaspoons of sugar, nutmeg, vanilla extract, and cinnamon. Dust the sugar coating over the flour and the cherries.

5. Bake in an air fryer that's preheated. Verify at 24 minutes; if still not golden brown, resume cooking and check till golden brown at five - minute intervals. Lock the drawer and turn the air fryer off. Leave it inside to collapse for 10 minutes. Stir and leave to cool slightly for 5 minutes or so.

9. Chocolate Cake in an Air Fryer

Ingredients

- ❖ White sugar ¼ cup
- ❖ Butter 3 ½ tablespoons
- ❖ Egg 1 large
- ❖ Cooking spray
- ❖ Apricot jam 1 tablespoon
- ❖ Flour 6 tablespoons
- ❖ Cocoa powder 1 tablespoon
- ❖ Salt

Steps

1. Heat up to 320 degrees F with an air fryer. Using cooking spray to spray a tiny fluted tube plate.

2. Using an electronic mixer to pound the butter and sugar with each other in a bowl until fluffy and smooth. Add the jam and egg, blend until mixed. Season with rice, salt, and cocoa powder; blend properly. Pour the batter into the pan that has been packed. Through the back of a spoon, level the top of the batter.

3. Place the pan in the basket of an air fryer. Cook for about 15 minutes, before a toothpick added into the middle of the cake, emerges out clean.

10. Air Fryer Sweet French Toast Sticks

Ingredients

- ❖ Eggs 2 large
- ❖ Thick bread 4 slices
- ❖ Parchment paper
- ❖ Milk ¼ cup
- ❖ Cinnamon 1 teaspoon
- ❖ Vanilla extract 1 teaspoon
- ❖ Nutmeg 1 pinch

Steps

1. To make sticks, cut each bread slice into thirds. To match the end of the air fryer bowl, cut a slice of parchment paper.

2. Heat the air fryer at 360-degree F.

3. Add the vanilla extract, eggs, milk, cinnamon, and nutmeg until well mixed. Dip a slice of bread into the mixture of eggs to ensure that each slice is well coated. To extract excess oil, shake a single bread stick and put in a thin piece in the air fryer's basket. To prevent overpopulating the fryer, cook in batches if appropriate.

4. Cook for 4-5 minutes, turn over the pieces of bread and cook for 5 more minutes.

11. Air-Fryer Cannoli

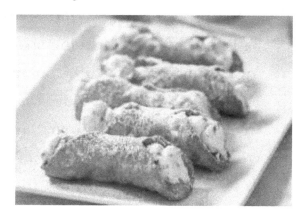

Ingredients

- ❖ Milk 1 package
- ❖ Powdered sugar ½ cup
- ❖ Orange zest 1 tablespoon
- ❖ Salt ½ teaspoon
- ❖ Turbinado sugar 1 cup
- ❖ Flour
- ❖ Freeze piecrusts 1 package
- ❖ Egg white 1 large
- ❖ Chocolate chips ½ cup
- ❖ Roasted pistachios ½ cup

Steps

1. Put the ricotta in a cheesecloth-lined strainer and push until the excess liquid drips out. In a medium cup, put the strained ricotta and whisk in the salt, orange zest, and powdered sugar. A pipe container or a zip-top container is spooned in. Before ready for usage, wait. Put on a plate of turbinado sugar. Put back.

2. To 1/16-inch length, roll out piecrusts on a finely floured board. Cut out 16 circles (3 1/2-inch). Wrap rings around cannoli molds, including some of the egg white to seal the scraping lip. Clean the whole wrapping lightly with some of the white shells. Roll to cover in turbinado sugar.

3. In a loosely sprayed with cooking oil bowl about 3/4-inch away, apply any at a time. Cook till crisp

and golden, 5 to 7 minutes, at 400 ° F. Remove with tongs carefully and chill for around 1 minute before taking the cannoli mold out of the shell gently. Let it cool absolutely for 10 minutes or so. Repeat for the shells left.

4. In different small containers, put chocolate chips and pistachios. Pipe the blend of ricotta into each cooled cannoli container. Dip 1 with either chocolate chips or pistachio chips. Dust with the sugar powder. Immediately, serve.

12. Double-Glazed Air-Fried Cinnamon Biscuit Bites

Ingredients

- ❖ Flour 2/3 cup
- ❖ Sugar 2 tablespoon
- ❖ Wheat flour 2/3 cup
- ❖ Cinnamon ¼ teaspoon
- ❖ Baking powder 1 teaspoon
- ❖ Salt ¼ teaspoon
- ❖ Cold salted butter 4 tablespoons
- ❖ Cooking spray
- ❖ Milk 1/3 cup
- ❖ Water 3 tablespoons
- ❖ Powdered sugar 2 cups

Steps

1. In a medium cup, whisk together the sugar, flour, cinnamon, baking powder, and salt. Add butter; use 2 blades or a pastry processor to cut through a mixture unless butter is well mixed with flour and coarse cornmeal resembles the mixture. Add the sugar and stir until the dough develops a ball. Put the dough on a flowery surface and knead for around 29-30 seconds before it is soft and develops a cohesive shape. Break the dough into 16 separate bits. Roll each piece softly into a flat surface.

2. Cover the air fryer bowl well with spray for frying. Put eight balls in the basket, leaving space for each one: spray with cooking oil spray on the donut balls. Cook till golden brown and whipped, 11-12 minutes at 350 ° F. Remove the donut nuts from the basket gently and put them over the foil on a wire rack. Enable 5 minutes to cool. Repeat with the donut balls that remain.

3. In a medium cup, whisk the water and powdered sugar

together until smooth. Enable 5 minutes to cool; glaze again, enabling the excess to trickle down.

13. Air Fryer Strawberry "Pop-Tarts"

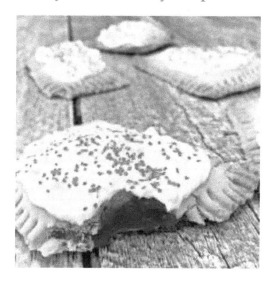

Ingredients

- ❖ Cooking spray
- ❖ Freeze piecrusts ½ package
- ❖ Sugar ¼ cup
- ❖ Strawberries 8 ounces
- ❖ Lemon 1 ½ teaspoons
- ❖ Powdered sugar ½ cup
- ❖ Candy sprinkles ½ ounce

Steps

1. In a medium microwaveable dish, whisk together using the sugar and strawberries. Allow standing for 15 minutes, sometimes stirring. Microwave on HIGH until polished and decreased, stirring midway through cooking for around 10 minutes. Total cooling, approximately 30 minutes.

2. On a well-floured board, roll the pie crust into a 12-inch shell. Break the dough into 12 rectangles, re-rolling scraps if required. Leaving a 1/2-inch edge, spoon around 2 teaspoons of the strawberry mixture into the middle of 6 of the dough rectangles. Rub the sides of the packed dough's rectangles with water; top with the remaining rectangles of the dough; push the sides with a fork to secure. Cover tarts well with spray for frying.

3. In an air fryer bowl, put 3 tarts in a single layer and cook at 350 ° F till golden brown, around 10 minutes. With the leftover tarts, repeat. Put it on a wire rack for about 30 minutes to cool down.

4. In a small cup, whisk the sugar and lemon juice together until smooth. Glaze the spoon over the cooled tarts and scatter generously with sprinkles of sweets.

14. Air Fryer Glazed Cake Doughnut Holes

Ingredients

- ❖ Sugar 2 tablespoons

- ❖ Flour 1 ¼ cups

- ❖ Salt ¼ teaspoon

- ❖ Baking powder 1 teaspoon

- ❖ Cooking spray

- ❖ Cold salted butter 4 tablespoons

- ❖ Milk 1/3 cup

- ❖ Water 3 tablespoons

- ❖ Powdered sugar 1 cup

Steps

1. In a medium dish, whisk together the sugar, baking powder, flour, and salt. Add butter; use 2 knives or a pastry cutter to cut into flour, till the butter is well mixed and appears like rough cornmeal. Add the milk and whisk till the dough is ball shaped. Place the dough on a flowery surface and knead for around 30 seconds before it is smooth and forms a cohesive shape. Break the dough into 14 identical shapes. Gently roll each to form uniformly smooth spheres.

2. Cover the bottom of the air-fryer basket completely with cooking oil. In the air fryer bowl, put 7 dough balls, distributed uniformly to prevent hitting. Spray the cooking spray for the dough balls. Cook until browned and puffed, around 10 minutes, at 350 ° F. Remove it gently from the basket and put it on a wire shelf.

3. In a medium cup, whisk the powdered sugar and water together until smooth. Place cooked balls of dough in a glaze, 1 at a time; roll to coat.

4. Repeat with the remaining dough and glaze process.

15. Peach Hand Pies in an Air Fryer

Ingredients

- ❖ Sugar 3 tablespoons

- ❖ Fresh peaches 2

- ❖ Lemon 1 tablespoon

- ❖ Salt ¼ teaspoon

- ❖ Cornstarch 1 teaspoon

- ❖ Vanilla extract 1 teaspoon

- ❖ Cooking spray

- ❖ Freeze piecrusts 1 package

Steps

1. In a medium cup, combine the lemon juice, peaches, pepper, sugar, and salt. Let stand for 15 minutes, sometimes stirring. Dump the peaches and leave 1 tablespoon of fluid. Whisk the

cornstarch into the allocated liquid; transfer to the peaches that have been drained.

2. Piecrusts are sliced into 8 circles. Put a filling of about 1 tsp in the middle of each circle. Rub water across the edges of the dough; fold the dough over the filling to create half-moons. Puncture the corners with a fork to grip; split the top of the pies with 3 narrow slits. Cover pies well with spray for frying.

3. In an air fryer bowl, put 3 pies in a single layer and cook at 350 ° F till lightly browned 13 to 15 minutes. Continue for the pies that remain.

16. Air Fryer Churros with Chocolate Sauce

Ingredients

- Salt ¼ teaspoon

- Water ½ cup

- Eggs 2 large

- Non-salted butter ¼ cup

- Flour ½ cup

- Cinnamon 2 teaspoons

- Sugar 1/3 cup

- Chocolate chips 4 ounces

- Vanilla kefir 2 tablespoons

- Cream 3 tablespoons

Steps

1. Take sugar, salt and 1/4 cup of butter to a medium-high boil in a shallow saucepan. Lower the heat; add flour and mix rapidly with a wooden spoon, around 30 seconds, until the dough is smooth. Continue to cook, stirring continuously, for 2 to 3 minutes before the dough continues to move away from the sides of the pan, and a film appears on the bottom of the plate. Place the dough into a medium dish. Stir continuously for around 1 minute until slightly cooled. Insert eggs, 1 at a time, mixing continuously with every addition until smooth. Move the mixture to a medium star tip designed piping container. Thirty-minute chill.

2. Pipe 6 single-layer bits in a basket of air fryers. Cook until crispy, around 10 minutes, at 380 ° F. Repeat for the dough that remains.

3. In a medium dish, whisk the sugar and cinnamon together. Brush the fried churros with the remaining 2 teaspoons of melted butter and cover them with the sugar mixture.

4. Put the cream and chocolate in a tiny, microwaveable dish. Microwave on HIGH for about 30 seconds, until molten and flat, swirling after 14 seconds. Stir the kefir in. Serve the churros with a sauce of cocoa.

17. Chocolate Orange Christmas Biscuits

Ingredients

- ❖ Flour 225 g
- ❖ Sugar 100 g
- ❖ Butter 100 g
- ❖ Orange juice 1 Large
- ❖ Egg 1 Large
- ❖ Cocoa Powder 2 Tbsp
- ❖ Vanilla Essence 2 Tsp
- ❖ Dark Chocolate

Steps

1. Heat the air fryer at 180c.

2. Add the flour and butter and massage the fat in a mixing bowl, so the products mimic breadcrumbs.

3. Insert the cinnamon, spice, orange and powdered cocoa and blend well.

4. Attach your egg and blend well until the dough it's just a little sticky, resembles the mixture.

5. Put some flour on your palms so that the combination doesn't adhere to you and create 8 equal-sized parts of the dough balls.

6. Flatten the dough balls and put inside each slice a rectangle of dark chocolate and then cover the dough above it so that the chocolate can't be seen.

7. Placed all 8 bits in the 180c air fryer for 15 minutes.

8. Only serve.

18. Air fryer Oat Sandwich Biscuits

Ingredients

- ❖ Flour 150 g
- ❖ Butter 100 g
- ❖ White Sugar 75 g
- ❖ Egg ½ Small
- ❖ Coconut ¼ cup
- ❖ Gluten-Free Oats ½ Cup
- ❖ White Chocolate 20 g
- ❖ Vanilla Essence 1 Tsp

Steps

1. Cream together the sugar and butter until it is nice and

fluffy. Add the nature of the recipe, chocolate, mint, and coconut. Add the flour and blend well.

2. Develop medium-sized biscuit forms then roll in the oats afterward.

3. Put 180c in an air fryer for 17 minutes.

4. Create the filling as they're cooling. Mix the butter and icing sugar until another fluffy mixture is perfectly ready. Stir in the lemon juice and vanilla, combine again and position on the one hand.

5. Apply the filling while the biscuits are cold and press them together because they represent a good sandwich.

19. Half Cooked Air Fryer Lemon Biscuits

Ingredients

- ❖ Butter 100 g
- ❖ Sugar 100 g
- ❖ Flour 225 g
- ❖ Lemon 1 Small
- ❖ Egg 1 Small
- ❖ Vanilla Essence 1 Tsp

Steps

1. Heat the air fryer to 180c.

2. Blend sugar and flour in a bowl. Add the butter and rub it in till the blend just look like breadcrumbs. Shake the cup periodically enough that the fatty pieces fall to the surface.

3. Mix the egg and lemon juice.

4. Integrate and whisk till getting lovely fluffy bread.

5. Stretch out and break down into medium-sized biscuits.

6. Put the biscuits into the air fryer on a baking tray and bake for 5 minutes at 180c.

7. Put on a cooling sheet and sprinkle icing sugar on it.

20. Melting Moments in The Air fryer

Ingredients

- ❖ Butter 100 g
- ❖ Sugar 75 g
- ❖ Flour 150 g
- ❖ Egg 1 Small
- ❖ White Chocolate 50 g
- ❖ Coconut 3 Tbsp
- ❖ Vanilla Essence 1 Tsp

Steps

1. Heat the air fryer till 180c.
2. In a big tub, cream the sugar and butter until they are nice and fluffy.
3. The eggs are broken, and then the vanilla essence is applied.
4. Use a rolling pin to beat the white chocolate such the huge and tiny bits are blended.
5. Insert the flour, and white chocolate then blend properly.
6. Using the coconut to roll into little balls and cover.
7. Place the balls on a baking sheet in the air fryer and bake at 180c for eight minutes. Lower the temperature for another 4 minutes to 160c.
8. Just serve.

21. Air Fryer Shortbread

Ingredients

- ❖ Flour 250 g
- ❖ Sugar 75 g
- ❖ Butter 175 g

Steps

1. Put your self-raised flour, butter, and caster sugar in a cup.
2. Rub the butter till it resembles dense breadcrumbs in the starch.
3. Marinate, and you'll have a dough ball of shortbread.
4. Slice into your favorite forms using cookie cutters.
5. Fry your shortbread within air fryer on either air freezer grill pan. Adjust the temperature to 181c/360f for 10 minutes and set the time.
6. Until serving, encourage it to cool a bit.

22. Air Fryer Cupcakes

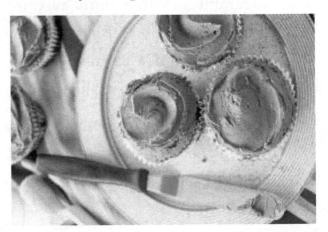

Ingredients

- ❖ Flour 400 g
- ❖ Sugar 450 g
- ❖ Cocoa Powder 50 g
- ❖ Butter 200 g
- ❖ Eggs 4 Medium
- ❖ Vanilla Essence 1 Tbsp
- ❖ Milk 480 ml
- ❖ Extra Virgin Olive Oil 1 Tbsp

Steps

1. Add the butter and sugar to a tub and blend the butter into the sugar with your hand mixer. Crack an egg in the cup, apply the vanilla extract, apply the extra virgin olive oil, and combine with the hand blender again. Add the cocoa powder, flour, and milk if it's fluffy and blend with a wooden spoon. Do not use a hand mixer since it can spill it all together. Change it with just a little more milk or water if it is too dense.

2. Pour in the muffin cups and cook chocolate cupcakes at 160c/320f in the air fryer for 12 minutes. Place it on one side and let it cool.

3. Get the chocolate buttercream as it cools. Blend the icing sugar into the butter using a hand mixer. Connect several ingredients and proceed to combine until you've got a smooth buttercream. When cupcakes cool, refrigerate it.

4. From the back, take your piping bag and build a fist. Then open your hand over it so that you have a funnel design. Then spoon the mixture with your other hand into the piping container.

5. So, when the top of the piping bag is almost fully grasped and twisted close, push softly to allow the air escape, so push with slight touch and swirl it on top.

23. Air Fryer Lemon Butterfly Buns

Ingredients

* Butter 100 g
* Sugar 100 g
* Eggs 2 Medium
* Flour 100 g
* Vanilla Essence ½ Tsp
* Cherries 1 Tsp
* Butter 50 g
* Icing Sugar 100 g
* Lemon juice ½ Small

Steps

1. Heat an air fryer till 170c.
2. Add the butter till it is light and fluffy in a big mixing bowl with the honey.
3. Add the meaning of Vanilla.
4. Beat the eggs and make sure that each one contributes a little starch.
5. Pull the remainder of the flour carefully in.
6. Cover the mixture with half of the tiny bun cases before you've run

out of containers. Place the first six in the Air fryer and then cook at 170c for 8 minutes.

7. Start preparing icing sugar because the buns are cooking. Cream the butter and add the icing sugar slowly. Attach the lemon and blend thoroughly. Add a little water if it is too dense.

8. Pick the top slice off onto the buns and chop in half and make butterfly shapes when the butterfly buns had already fully cooked. Put the icing sugar in the center. Then put on top of 1/3 of cherry and sieve with a little icing sugar.

9. Just serve.

24. Air Fryer Apple Crisp

Ingredients

- ❖ Apples 6 Medium
- ❖ Sugar 1 Tbsp
- ❖ Cinnamon 1 Tbsp
- ❖ Flour 120 g
- ❖ Sugar 40 g
- ❖ Butter 50 g
- ❖ Oats 60 g

Steps

1. Peel and dice the apples, then put them in a mixing bowl. Toss in the sugar and cinnamon from the caster. Move to Ramekins.

2. In a cup, stack the flour and butter and mix the fat into the flour unless coarse breadcrumbs appear.

3. Combine. When it is fully blended, incorporate sugar and oats.

4. Cover. Apply topping to the apples and place the ramekins into the basket of the air fryer.

5. Only cook. Begin with 8 minutes of 160c/320f, followed by 5 minutes of 200c/400f and serve.

25. Chocolate Mug Cake

Ingredients

- ❖ Flour ¼ Cup
- ❖ Sugar 5 Tbsp
- ❖ Cocoa Powder 1 Tbsp
- ❖ Milk 3 Tbsp
- ❖ Coconut Oil 3 Tsp

Steps

1. In the cup, combine all the ingredients properly. But make sure that they are blended correctly, or one time you could probably wind up with a cake

with barely any chocolate and then fill the next one.

2. Put the mug in the fridge and cook at 200c for 10 minutes. For the other mugs, rinse and repeat until everybody has already had their chocolate strike.

3. Serve it.

26. Air Fryer Blueberry Jam Tarts

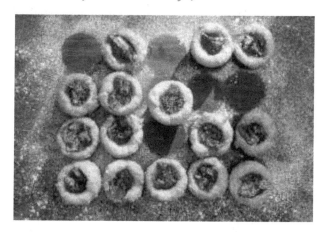

Ingredients

* Pie crust 350 g

* Instant Pot Blueberry Jam 500 g

Steps

1. To prevent the pastry from binding, flour tart tins.

2. On a worktop, roll the pie crust out and layer over tart tins.

3. Break the tart tins around them so that with each one, you have a pie crust.

4. Load your tarts with blueberry jam to 3/4 full.

5. Put in the air fryer or air fryer oven basket and cook at 180c/360f for 10 minutes.

6. Only serve.

27. Chocolate Orange Chocolate Fondant

Ingredients

* Flour 2 Tbsp

* Sugar 4 Tbsp

* Dark Chocolate 115 g

* Butter 115 g

* Orange 1 Medium

* Eggs 2 Medium

Steps

1. Heat the fridge to 180c.

2. In a glass dish over a wide pan of hot water, melt the butter and chocolate. Stir until the color is smooth and creamy.

3. The eggs and sugar are whisked and pounded until they are yellow and frothy.

4. Connect the orange to the chocolate, along with the egg and sugar combination. Finally, whisk in the flour and thoroughly blend all.

5. Complete the mixture with the ramekins 75 percent complete and bake for 11 minutes.

6. Remove from the fridge and enable you to cook for 2 minutes in the ramekins. Place the ramekins (gently) upside down on a serving plate with a blunt knife to rub the bottom as this loosens the tips.

7. You will release the fondant from the middle and have a lovely pudding with a fluffy core.

8. Serve with ice cream or hot syrup of milk.

28. Air Fryer Pumpkin Pie

Ingredients

- ❖ Flour 225 g
- ❖ Butter 100 g
- ❖ Sugar 25 g
- ❖ Cinnamon 1 Tbsp
- ❖ Nutmeg 1 Tsp

Steps

1. Get the traditional crust of the sandwich. Mix the sliced butter into the flour in a dish until it appears like breadcrumbs. Add in the cinnamon, sugar, and nutmeg. Blend, so you have a dry pie crust, incorporating a little water at a time. Take out the crust of your pie and put it in the pie pan.

2. Put your cubed pumpkin and cubed ginger and put 1 cup of water. Set to cook for 4 minutes under manual pressure/pressure. Use accelerated pressure release and pressure release manually.

3. Wash your Pot Instant. Flush the fluid from your Instant Pot using a sieve and then rinse it with a milky cloth. As the pumpkin contains a number, this can eliminate any extra liquid because it will interrupt your pumpkin pie's arrangement if you don't.

4. Create a topping for pumpkin pie. In the Instant Cup, bring the washed pumpkin and ginger back in and incorporate all the pumpkin filling ingredients other than the milk. Mix the eggs and remaining ingredients into the pumpkin using a hand mixer until you have a creamy, thin pumpkin sauce. Whisk and blend well in the double milk.

5. Put the filling of the pumpkin pie in the pie crust and ensure it doesn't go more than 1 cm off the end since it will otherwise be

impossible to manage and prone to bubble over the surface.

6. In an air fryer, prepare the pumpkin pie. Put the pumpkin pie on the center shelf and bake it at 180c/360f for 24 minutes.

7. Put it in the fridge and leave it to cool the whole night. It will make the pumpkin pie firm up, and then it will be ready for slicing the next day.

29. Leftover Coconut Sugar Recipes

Ingredients

- ❖ Flour 500 g
- ❖ Butter 350 g
- ❖ Cheese 100 g
- ❖ Coconut Sugar 200 g
- ❖ Honey 2 Tbsp
- ❖ Vanilla Essence 1 Tsp
- ❖ Cinnamon 1 Tsp

Steps

1. The air fryer should be heated up to 180c.

2. Mix the rice, butter, and sugar in a mixing dish. Rub the fat into the flour and sugar using the rubbing process, until it resembles breadcrumbs.

3. Add the cinnamon and honey and keep baking it until a smooth dough emerges.

4. Divide it into 3 parts. 1/5 on a work surface ready for next usage, then 2/5 for the middle in a bowl and finally the remaining 2/2 for the covering.

5. At the bottom of your air fryer, put a baking pad.

6. Line a very thin layer of the dough with the bottom of the air fryer (using the fingertips rather than a rolling pin) such that it would be like a cheesecake rim.

7. Place the fryer in the air and cook at 180c for 5 minutes.

8. Place the air fryer to one foot. Create the fluffy filling as it is refrigerating. Add the cheese and combine well in the bowl with 2/5 of the dough until you have a wonderful cheesecake-style combination that is richer than a typical cheesecake, but also light and fluffy. Add the blackberries to it and put them on top of the crust in the air fryer.

9. Use your hands to spread it on top of your shortbread spread of cheesecake so that it can shape like your top crumble.

10. Place the 180c in the air-fryer for 15 minutes. Cook before you're on top of a beautiful crumble.

11. Take the shortbread strips from the air fryer and put them in the fridge on a wide plate so that the cheesecake's center can be completely placed.

12. Cut into bars and serve.

30. Air Fryer Mince Pies

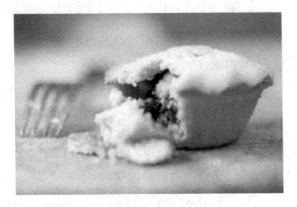

Ingredients

- ❖ Pie Crust 500 g
- ❖ Jar Mince Meat 350 g
- ❖ Egg 1 Small
- ❖ Icing Sugar 50 g
- ❖ Flour

Steps

1. In a mixing bowl, add the pie ingredients. Rub the flour with the fat and stir in the sugar. Insert a little more virgin olive oil and blend even if you have a pastry with a little water.

2. Flour a rolling pin and a clean worktop with flour. Roll out the pastry and cut out to the desired size using pastry cutters.

3. Pack the pastry into muffins pastry and add each one with a dollop of chopped meat.

4. Using your hands to push down and cover, apply another sheet of pastry over the top such that no thin meat escapes while preparation.

5. Using a pastry brush to apply an egg glaze to your thin pies' surface and move it to the air fryer. In your air-fryer oven, fried air for 14 minutes at 180c/360f.

6. Eat hot or save later. A splashing of icing sugar surrounded by pies can also be added.

31. Air Fryer Brownies

Ingredients

- ❖ Flour 100 g
- ❖ Butter 100 g
- ❖ Eggs 2 Large
- ❖ Cocoa Powder 30 g
- ❖ Brown Sugar 175 g
- ❖ Golden Syrup 1 Tbsp

❖ Vanilla Essence 2 Tsp

Steps

1. Fill up the butter into the baking pan of air fryer and break it into bite-size pieces. Put the baking pan in the air fryer's basket and cook at 140c/280f for 2 minutes or until melted.

2. To be able to touch causes it to cool sufficiently.

3. Fill up the sugar, eggs, cocoa powder, golden syrup, and vanilla essence into your air-fryer baking pan. Mix well with the whisk in your hand.

4. Add the flour and blend with a fork until everything is completely mixed.

5. Put the baking pan down in the air fryer bowl and cook for 14 minutes at 180c/360f till a cocktail string comes out clean when placed in the middle of the brownies.

6. Offer with whipped cream, caramel sauce of favorite toppings.

32. Chocolate Eclairs in The Air Fryer

Ingredients

❖ Butter 50 g
❖ Flour 100 g
❖ Eggs 3 medium
❖ Water 150 ml

Steps

1. Heat an air fryer till 180c.

2. Put the fat in the water as it is heating up, melt it in a wide pan over medium heat and then bring it to a boil.

3. Take it from the heat and substitute the flour and whisk.

4. Transfer the pan to the heat and swirl in the pan's center to create a medium disc.

5. To encourage it to cool, move the dough to a cold plate once the eggs are mixed until you have a nice mixture.

6. Then render and put in the Air fryer in éclair designs. Cook on 180 for 10 minutes and on 160 for a further 8 minutes.

7. Make the cream filling when the dough is cooking, combine the vanilla essence, icing sugar, and whipped cream until soft and dense with a fork.

8. Left the eclairs to cool and create the chocolate topping as they are cooling. Put in a glass bowl the milk chocolate, butter, and cream. Put it over a pan of warm water

and blend well before the chocolate is melted.

9. Fill the tops with molten chocolate and serve.

33. Air Fryer Chocolate Profiteroles

Ingredients

- ❖ <u>Butter </u>100 g
- ❖ <u>Flour </u>200 g
- ❖ Eggs 6 Medium
- ❖ Water 300 ml

Steps

1. Heat an air fryer till 170c.
2. Put the fat in water in a wide pan and fry on medium heat to make sure you get it to the boil.
3. Take it from the heat and blend in the flour and then place it again on the heat until it forms a large dough in the plate's center.
4. Adjust the dough from one side to cool it down. Put in the eggs and blend before you have a nice combination.
5. Create profiterole shapes and bake for 8-10 minutes on 180c.
6. When the eclairs are making for the cream filling – combine with vanilla essence, icing sugar and whipped cream until smooth and heavy.

7. While the profiteroles are frying, create the chocolate coating – put the chocolate, cream, and butter in a glass cup, over a pan of boiling water. Mix before you have molten chocolate.
8. Finish the profiteroles of dark chocolate on the outer surface.

34. Air Fryer Doughnuts from Scratch

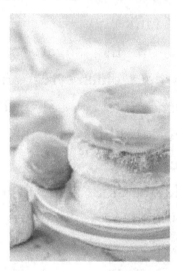

Ingredients

- ❖ <u>Bread Maker Doughnut Dough</u> 500 g
- ❖ <u>Icing Sugar </u>240 ml
- ❖ <u>Milk </u>40 ml
- ❖ <u>Vanilla Essence </u>1 Tsp
- ❖ <u>Extra Virgin Olive Oil Spray</u>
- ❖ <u>Flour for rolling</u>
- ❖ <u>Food Coloring</u>

Steps

1. Remove the bread maker from the doughnut dough and lay it on a floured work surface. To keep it from sticking, add flour into it.

2. Print out the large doughnut forms with your biscuit cutters. Cut out the doughnut holes with a smaller knife. Place the holes in the doughnut to one hand.

3. Only cook. Load up to 4 donuts into the air fryer's basket and cook at 180c/360 for 8 minutes. However, spray with olive oil after 4 minutes to help with the soft glow.

4. Terminate. In a cup, mix the icing sugar and milk, so you have a strong glaze. For using various colored doughnuts, apply food coloring or break into ramekins. Sprinkle and eat with the 100's and 1000's.

35. Air Fryer Baking for Easter

Ingredients

- Milk Chocolate 225 g

- Butter 50 g

- Corn 75 g

- Golden Syrup 1 Tbsp

- A packet of Cadburys Mini Eggs 200 g

Steps

1. Break down the milk chocolate into squares and fill it with butter and golden syrup into the air fryer baking tray. Cook at 140c/280f for 5 minutes and mix until the butter and chocolate are completely melted and blended. Add the corn flakes and mix well before all the corn flakes are covered in chocolate. Load a few mini eggs on top of each cake into the baking cups and refrigerator. Remove it from the fridge after an hour and feed.

2. Secondly, create the cake batter. Beat the butter and the sugar in a bowl with a hand mixer until smooth and fluffy. Add the eggs and combine again on low and whisk in the cake batter's remaining ingredients and blend very well in a fork. Load the cake batter into cupcakes made of silicone or identical containers and put in the air fryer's basket. Cook it at 180c/360f for 10 minutes. Remove and allow to cool from the air fryer.

3. When the cupcakes are cooling, render the cupcake frosting. Mix the icing sugar into the cream

cheese in a cup and use your hand blender again. When it's smooth and fluffy, the vanilla essence is applied to the icing sugar lumps and combined softly with a fork.

4. The cupcake frosting covering is filled while cold. Wait until the cupcakes have reached room temperature and swirl over the cupcakes with the cupcake frosting. Attach and feed the mini chickens.

36. Molten lava cake

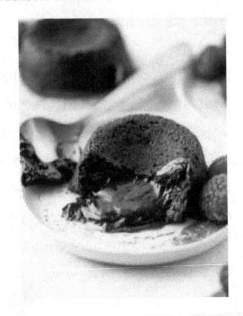

Ingredients

- ❖ Egg yolk 1
- ❖ Egg 1
- ❖ Unsalted butter 2 tablespoons
- ❖ White caster sugar 3 tablespoons
- ❖ Vanilla extract ½ tablespoon

- ❖ Flour 3 tablespoons
- ❖ Chocolate 30g
- ❖ Salt 1 pinch

Steps

1. In a big cup, add the vanilla extract, butter, sugar, and whisk till the mixture becomes soft and fluffy.

2. Beat the yolk of the egg and whites and apply it to the mixture of butter and sugar. Whisk until there is a creamy consistency in the mixture.

3. Add flour and salt to the mixture and use a spatula to fold onto the mixture.

4. In the microwave, heat the chocolate for around a minute or molten, then add the chocolate into the batter and blend well easily.

5. Move this mixture and fill it to the full in a greased ramekin or another air-freezer-safe bowl.

6. For 8-10 minutes, put the bowls into an air fryer at 180 ° C.

37. Basque Burnt Cheesecake

Ingredients

- ❖ Cheese 250g
- ❖ Egg yolk 1

❖ Eggs 2

❖ Sugar 70 g

❖ Vanilla extract 0.5g

❖ Whipping cream 170g

❖ Cake flour 6g

Steps

1. At 200 ° C, heat the air fryer.
2. Shake the cream cheese along with the sugar, using a mixer or whisk.
3. Bit by bit, incorporate egg yolk and whole eggs and blend until the mixture has a moist, soupy texture.
4. Pour in the milk and vanilla extract from the whipping and mix to mix.
5. Sift the cake flour into the mixture and whisk until smooth.
6. With non-stick baking paper, line a pan and dump the mixture in.
7. Bake for 18 minutes at 180 ° C, then for another 3-5 minutes at 200 ° C, till the cake layer is black.
8. Serve chilled or hot.

38. Cinnamon Rolls

Ingredients

❖ Cinnamon 1 tablespoon

❖ Unsalted butter 80g

❖ Brown sugar 6 tablespoons

❖ Puff pastry 1 sheet

❖ Powdered sugar ½ cup

❖ Milk 1 tablespoon

❖ Lemon juice 2 teaspoons

Steps

1. In a cup, add the butter, cinnamon, and brown sugar and whisk.
2. Roll out the rectangular outline of the puff pastry sheets and scatter the cinnamon mixture evenly over it.
3. To make the cinnamon swirls, carefully roll the sheet up loosely.
4. Break the roll into bits that are 2.5CM long.
5. Place it in a preheated 200 ° C air fryer and bake for 6 minutes or until browned.
6. Integrate the lemon juice, sugar, and milk to create the coating.
7. Pour over the baked cinnamon rolls with icing and serve nice.

39. Nutella-stuffed Kodiak Balls

Ingredients

❖ Kodiak Cakes Whole Wheat Honey Oat Flapjack and Waffle Mix 110g

❖ Non-fat Yoghurt 110g

- ❖ Nutella 30g
- ❖ Sugar 1 tablespoon
- ❖ Cinnamon 1 teaspoon

Steps

1. In a basket, combine the yogurt and Kodiak.
2. Roll it out and split it into 6 identical rectangles.
3. Scoop around a tbsp of Nutella and put it in the center of the dough that has been cut out.
4. Cover the dough across the Nutella and mound it into a ball, using your hands.
5. If you're done with all 6 spheres, put them for 5 minutes in a hot oven air fryer at 160 ° C.
6. Until eating, combine the sugar and cinnamon and wrap the baked balls in it.

40. Cinnamon-coated donuts

Ingredients

- ❖ Milk 1 cup
- ❖ Instant yeast 2½ teaspoon
- ❖ Sugar ¼ cup
- ❖ Salt ½ teaspoon
- ❖ Egg 1
- ❖ Unsalted butter ¼ cup
- ❖ Flour 3 cups
- ❖ Cooking spray

Steps

1. Mix the sugar, milk, and yeast in a wide bowl and let the mixture rest for 10 minutes.
2. Add egg, cinnamon, butter, and flour and stir until a fluffy dough develops.
3. Grease a bowl and put it with the dough. Cover and let it grow for 11/2 hours, or until it is double in height, with a cling wrap.
4. 1-On a floured board spread out the dough and cut out 13 donuts into 8CM-wide circles. Then, carve out a middle 2.5CM-wide.
5. Put these cut donuts on a parchment paper sheet and let them grow for another 25-30 minutes.
6. The air fryer is heated up to 180 ° C. Spray with cooking spray on the air fryer basket and put the donuts in without combining.
7. Wait for 4 minutes, then flip and cook for 4 minutes more.
8. Rub the donut with molten butter to incorporate the toppings and flip it into the topping

combination with sugar and cinnamon on both sides to cover.

41. Portuguese Egg Tarts

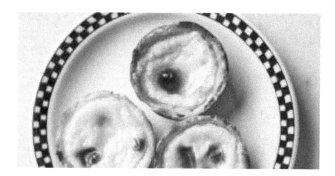

Ingredients

- ❖ Sugar 10 g
- ❖ Milk 45 g
- ❖ Egg 1
- ❖ Puff pastry 1 sheet

Steps

1. Stir the sugar and milk in a saucepan and carry it to a boil. Put aside to cool down.
2. In a wide tub, stir in the liquid.
3. Throw in the mixture of milk and whisk. Then, strain it to get rid of bubbles using a sieve.
4. Unroll the sheet of pastry and cut out 10-12CM circles in diameter.
5. Gently push the dough down to match, then add the mixture into it until it is 80 percent finished.
6. Bake at 150 ° C for 15 minutes in a preheated air fryer. Take the fryer from the air and cook.

42. Banana muffin

Ingredients

- ❖ Bananas 2
- ❖ Olive oil ⅓ cup
- ❖ Egg 1
- ❖ Sugar ½ cup
- ❖ Vanilla extract 1 teaspoon
- ❖ Cinnamon 1 teaspoon
- ❖ Flour ¾ cup

Steps

1. Mash the bananas in a big bowl and then add the sugar, bacon, vanilla extract, and olive oil. Mix well.
2. Add the cinnamon and flour then fold the mixture in until it is mashed together.
3. Divide this mixture uniformly into muffin cake.
4. Pop this for about 15 minutes into a hot oven air fryer at 160 ° C.

43. Chocolate Chip Brownies

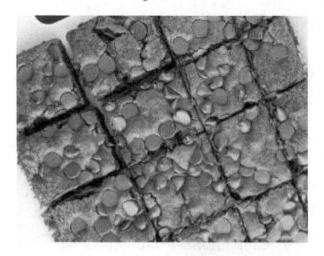

Ingredients

- ❖ Flour ½ cup
- ❖ Cocoa powder 6 tablespoons
- ❖ Chocolate chips ¼ cup
- ❖ Sugar ½ cup
- ❖ Unsalted butter ¼ cup
- ❖ Eggs 2
- ❖ Vegetable oil 1 tablespoon
- ❖ Vanilla extract ½ teaspoon
- ❖ Salt ¼ teaspoon
- ❖ Baking powder ¼ teaspoon

Steps

1. Combine all the ingredients in a large bowl and blend well.
2. Grease a buttery baking sheet and pour the mixture in.

3. Put this for 15 minutes in a preheated 160 ° C air fryer.
4. Enable it to refrigerate and eat.

44. Cassava cake

Ingredients

- ❖ Grated cassava 450g
- ❖ Coconut cream 200ml
- ❖ Egg 1
- ❖ Sugar ½ cup
- ❖ Butter 1 tablespoon

Steps

1. Mix all the ingredients in a bowl.
2. Switch to a baking sheet and use foil to protect the dish.
3. Put it at 180 ° C in a hot oven air fryer and cook for 34 minutes. Remove the foil and cook for another 14 minutes or until it is browned across the cake surface.
4. Before serving, set aside to cool.

45. Roti boy's Coffee Bun

Ingredients

- ❖ Milk 150g
- ❖ Wheat flour 250g
- ❖ Sugar 50g
- ❖ Instant yeast 1 tablespoon
- ❖ Egg yolk 1

❖ Butter 30g

Steps

1. Add the egg, sugar, flour, milk, and yeast to a big bowl and combine well.
2. Add knead and butter once soft and elastic in the dough.
3. Enable the dough under a moist cloth to rise for 35-40 minutes. Break it into 2 sections and enable it to increase for 10 more minutes.
4. Beat the sugar and butter together to create the icing. Put flour, coffee, and egg and combine properly.
5. In a piping container, move the topping and roll it on the elevated dough.
6. Cook for 25 minutes in an oven and bake at 160 ° C.
7. Serve it as a sweet.

46. Air-Fryer Bread Pudding

Ingredients

❖ Chocolate 2 ounces

❖ Half-and-half cream 1/2 cup

❖ Sugar 2/3 cup

❖ 2% milk 1/2 cup

❖ Egg 1 large

❖ Vanilla extract 1 teaspoon

❖ Salt 1/4 teaspoon

❖ Sliced bread 3 cups

Steps

1. Melt the chocolate in a shallow microwave-safe bowl, mix until smooth. Using a cream to stir; set aside.
2. Mix the oil, vanilla, salt, and egg in a big cup. Stir in a blend of cocoa. Attach bread cubes and cover with a flip. Let the 15 minutes stand.
3. Heat a 325 ° air fryer.
4. Place the air-fryer basket on a plate. Cook until 12-15 minutes, a knife inserted in the middle comes out clean.

47. Air-Fryer Carrot Coffee Cake

Ingredients

❖ Buttermilk ½ cup

❖ Sugar 1/3 cup

❖ Egg 1 large

❖ Canola oil 3 tablespoons

❖ Vanilla extract 1 teaspoon

❖ Grated orange 1 teaspoon

❖ Brown sugar 2 tablespoons

❖ Flour 2/3 cups

❖ Baking powder 1 teaspoon

- ❖ Chopped walnuts 1/3 cup
- ❖ Cranberries ¼ cup
- ❖ Carrots 1 cup
- ❖ Baking soda ¼ cup
- ❖ Salt ¼ teaspoon
- ❖ Pie spice 2 teaspoons

Steps

1. Heat the fryer to 350 degrees. 6-in, grease and starch. Take a rectangular pan for baking. Whisk together all the ingredients in a big bowl. Beat in the egg mixture steadily. Fold in the dried cranberries and carrots. In the prepared cup, pour.

2. Combine the walnuts, the remaining 2 teaspoons of sugar and 1 teaspoon of pumpkin spice in a shallow cup. Sprinkle the batter equally over it. Place the pan softly in the basket of a major air fryer.

3. Cook for 35-40 minutes before a toothpick inserted in the middle comes out clean.

48. Air-Fryer S' mores Crescent Rolls

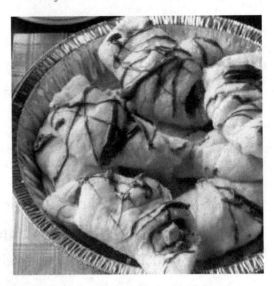

Ingredients

- ❖ Freeze crescent rolls 8 ounces
- ❖ Graham crackers 2
- ❖ Chocolate chips 2 tablespoons
- ❖ Nutella ¼ cup
- ❖ Marshmallows 2/3 cup

Steps

1. Heat the 300 ° air fryer. Unroll the crescent dough; break it into eight triangles. Put 1 teaspoon of Nutella at each triangle's broad end. Sprinkle with marshmallows, chocolate chips and graham crackers; rollback.

2. Organize rolls in batches, in a single sheet on a greased tray in the air-fryer bowl. Curve for crescents to shape. Cook for 8-10 minutes until it is golden brown.

Heat remaining Nutella in a microwave to achieve a muggy uniformity, spoon over rolls. Represent it as a sweet.

49. Air Fryer Donuts

Ingredients

- ❖ Milk ½ cup
- ❖ Cooking spray
- ❖ Sugar ¼ cup
- ❖ Dry yeast 1 packet
- ❖ Flour 2 cup
- ❖ Salt ½ teaspoon
- ❖ Butter 4 tablespoon
- ❖ Egg 1 large
- ❖ Vanilla extract 1 teaspoon

Steps

1. Grease a large bowl with spray for frying. Add milk into a thin, microwave-safe bowl. Microwave for 40 seconds until lukewarm. Add a teaspoon of sugar and mix to dissolve, then sprinkle with the yeast and allow to rest for around 8 minutes until frothy.

2. Whisk the salt and flour together in a medium dish. Whisk together the remaining half a cup of sugar, egg, butter, and vanilla in a big bowl. Pour in the combination of yeast, blend to incorporate, add to the dry ingredients, and stir it.

3. Switch to a lightly floured surface and knead for around 5 minutes until elastic and just slightly tacky, adding a teaspoon of more flour at a time as required. Put the dough in an oiled bowl and cover it with a clean dishtowel. Let the dough rise for around 1 hour in a warm place until it has doubled in size.

4. Cover a broad baking sheet with cooking spray with parchment paper and gently grease it. Punch down the dough, then transform it onto a finely floured work surface and stretch it out into a 1/2' wide rectangle.

5. Punch the doughnuts out with a doughnut cutter or 3 'and 1' biscuit cutters. Knead some scraps together and punch more doughnuts or holes out. Put doughnuts and holes on baking sheets, cover with a dishcloth, and rise again, another 40 minutes to 1 hour.

6. Grease the air fryer basket with olive oil spray and add 2 doughnuts and 2 doughnut holes at a time to guarantee that the doughnuts do not strike. Cook until deeply golden at 375 ° for 6 minutes. Put on the cooling rack

and repeat for the remaining dough.

7. Return to the cooling rack and allow to set before serving for 5 minutes.

50. Air Fryer & Campfire Nutella S'mores

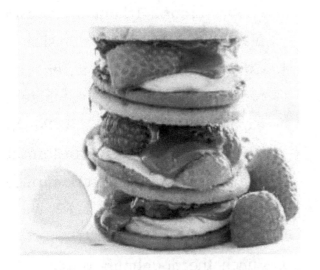

Ingredients

- ❖ Biscuits 8
- ❖ Marshmallows 4 large
- ❖ Nutella 4 teaspoon
- ❖ Raspberries or strawberries

Steps

1. Heat the air fryer at 180-degree C.
2. Put 4 biscuits in the air fryer.
3. Place 1 marshmallow on every half.
4. Cook for 5 minutes till lightly browned.
5. Add Nutella and the berries.

6. Do toppings with leftover biscuits and serve.

51. Air Fryer Cinnamon Sugar Doughnuts

Ingredients

- ❖ Butter ¼ cup
- ❖ White Sugar ½ cup
- ❖ Brown sugar ¼ cup
- ❖ Cinnamon 1 teaspoon
- ❖ Nutmeg ¼ teaspoon
- ❖ Flaky biscuit dough 1 package

Steps

1. In a bowl, put together 1/2 cup of white sugar and butter until crumbly. Add the egg yolks and whisk until they are well blended.
2. In a separate cup, sift the baking powder, flour, and salt. Put 1/3 of the flour mixture into the egg-sugar mixture and 1/2 of the sour cream; stir until mixed. Using the leftover flour and sour cream to mix in. Cool the dough until it's fit for use.
3. In a bowl, add 1/3 of a cup of sugar and cinnamon.
4. Roll the dough to 1/2-inch thickness on a well-floured work surface. Break the dough into 9 wide circles; break a tiny circle

from the middle of each large circle to establish a doughnut.

5. Heat the air fryer at 350 degrees F.
6. Run 1/2 of the molten butter over the doughnuts on both ends.
7. Put 1/2 of the donuts in the air fryer's basket; cook for 8 minutes.

With the leftover melted butter, color fried donuts and quickly dip into the mixture of cinnamon-sugar. Repeat for the doughnuts that remain.

Conclusion

A reason is why the air fryer diet is so popular: it works, and weight reduction is merely only the beginning. Research has been conducted on-air fryer diet that is gluten-free and low carbs containing diet. Studies have shown that this diet enhances energy levels, stabilizes mood, controls sugar in the blood, boosts cholesterol, lowers blood pressure, and more. Despite its long history, though, much remains uncertain about the diet, including its modes of operation, the right therapy, and the broad reach of its applicability. However, the inappropriate implementation of the diet may have significant health consequences and may not be the safest solution for maintaining good well-being. It takes at least two weeks for the body to react to the drastic carbohydrate loss, and occasionally four times as much.

The air fryer low carbs and gluten-free diet usually have unique effects on the body and cells that have benefits beyond what nearly every diet can offer. Carbohydrate restriction and ketone output mixtures reduce insulin rates, activate autophagy (cell clean-up), improve mitochondrial chemicals' development and productivity, reduce inflammation, and burn fat.

CPSIA information can be obtained
at www.ICGtesting.com
Printed in the USA
BVHW062345010621
608546BV00013B/1974

9 781802 592023